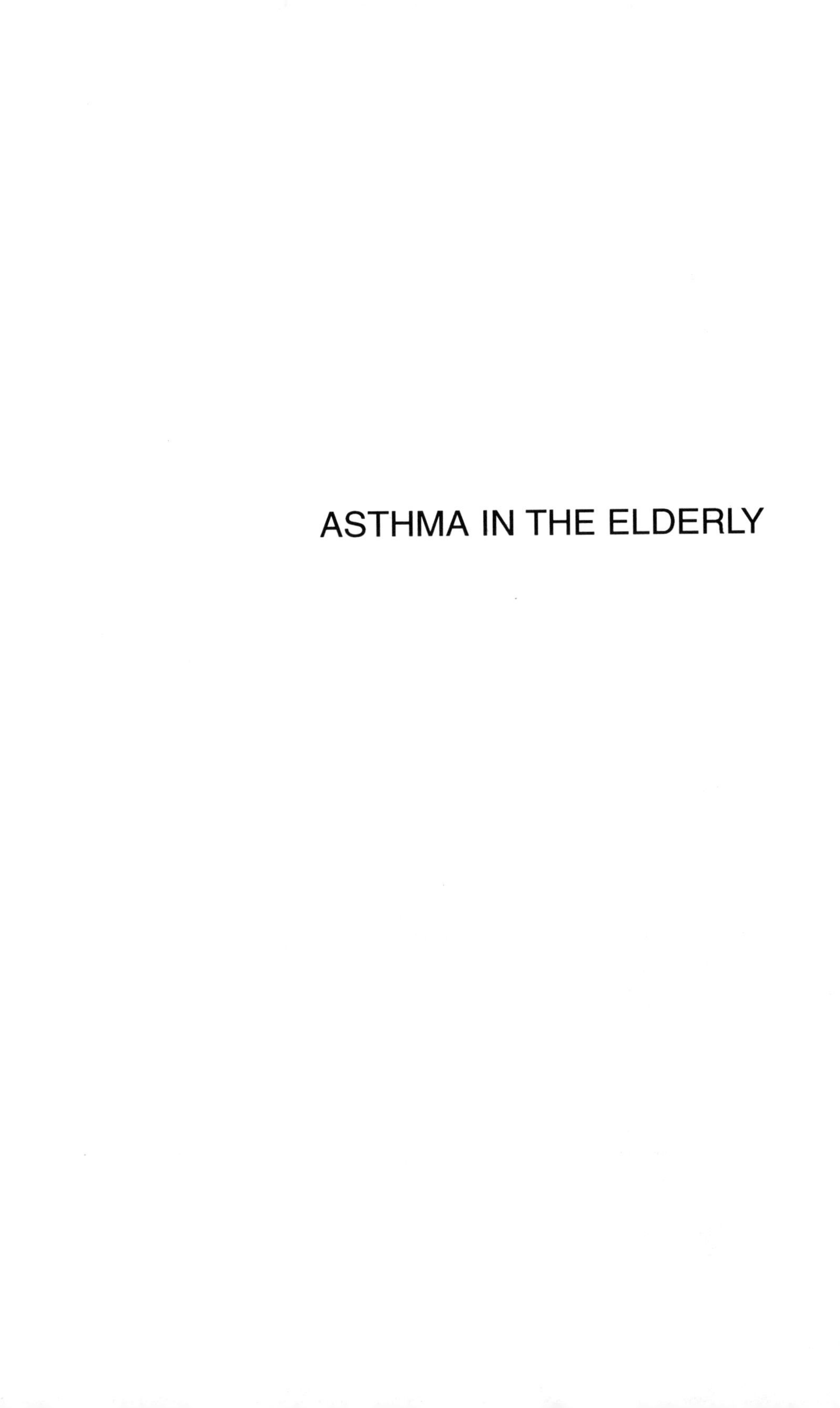

ASTHMA IN THE ELDERLY

LUNG BIOLOGY IN HEALTH AND DISEASE

Executive Editor

Claude Lenfant
Director, National Heart, Lung and Blood Institute
National Institutes of Health
Bethesda, Maryland

1. Immunologic and Infectious Reactions in the Lung, *edited by Charles H. Kirkpatrick and Herbert Y. Reynolds*
2. The Biochemical Basis of Pulmonary Function, *edited by Ronald G. Crystal*
3. Bioengineering Aspects of the Lung, *edited by John B. West*
4. Metabolic Functions of the Lung, *edited by Y. S. Bakhle and John R. Vane*
5. Respiratory Defense Mechanisms (in two parts), *edited by Joseph D. Brain, Donald F. Proctor, and Lynne M. Reid*
6. Development of the Lung, *edited by W. Alan Hodson*
7. Lung Water and Solute Exchange, *edited by Norman C. Staub*
8. Extrapulmonary Manifestations of Respiratory Disease, *edited by Eugene Debs Robin*
9. Chronic Obstructive Pulmonary Disease, *edited by Thomas L. Petty*
10. Pathogenesis and Therapy of Lung Cancer, *edited by Curtis C. Harris*
11. Genetic Determinants of Pulmonary Disease, *edited by Stephen D. Litwin*
12. The Lung in the Transition Between Health and Disease, *edited by Peter T. Macklem and Solbert Permutt*
13. Evolution of Respiratory Processes: A Comparative Approach, *edited by Stephen C. Wood and Claude Lenfant*
14. Pulmonary Vascular Diseases, *edited by Kenneth M. Moser*
15. Physiology and Pharmacology of the Airways, *edited by Jay A. Nadel*
16. Diagnostic Techniques in Pulmonary Disease (in two parts), *edited by Marvin A. Sackner*
17. Regulation of Breathing (in two parts), *edited by Thomas F. Hornbein*
18. Occupational Lung Diseases: Research Approaches and Methods, *edited by Hans Weill and Margaret Turner-Warwick*
19. Immunopharmacology of the Lung, *edited by Harold H. Newball*
20. Sarcoidosis and Other Granulomatous Diseases of the Lung, *edited by Barry L. Fanburg*
21. Sleep and Breathing, *edited by Nicholas A. Saunders and Colin E. Sullivan*

22. *Pneumocystis carinii* Pneumonia: Pathogenesis, Diagnosis, and Treatment, *edited by Lowell S. Young*
23. Pulmonary Nuclear Medicine: Techniques in Diagnosis of Lung Disease, *edited by Harold L. Atkins*
24. Acute Respiratory Failure, *edited by Warren M. Zapol and Konrad J. Falke*
25. Gas Mixing and Distribution in the Lung, *edited by Ludwig A. Engel and Manuel Paiva*
26. High-Frequency Ventilation in Intensive Care and During Surgery, *edited by Graziano Carlon and William S. Howland*
27. Pulmonary Development: Transition from Intrauterine to Extrauterine Life, *edited by George H. Nelson*
28. Chronic Obstructive Pulmonary Disease: Second Edition, Revised and Expanded, *edited by Thomas L. Petty*
29. The Thorax (in two parts), *edited by Charis Roussos and Peter T. Macklem*
30. The Pleura in Health and Disease, *edited by Jacques Chrétien, Jean Bignon, and Albert Hirsch*
31. Drug Therapy for Asthma: Research and Clinical Practice, *edited by John W. Jenne and Shirley Murphy*
32. Pulmonary Endothelium in Health and Disease, *edited by Una S. Ryan*
33. The Airways: Neural Control in Health and Disease, *edited by Michael A. Kaliner and Peter J. Barnes*
34. Pathophysiology and Treatment of Inhalation Injuries, *edited by Jacob Loke*
35. Respiratory Function of the Upper Airway, *edited by Oommen P. Mathew and Giuseppe Sant'Ambrogio*
36. Chronic Obstructive Pulmonary Disease: A Behavioral Perspective, *edited by A. John McSweeny and Igor Grant*
37. Biology of Lung Cancer: Diagnosis and Treatment, *edited by Steven T. Rosen, James L. Mulshine, Frank Cuttitta, and Paul G. Abrams*
38. Pulmonary Vascular Physiology and Pathophysiology, *edited by E. Kenneth Weir and John T. Reeves*
39. Comparative Pulmonary Physiology: Current Concepts, *edited by Stephen C. Wood*
40. Respiratory Physiology: An Analytical Approach, *edited by H. K. Chang and Manuel Paiva*
41. Lung Cell Biology, *edited by Donald Massaro*
42. Heart–Lung Interactions in Health and Disease, *edited by Steven M. Scharf and Sharon S. Cassidy*
43. Clinical Epidemiology of Chronic Obstructive Pulmonary Disease, *edited by Michael J. Hensley and Nicholas A. Saunders*
44. Surgical Pathology of Lung Neoplasms, *edited by Alberto M. Marchevsky*
45. The Lung in Rheumatic Diseases, *edited by Grant W. Cannon and Guy A. Zimmerman*
46. Diagnostic Imaging of the Lung, *edited by Charles E. Putman*

47. Models of Lung Disease: Microscopy and Structural Methods, *edited by Joan Gil*
48. Electron Microscopy of the Lung, *edited by Dean E. Schraufnagel*
49. Asthma: Its Pathology and Treatment, *edited by Michael A. Kaliner, Peter J. Barnes, and Carl G. A. Persson*
50. Acute Respiratory Failure: Second Edition, *edited by Warren M. Zapol and Francois Lemaire*
51. Lung Disease in the Tropics, *edited by Om P. Sharma*
52. Exercise: Pulmonary Physiology and Pathophysiology, *edited by Brian J. Whipp and Karlman Wasserman*
53. Developmental Neurobiology of Breathing, *edited by Gabriel G. Haddad and Jay P. Farber*
54. Mediators of Pulmonary Inflammation, *edited by Michael A. Bray and Wayne H. Anderson*
55. The Airway Epithelium, *edited by Stephen G. Farmer and Douglas Hay*
56. Physiological Adaptations in Vertebrates: Respiration, Circulation, and Metabolism, *edited by Stephen C. Wood, Roy E. Weber, Alan R. Hargens, and Ronald W. Millard*
57. The Bronchial Circulation, *edited by John Butler*
58. Lung Cancer Differentiation: Implications for Diagnosis and Treatment, *edited by Samuel D. Bernal and Paul J. Hesketh*
59. Pulmonary Complications of Systemic Disease, *edited by John F. Murray*
60. Lung Vascular Injury: Molecular and Cellular Response, *edited by Arnold Johnson and Thomas J. Ferro*
61. Cytokines of the Lung, *edited by Jason Kelley*
62. The Mast Cell in Health and Disease, *edited by Michael A. Kaliner and Dean D. Metcalfe*
63. Pulmonary Disease in the Elderly Patient, *edited by Donald A. Mahler*
64. Cystic Fibrosis, *edited by Pamela B. Davis*
65. Signal Transduction in Lung Cells, *edited by Jerome S. Brody, David M. Center, and Vsevolod A. Tkachuk*
66. Tuberculosis: A Comprehensive International Approach, *edited by Lee B. Reichman and Earl S. Hershfield*
67. Pharmacology of the Respiratory Tract: Experimental and Clinical Research, *edited by K. Fan Chung and Peter J. Barnes*
68. Prevention of Respiratory Diseases, *edited by Albert Hirsch, Marcel Goldberg, Jean-Pierre Martin, and Roland Masse*
69. *Pneumocystis carinii* Pneumonia: Second Edition, Revised and Expanded, *edited by Peter D. Walzer*
70. Fluid and Solute Transport in the Airspaces of the Lungs, *edited by Richard M. Effros and H. K. Chang*
71. Sleep and Breathing: Second Edition, Revised and Expanded, *edited by Nicholas A. Saunders and Colin E. Sullivan*
72. Airway Secretion: Physiological Bases for the Control of Mucous Hypersecretion, *edited by Tamotsu Takishima and Sanae Shimura*
73. Sarcoidosis and Other Granulomatous Disorders, *edited by D. Geraint James*

74. Epidemiology of Lung Cancer, *edited by Jonathan M. Samet*
75. Pulmonary Embolism, *edited by Mario Morpurgo*
76. Sports and Exercise Medicine, *edited by Stephen C. Wood and Robert C. Roach*
77. Endotoxin and the Lungs, *edited by Kenneth L. Brigham*
78. The Mesothelial Cell and Mesothelioma, *edited by Marie-Claude Jaurand and Jean Bignon*
79. Regulation of Breathing: Second Edition, Revised and Expanded, *edited by Jerome A. Dempsey and Allan I. Pack*
80. Pulmonary Fibrosis, *edited by Sem Hin Phan and Roger S. Thrall*
81. Long-Term Oxygen Therapy: Scientific Basis and Clinical Application, *edited by Walter J. O'Donohue, Jr.*
82. Ventral Brainstem Mechanisms and Control of Respiration and Blood Pressure, *edited by C. Ovid Trouth, Richard M. Millis, Heidrun F. Kiwull-Schöne, and Marianne E. Schläfke*
83. A History of Breathing Physiology, *edited by Donald F. Proctor*
84. Surfactant Therapy for Lung Disease, *edited by Bengt Robertson and H. William Taeusch*
85. The Thorax: Second Edition, Revised and Expanded (in three parts), *edited by Charis Roussos*
86. Severe Asthma: Pathogenesis and Clinical Management, *edited by Stanley J. Szefler and Donald Y. M. Leung*
87. *Mycobacterium avium*–Complex Infection: Progress in Research and Treatment, *edited by Joyce A. Korvick and Constance A. Benson*
88. Alpha 1–Antitrypsin Deficiency: Biology • Pathogenesis • Clinical Manifestations • Therapy, *edited by Ronald G. Crystal*
89. Adhesion Molecules and the Lung, *edited by Peter A. Ward and Joseph C. Fantone*
90. Respiratory Sensation, *edited by Lewis Adams and Abraham Guz*
91. Pulmonary Rehabilitation, *edited by Alfred P. Fishman*
92. Acute Respiratory Failure in Chronic Obstructive Pulmonary Disease, *edited by Jean-Philippe Derenne, William A. Whitelaw, and Thomas Similowski*
93. Environmental Impact on the Airways: From Injury to Repair, *edited by Jacques Chrétien and Daniel Dusser*
94. Inhalation Aerosols: Physical and Biological Basis for Therapy, *edited by Anthony J. Hickey*
95. Tissue Oxygen Deprivation: From Molecular to Integrated Function, *edited by Gabriel G. Haddad and George Lister*
96. The Genetics of Asthma, *edited by Stephen B. Liggett and Deborah A. Meyers*
97. Inhaled Glucocorticoids in Asthma: Mechanisms and Clinical Actions, *edited by Robert P. Schleimer, William W. Busse, and Paul M. O'Byrne*
98. Nitric Oxide and the Lung, *edited by Warren M. Zapol and Kenneth D. Bloch*
99. Primary Pulmonary Hypertension, *edited by Lewis J. Rubin and Stuart Rich*
100. Lung Growth and Development, *edited by John A. McDonald*

101. Parasitic Lung Diseases, *edited by Adel A. F. Mahmoud*
102. Lung Macrophages and Dendritic Cells in Health and Disease, *edited by Mary F. Lipscomb and Stephen W. Russell*
103. Pulmonary and Cardiac Imaging, *edited by Caroline Chiles and Charles E. Putman*
104. Gene Therapy for Diseases of the Lung, *edited by Kenneth L. Brigham*
105. Oxygen, Gene Expression, and Cellular Function, *edited by Linda Biadasz Clerch and Donald J. Massaro*
106. Beta$_2$-Agonists in Asthma Treatment, *edited by Romain Pauwels and Paul M. O'Byrne*
107. Inhalation Delivery of Therapeutic Peptides and Proteins, *edited by Akwete Lex Adjei and Pramod K. Gupta*
108. Asthma in the Elderly, *edited by Robert A. Barbee and John W. Bloom*

ADDITIONAL VOLUMES IN PREPARATION

Dyspnea, *edited by Donald A. Mahler*

Asthma and Immunological Diseases in Pregnancy and Early Infancy, *edited by Michael Schatz, Robert S. Zeiger, and Henry Claman*

Inflammatory Mechanisms in Asthma, *edited by Stephen T. Holgate and William W. Busse*

Self-Management of Asthma, *edited by Harry Kotses and Andrew Harver*

Physiological Basis of Ventilatory Support, *edited by John J. Marini and Arthur S. Slutsky*

Treatment of the Hospitalized Cystic Fibrosis Patient, *edited by David M. Orenstein and Robert C. Stern*

Proinflammatory and Antiinflammatory Peptides, *edited by Sami L. Said*

Biology of Lung Cancer, *edited by Madeleine A. Kane and Paul Bunn, Jr.*

The opinions expressed in these volumes do not necessarily represent the views of the National Institutes of Health.

ASTHMA IN THE ELDERLY

Edited by

Robert A. Barbee
John W. Bloom

University of Arizona College of Medicine
Tucson, Arizona

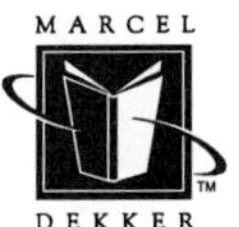

MARCEL DEKKER, INC.   NEW YORK · BASEL · HONG KONG

Library of Congress Cataloging-in-Publication Data

Asthma in the elderly / edited by Robert A. Barbee, John W. Bloom.
       p. cm. -- (Lung biology in health and disease ; v. 108)
    Includes bibliographical references and index.
    ISBN 0-8247-9870-8 (hardcover : alk. paper)
    1. Asthma in old age.   I. Barbee, Robert A. II. Bloom, John W. III. Series
    [DNLM: 1. Asthma--in old age. W1 LU62 v.108 1197 / WF 553 A8542
  1997]
    RC591.A818113 1997
    618.97'238--dc21
DNLM/DLC
for Library of Congress   97-22376
                                                           CIP

The publisher offers discounts on this book when ordered in bulk quantities. For more information, write to Special Sales/Professional Marketing at the address below.

This book is printed on acid-free paper.

MARCEL DEKKER, INC.
270 Madison Avenue, New York, New York 10016
http://www.dekker.com

Current printing (last digit):
10 9 8 7 6 5 4 3 2 1

PRINTED IN THE UNITED STATES OF AMERICA

INTRODUCTION

In this hearth made of clay
We will rekindle fire out of the embers
Blow on it once or twice
And flames will leap out of a half-burnt log.
And in the cauldron of my body
My heart's water will come to boil.

–Amrita Pritam

This poem, by a contemporary Indian writer from the state of Punjab, is a true recipe for how to approach the care of the elderly.

We now know that the prevalence of asthma is almost as high in people 65 years of age and older as it is in those younger than 18 years of age. Demographers have rightfully impressed upon us that the elderly constitute an ever-increasing segment of the population. It should therefore be obvious that attacking chronic diseases—especially very prevalent ones—up front in these people is critical. This is good common sense and good economy!

But there is really much more to it. As Amrita Pritam's verse implies, there is also the matter of the quality of life. The Roman orator Cicero pointed out, "No one is so old to think that he cannot live one additional year." Considering that today's average longevity is approaching 80 years, it is evident that the elderly, asthmatic or not, are anticipating a good number of additional years. The expectation is obvious: these years must be enjoyable. Thus, asthma in the elderly must be treated with the same vigor as is asthma in the young. However, as we well know, diseases and their treatment must often be approached differently in the elderly because of the interacting effects of aging, coexisting diseases, and drug interactions.

In 1992, this series of monographs presented *Pulmonary Disease in the Elderly Patient*, edited by Donald A. Mahler. In it, dyspnea and wheezing in the elderly were discussed authoritatively, but asthma was not the subject of any chapter. Was this an omission? Absolutely not! At that time—albeit not so long ago—the concepts about asthma and its treatment were not what they are today. Research on this disease has grown exponentially and has been remarkably successful in bringing immense benefits to patients. Thanks to the effort of the editors—Dr. Barbee and Dr. Bloom—and their outstanding contributors, this volume represents an important vehicle by which elderly patients in particular can receive these benefits. It is a scholarly and practical guide to the treatment of asthma in these patients.

The editors and authors of this book are well recognized for their expertise, and I, as the Executive Editor of this series of monographs, am most appreciative of the opportunity to introduce this volume.

Claude Lenfant, M.D.
Bethesda, Maryland

PREFACE

The last 15 years have witnessed an extraordinary increase in our understanding of the basic mechanisms that characterize asthma. It is now clear that the pathological airway lesion is the product of a unique inflammatory process involving a wide variety of cells and mediators. Despite this greater insight into the underlying mechanisms of the disease, there has been a significant increase in the morbidity and mortality of asthma. Much of this increase has been in older adults, a population that will increase dramatically as the "baby boomers" progress from middle to old age. Unfortunately, neither the underlying mechanisms nor the pathological features of asthma in the eldery has been studied in any depth. While it is clear that the allergic factors that characterize the disease in children and young adults are less prominent in older patients, the nature of the inflammatory process and the pathology that results are not well understood. Nor is it possible in many instances to make a clear distinction between asthma and chronic obstructive pulmonary disease, except by arbitrary smoking criteria.

If the basic mechanisms of asthma in the elderly are not well understood, the clinical and physiological aspects of the disease are equally obscure. Anatomic changes in the aging lung alter both its clinical presentation and the therapeutic responses to bronchodilators. Comorbid conditions and changes in drug metabolism combine to make pharmacological management more challenging. Socioeconomic factors contribute to lower rates of medication adherence and less success with patient-education efforts. Finally, the list of differential diagnostic possibilities is longer and more compex.

Because the literature that deals specifically with asthma in the eldery is quite limited, several authors in this volume have drawn on studies of younger asthma patients and applied their findings to the older population. For example, longitudinal epidemiological studies of childhood asthma that have followed cohorts into adulthood provide insight into the evolutionary changes that may occur with those who experience adult onset of disease that persists into old age. Management principles that are applicable in caring for younger patients with acute exacerbations have been modified to accommodate the narrower therapeutic window of the elderly patient.

It is our hope that this volume will be of value to all clinicians who care for the increasingly large elderly patient population: internists, family practioners, geriatricians, and pulmonologists. By emphasizing the relatively high prevalence of this "childhood" disease among the older population, our goal is not only to increase the recognition of asthma in the elderly, but also to stimulate studies that will provide answers to the many questions for which only conjecture and speculation are currently available.

We would like to express our sincere thanks and appreciation to the chapter authors who have contributed to this volume. Their dedication to a difficult task has been exceptional. Finally, we would like to thank Dr. Claude Lenfant for his support and encouragement.

Robert A. Barbee
John W. Bloom

CONTRIBUTORS

Tahir Ahmed, M.D. Professor of Medicine, University of Miami School of Medicine, and Division of Pulmonary Diseases, Mount Sinai Medical Center, Miami Beach, Florida

William C. Bailey, M.D. Professor of Medicine, Division of Pulmonary and Critical Care Medicine, and Director, Lung Health Center, School of Medicine, University of Alabama at Birmingham, Birmingham, Alabama

Robert A. Barbee, M.D. Professor of Medicine, Pulmonary/Critical Care Division, University of Arizona College of Medicine, Tucson, Arizona

John W. Bloom, M.D. Associate Professor, Departments of Pharmacology and Medicine, University of Arizona College of Medicine, Tucson, Arizona

Paul L. Enright, M.D. Assistant Research Professor of Medicine, Respiratory Sciences Center, University of Arizona, Tucson, Arizona

E. A. Gallagher, M.S.P.H. Research Assistant and Doctoral Student, Department of Health Behavior, School of Public Health, University of Alabama at Birmingham, Birmingham, Alabama

Henry Gong, Jr., M.D.   Professor of Medicine, University of Southern California School of Medicine, Los Angeles, and Chairman, Department of Medicine, and Chief, Environmental Health Service, Rancho Los Amigos Medical Center, Downey, California

Connie L. Kohler, Dr.P.H.   Assistant Professor, Department of Health Behavior, School of Public Health, University of Alabama at Birmingham, Birmingham, Alabama

Bruce P. Krieger, M.D.   Professor of Medicine, University of Miami School of Medicine, and Pulmonary Division, Mount Sinai Medical Center, Miami Beach, Florida

Susan K. Pingleton, M.D.   Professor of Medicine and Director, Division of Pulmonary and Critical Care Medicine, Department of Internal Medicine, University of Kansas Medical Center, Kansas City, Kansas

Rick Player, M.D.   Assistant Professor, Division of Pulmonary and Critical Care Medicine, Lung Health Center, School of Medicine, University of Alabama at Birmingham, Birmingham, Alabama

Charles E. Reed, M.D.   Emeritus Professor of Medicine, Mayo Medical School, Rochester, Minnesota

Joseph R. Rodarte, M.D.   Professor and Chief, Pulmonary and Critical Care Section, Department of Medicine, Baylor College of Medicine, Houston, Texas

Richard E. Sobonya, M.D.   Professor of Pathology, University of Arizona Health Sciences Center, Tucson, Arizona

Gayle A. Traver, R.N., M.S.N.   Clinical Assistant Professor of Medicine, College of Medicine, and Associate Professor, College of Nursing, University of Arizona, Tucson, Arizona

Adam Wanner, M.D.   Joseph Weintraub Professor of Medicine and Chief, Division of Pulmonary and Critical Care Medicine, University of Miami School of Medicine, Miami, Florida

CONTENTS

Introduction   Claude Lenfant   *iii*
Preface   *v*
Contributors   *vii*

1. Epidemiology and Natural History   **1**
Robert A. Barbee

    I. Introduction   1
   II. What Is Asthma?   2
  III. Epidemiological Tools for the Diagnosis of Asthma   4
  IV. Studies of Asthma Prevalence   6
   V. Morbidity and Mortality   9
  VI. The Semantics and Diagnostic Labeling of Chronic
       Airflow Obstruction   13
 VII. The Clinical Characteristics and Natural History of Asthma
       in the Elderly   17
VIII. Summary   23
       Abbreviations   25
       References   26

2. The Role of Allergy and Airway Inflammation   **33**
Charles E. Reed

I.	Introduction	33
II.	Asthma from Environmental Allergens	33
III.	Allergic Inflammation	35
IV.	Summary and Conclusions	46
	Abbreviations	47
	References	47

3. Pathology of Asthma in the Elderly   **53**
Richard E. Sobonya

I.	Introduction	53
II.	Comparative Pathology of Asthma, Simple Chronic Bronchitis, and Chronic Obstructive Bronchitis (Small Airways Disease) as Part of Chronic Obstructive Pulmonary Disease	54
III.	Effects of Aging: Asthmatic Bronchitis	60
IV.	Remodeling of Asthmatic Airways	61
V.	Summary	63
	Abbreviations	63
	References	63

4. Physiology of the Aging Lung   **69**
Paul L. Enright and Joseph R. Rodarte

I.	Introduction	69
II.	Static Lung Volumes	70
III.	Maximal Expiratory Flow	72
IV.	Nonuniform Regional Ventilation	73
V.	Spirometry	74
VI.	Respiratory Muscle Strength	75
VII.	Arterial Blood Gases	77
VIII.	Diffusing Capacity	77
IX.	Bronchodilator Response	79
X.	Nonspecific Airways Hyperreactivity	80
XI.	Pulmonary Function Tests to Assist in the Diagnosis of Asthma	82
XII.	Pulmonary Function Tests to Assess Asthma Therapy in the Eldery	85
XIII.	Summary	88

Abbreviations 89
References 89

5. Differential Diagnosis of Asthma in the Elderly **93**
Tahir Ahmed, Bruce P. Krieger, and Adam Wanner

I. Introduction 93
II. Definitions 95
III. Pathophysiological Characteristics 96
IV. Clinical Presentation of Asthma in the Elderly 101
V. Near Fatal Asthma 113
VI. Economic Impact 114
References 115

6. Management Overview: Special Considerations for the Elderly **121**
Connie L. Kohler, E. A. Gallagher, Rick Player,
and William C. Bailey

I. Introduction 121
II. Characteristics of Older Adults and Other Factors that Can
Influence Successful Management 122
III. Management Considerations for Older Patients 125
IV. Summary: Asthma Management via Stepped Care 129
References 131

7. Pharmacological Management of Asthma in the Elderly **135**
John W. Bloom

I. Introduction 135
II. Bronchodilators 136
III. Anti-Inflammatory Agents 152
IV. Approach to Therapy 162
V. Conclusions 165
Abbreviations 165
References 165

8. Management of Acute Exacerbations in the Elderly Asthmatic **183**
Susan K. Pingleton

I. Introduction 183
II. Pathophysiology 184
III. Etiology of Acute Exacerbation 186

	IV.	Differential Diagnosis	187
	V.	Assessment	188
	VI.	Management	191
	VII.	Summary	199
		Abbreviations	199
		References	199

9. Patient Education: Creating Partnership Care   **203**
Gayle A. Traver

	I.	Changes with Aging that Affect Educational Programs	204
	II.	Patient Education	206
	III.	The Integrated Plan of Care	214
		Abbreviations	215
		References	215

10. Coexisting Conditions that Complicate Asthma Management in the Elderly   **219**
Henry Gong, Jr.

	I.	Introduction	219
	II.	Overview	220
	III.	Limitations of this Review	225
	IV.	Comorbid Conditions in Elderly Asthmatics	225
	V.	Summary	247
		Abbreviations	247
		References	248

Author Index   *259*
Subject Index   *285*

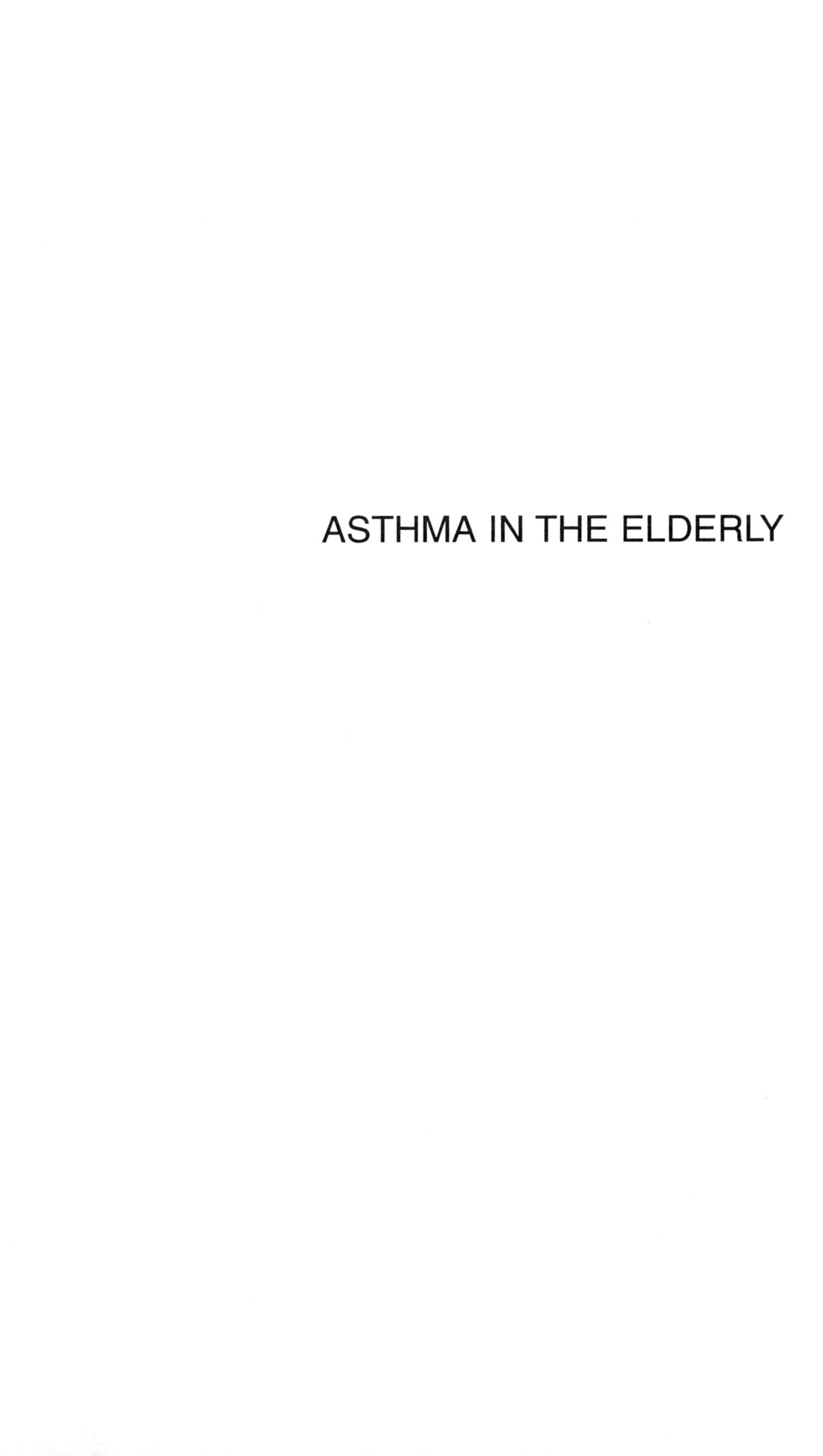

ASTHMA IN THE ELDERLY

1

Epidemiology and Natural History

ROBERT A. BARBEE

University of Arizona College of Medicine
Tucson, Arizona

I. Introduction

For most of us, the image which comes to mind when we hear of someone with asthma is that of a child or young adult with episodic wheezing and shortness of breath. Among the elderly, similar symptoms are more likely to be attributed to chronic bronchitis, emphysema, or perhaps, more generically, chronic obstructive pulmonary disease (COPD). However, in recent years, a diagnosis of asthma has been applied to this older population, both with and without an accompanying COPD diagnosis. Epidemiological studies that previously targeted childhood asthma have expanded to include the entire age range, encompassing not only those whose childhood disease continues into adulthood but also those whose initial diagnosis occurs in late middle age or beyond. Along with this increased focus on the older individual with asthma has come a diagnostic question that is critical in the assessment of chronic airflow obstruction in the elderly: "What are the criteria that allow the epidemiologist to distinguish among the diagnostic categories that make up the spectrum of chronic airflow obstruction in this age group?"

How, for example, is one to distinguish between asthma and what is often referred to as COPD with an asthmatic component? If physiological reversibility is limited in the elderly patient with asthma, what are the features of this diagnostic label that distinguish it from COPD or chronic bronchitis? Given a similar set of symptoms and clinical findings, should a different diagnosis be applied to a patient with airflow obstruction who has never smoked than to a second patient with a smoking history, however slight or remote? How important diagnostically is a history of allergies, present many years previously, when those allergic markers no longer exist?

For the clinician, diagnostic disease labels are applied to individual patients after a large amount of historical, physical, and laboratory data is collected. Even in this setting, the relationship of asthma to chronic obstructive lung disease is often uncertain. Not uncommonly, both diagnostic labels are given to the same patient. For epidemiologists, this diagnostic dilemma is even more difficult. By definition, their task is to observe the occurrence of disease, usually identified by the presence of specific symptoms, in large populations and to determine the condition's frequency, changing attack rates, and relationships to a variety of factors that may affect both. Of necessity, the database for each individual subject is quite limited, often including only the responses to a structured questionnaire. Despite these differences, the dilemma for both clinicians and epidemiologists is similar: The lack of universally accepted criteria upon which to make a specific diagnosis. In the case of older patients, this dilemma is even greater, as the clinical markers of allergy that characterize the disease and provide help in diagnosis for the younger individual are less apparent (1–3), and the symptoms characterizing asthma may be produced by a large number of diagnostic entities, some of which are not even of pulmonary origin.

The following discussion focuses on this diagnostic problem as it relates to the epidemiological identification of asthma in the elderly. Because of the paucity of epidemiological data relating specifically to this age group, studies throughout the age range are reviewed and, whenever possible, applied to the older asthma population.

II. What Is Asthma?

For a disease initially described over two thousand years ago and affecting millions of people worldwide, a precise definition of asthma has been extremely difficult to produce. In large measure, it has been this lack of a clear definition that has made epidemiological studies of asthma difficult. In his 1837 treatise *The Practice of Medicine*, Armstrong, an English physician, used descriptive terms to characterize asthma (4). He observed that it was a disease that affected men more often than women and was worse both in the heat of the summer and in winter, when fog and sharp winds were common in London. By implication, he was emphasizing the major impact of environmental conditions on asthma severity without describing its symptoms. Throughout the first half of this century, authors continued to emphasize environmental and/or allergic factors in the definition of asthma. In 1947, Rackemann expanded the definition of the disease by dividing it into "extrinsic" and "intrinsic" forms (5). The former was provoked by some foreign, usually environmental allergic stimulus, and the latter was characterized by airway reactivity to such things as infection or physical or psychological stimuli. Because a majority of asthmatic episodes were felt to be associated with allergic triggers, the perceived incidence of disease in older individuals, in whom allergic markers are much less prominent, was felt to be low. Confirmation of this age relationship between extrinsic and intrinsic asthma was provided in a report by Ford (6). More than ten thousand asthma patients in South Australia were surveyed to determine the principal causes of their disease. These patients were divided by age into extrinsic and intrinsic categories, using Rackemann's criteria (5). Between ages 15 and 45, almost 80% were felt to belong to the extrinsic category. Over age 60, some 88% were classified as intrinsic. Less than 3% of asthma patients in this population had the onset of their disease after age 60.

In the 1960s two primary features were incorporated into the definition of asthma: bronchial hyperresponsiveness to a variety of stimuli, and, in response to such stimuli, a widespread narrowing of the airways that was either partially or totally reversible, either spontaneously or in response to treatment (7). Little was known about the bronchial pathology involved in either of these features except as determined by the study of autopsy material from patients dying in status asthmaticus (8). In such patients the airways were characterized by inflammation, edema, epithelial sloughing, and mucous plugging. It was not until the 1980s that biopsy and bronchoalveolar lavage material from healthy young patients with mild asthma were obtained bronchoscopically, and made available for study. In 1985, Laitinen et al. (9) were among the first to describe the presence of a desquamative eosinophilic inflammatory infiltrate in the bronchi of patients with mild, stable asthma. Shortly thereafter, a large number of reports confirmed, by both biopsy and bronchoalveolar lavage analysis, the presence of airways inflammation as a constant feature, even in the mildest forms of asthma (10–14). Shortly thereafter, a number of authors correlated the severity of the bronchial hyperresponsiveness with the intensity of this inflammatory infiltrate (15–18).

As a result of these studies and others, which have documented the increasingly complex interactions of inflammatory cells, mediators, and cytokines in the asthmatic airways, the definition of asthma in the 1990s has been expanded to include three primary features (19):

1. Chronic airways inflammation that, in susceptible individuals, causes recurrent episodes of wheezing, breathlessness, chest tightness, and cough
2. Widespread but variable airflow limitation that is at least partially reversible, either spontaneously or with treatment
3. Bronchial hyperresponsiveness to a variety of stimuli

Unfortunately, from both a clinical and epidemiological standpoint, only the latter two criteria can be utilized in attempting to identify individuals with asthma.

III. Epidemiological Tools for the Diagnosis of Asthma

In spite of the progress that has been made in documenting the inflammatory airways lesion in asthma, the search for an epidemiological "gold standard" that would simplify the process of making that diagnosis in large populations has not been successful. As a result, the identification of individuals with asthma has depended primarily on symptom data, collected by standardized respiratory questionnaires. A number of such questionnaires have been developed for this purpose.

The first was produced by the British Research Council in 1960. Although its primary focus was to identify individuals with bronchitis, later versions added questions related to wheezing and chest tightness. Subsequently, questionnaires have been developed by the National Heart, Lung and Blood institute (NHLBI), the American Thoracic Society (ATS), and the investigators involved in the Tucson epidemiological study of airways obstructive disease. With each new version, the objective has been to produce a more discriminating sequence of questions that would increase the sensitivity of the data obtained. In addition to questions concerning the presence of wheeze, cough, and shortness of breath, most current instruments ask directly whether a physician has ever made a diagnosis of asthma by asking, for example: "Has a doctor ever told you that you have asthma?" The questionnaires also ask whether the asthma symptoms are current and whether medications have been prescribed: "Have you had these symptoms within the past year?" "Have you required medication?" In 1993, Toren et al. (20) reviewed the status of questionnaire-derived asthma epidemiologic data. In so doing, they estimated their sensitivity and specificity. *Sensitivity* is defined as the fraction of true or actual asthma that is identified by questionnaire. Simply stated, it is the percentage of the total asthma population in the study area that is identified by the instrument. *Specificity* is a measure of the fraction of healthy (nonasthmatic) subjects who are identified as healthy and not mistakenly given an asthma label. In addition to the sensitivity and specificity requirements, questionnaires must also satisfy *reliability* and *validity* criteria. A reliable tool is one in which the respondents answer to questions are the same when the questionnaire is repeated after a period of time. This can be tested quite readily. Validity measures are more difficult and are dependent upon the definition of the disease in question—in this case, asthma. Because the definitions used, although they employ much of the same symptom data, have often not been standardized, validation can only be measured against the definition that is being used in that particular study. In some cases the definitions involve symptoms alone. In others, a physiological measure of bronchial hyperresponsiveness is included in an attempt to produce a more valid asthma diagnosis. Some investigators have achieved increased validity by comparing the answers to their questionnaire with data obtained from previously validated instruments. Despite all of these efforts, none of the above methods have achieved levels of sensitivity or specificity that are completely satisfactory. Epidemiological problems in the determination of asthma prevalence were emphasized by Speizer in a 1974 review (21). He concluded: "The lack of uniformity of diagnostic criteria as applied to clinical practice, the secondhand nature of the information-gathering system, and the potential for selection bias implicit in the way in which patients are selected result in very variable estimates of risk of disease." Even when questions of physician diagnosis are included, it is necessary to accept the fact that doctors do not necessarily use the same criteria to make an asthma diagnosis.

Many authors have collected and correlated clinical markers of allergy with their questionnaire data in an attempt to increase the validity of their asthma diagnoses. The most common of these have been allergen skin-test reactivity, the presence of eosinophilia in either blood or sputum, and measurements of serum immunoglobulin E (IgE) (22–25). Because of the rather sharp age-related declines in skin-test reactivity and IgE levels, especially over age 55, these markers are of much less value in studies of older populations (2,3). Burrows, et al. (26) have attempted to control for this age-related decline by using age- and sex-corrected IgE levels to conclude that even in the elderly, the presence of asthma is correlated with IgE levels. Others have not confirmed such a relationship (27).

In an attempt to increase the validity of epidemiological asthma prevalence data, Woolcock and others have used abbreviated histamine or methacholine bronchoprovocation protocols to identify subjects with bronchial hyperresponsiveness (28–34). As a rule, asthmatics are 100 to 1000 times more sensitive than nonasthmatics to the bronchoconstrictive effects of such agents (35–37). Reed and others (38,39) have used that difference to establish criteria by which one can identify not only active asthma but also those whose disease is in clinical remission. Utilizing these background data, Pratter et al. have emphasized the increased asthma specificity that can be achieved by combining symptom data with data obtained by methacholine inhalation challenge (40). Woolcock et al. (41) used a combination of intermittent breathlessness determined by questionnaire and histamine responsiveness to determine the prevalence of asthma in a native population from Papua, New Guinea. However, even with this combination, they were unable to separate asthma from COPD in patients with more severe airflow obstruction. Similarly, Enarson et al. (42) found significant overlap in bronchial responsiveness to methacholine when they attempted to separate asthmatics from those with chronic bronchitis in a large population of male factory workers. Although they noted that a combination of symptoms plus bronchial responsiveness was more closely associated with asthma than with chronic bronchitis, the overlap was such that separation of the two entities was not at all clear-cut. Additional confusion concerning the value of bronchial inhalation challenge in epidemiological studies was provided by Sears et al., when they reported that a significant percentage of children with no respiratory symptoms demonstrated bronchial hyperresponsiveness, which correlated with serum IgE levels (34).

Clearly, a gold standard for the epidemiological diagnosis of asthma has not been found. However, by using a combination of traditional asthma symptoms, physician confirmation of an asthma diagnosis, and hyperresponsiveness to bronchial challenge, it is possible to make reasonable estimates of disease prevalence in most epidemiological populations. Unfortunately, the prevalence data in one population cannot generally be applied to another, either because the methods used are not the same, the population base is different, or the environmental conditions are not similar. This is particularly true in the elderly population, where, in addition to these factors, the confounding variables related to underlying chronic airflow obstruction are even greater than in younger populations.

IV. Studies of Asthma Prevalence

Despite the lack of a gold standard for the identification of asthma in epidemiological studies and the methodological problems noted previously, reports of disease prevalence from a number of geographic areas have been available for many years. Unfortunately, for the purpose of this review, most of them have been carried out on populations of schoolchildren or young adults. Because many of the problems of asthma identification occurring in older adults are also present in the young, a sample of childhood studies is reviewed, followed by a discussion of the few reports that deal solely with the elderly. Throughout this discussion, several confounding variables that affect prevalence rates will be apparent. Two types of prevalence are considered: point prevalence, or the frequency of disease found at a single point in time, and cumulative prevalence, or the total amount of disease that can be identified over time—usually a period of years. The latter includes those who may have had active disease in the past but are currently in remission.

In 1969, Williams and McNicol reported a study of 3000 Australian schoolchildren. In this population, the point prevalence of asthma among 10-year-olds was 3.7%, with a cumulative prevalence of 11.7% (24). In addition to their determination of asthma prevalence, these investigators also addressed the question of disease labeling. They concluded that there was no significant difference between what many physicians labeled "wheezy bronchitis" and asthma. In their view, the relatively large number of children who were given a bronchitis label were in fact suffering from asthma. As noted below, a similar labeling problem adds confusion to the diagnosis of asthma in the elderly. In her report, Smith found that the prevalence of wheezing without an asthma diagnosis was over twice that of diagnosed asthma, emphasizing the problem of making a specific disease diagnosis from symptoms alone (43). What percentage of Smith's total population with wheezes truly had asthma is not clear, but the lack of specific diagnostic criteria significantly affects asthma prevalence. This dilemma was emphasized by Speight et al. from Tyneside, England. In a survey of third-grade children, 11% reported having wheezing episodes since beginning school, most of which had occurred within the previous year. Only 12.7% of these children were given a diagnosis of asthma. Most of the others were said by their physicians to have allergic bronchitis, recurrent bronchitis, recurrent colds, or wheezy bronchitis (44). Even a minor change in diagnostic labeling in this population would have had a significant effect on asthma prevalence.

In contrast with the relatively high asthma prevalence rate found by Williams and McNicol in Australia, the point prevalence of physician-diagnosed asthma among schoolchildren in Oslo was only 1.6%. At the same time, the prevalence of those with occasional wheezing was 9.5%, and of those with attacks of breathlessness, 4% (45). Somewhere between these two extremes, Auerbach et al. reported that the point prevalence of asthma in 17-year-old Israeli males who were examined to determine their eligibility for military service was 5.0%, with a cumulative prevalence of 7.9% (46).

When a similar cohort of 17-year-old males was examined 4 years later, the prevalence rates were 5.9% and 9.6%, respectively. Auerbach et al. concluded that the increased rates were real and that in this population, the prevalence of asthma was increasing rather rapidly. In a similarly aged population of Finnish young men, Haahtela et al. reported a sixfold increase in asthma prevalence over a 23-year period (47). Both Auerbach and Haahtela et al. felt that this increase in prevalence was probably related to an increase in environmental triggers or stimuli. Other investigators have noted a similar increase in asthma prevalence and, in general, have also attributed the increase to environmental factors (48–51). When a broad range of ages were studied, the increases were generalized, but greater in younger subjects. In racially mixed populations, increases among blacks have been greater than among Caucasians.

Perhaps because asthma is more readily identified in the younger populations, where allergic markers are more prominent, it has generally been found that prevalence rates are lower in older adults. This was indeed the case in a number of reports (6,51,52). Contrary to this impression, Ross reported that in his Malaysian study population, adults had a higher rate of asthma onset and prevalence than children (53). A similar finding was reported by Turner et al. in a New Guinea population study (48). It is possible that these reports from Asia may reflect population samples that are somewhat atypical. However, both studies illustrate the problems that exist when one attempts to compare asthma prevalence from one country to another. Even within the same country, it is not uncommon to see significant differences from one locale to another. Peat et al. related these differences to the type and intensity of local environmental allergen exposure in their study of two communities in Australia (54). Similar geographic variability has been noted in the United States. According to data from the National Health Interview Study, published in 1989 (55), the overall prevalence of asthma was 4.8%. Included in this average is a rate of approximately 3% in Tecumseh, Michigan (56) and over 6% in Tucson, Arizona (22).

One of the first studies to specifically examine the occurrence of asthma in the older adult was reported by Ford in 1969 (6). In a survey of 11,000 asthma sufferers from Australia, he found that only 15% of the population dated the onset of their disease between ages 45 and 59. Less than 3% had their initial diagnosis made past age 60. Shortly thereafter, Derrick confirmed his findings in Australians of all ages who were hospitalized for their disease (57). In this apparently more severely affected population, well over 50% dated the onset of their disease to the first decade of life. Only 3% had their initial diagnosis made after age 60, less than 1% over 70.

Perhaps because of greater interest or awareness of asthma in the elderly in recent years, a number of authors have emphasized the importance of performing pulmonary function studies in this population so that those with reversible airflow obstruction can be identified. During a random survey of elderly men and women in England, Banerjee et al. (58) found a high percentage with significantly decreased peak expiratory flow (PEF) rates. Sixty-four of these had an improvement of 15% or more in their flows following the inhalation of a bronchodilator; only a small minority of them were receiving respiratory-related medication. The investigators suggested that in old age, potentially reversible airways obstruction is often overlooked or misdiagnosed. Similarly, Allen identified 13 elderly patients with asthma in whom the diagnosis was either missed or delayed because the possibility of reversible disease had been overlooked (59). Both studies stress that the true prevalence of asthma in the elderly may be significantly greater than that reported in epidemiological studies.

In a report from the United States, Dodge and Burrows (22) also suggest that both the prevalence and incidence of asthma in the elderly is much higher than reported by Ford (6) and Derrick (57). During a 4-year follow-up of their community-based population of nearly three thousand subjects, 1.4% were given a new physician diagnosis of asthma. The point prevalence of disease in this population was 6.6%. Among subjects over age 60, both males and females had prevalence rates exceeding 6%, with the male rate slightly higher than that of females. The incidence of new disease was highest in children under age 10 and adults over age 60. At about the same time, Burr et al. reported similar findings in a random survey of the older population from Wales (60). The prevalence of asthma in this population was 6.5%.

The data from the National Health Interview Survey, shown in Fig. 1, would appear to confirm these findings. Although the highest prevalence, 6.1%, was

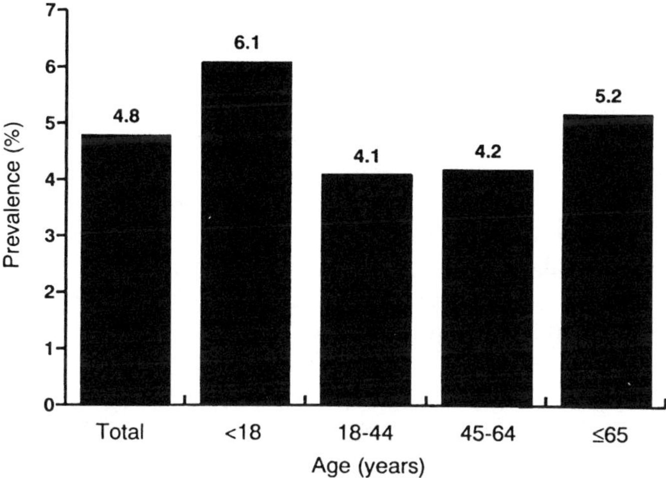

Figure 1 The prevalence of asthma in the United States by age: 1989 National Health Interview Study. For all age groups, asthma prevalence is 4.86%. The 5.2% prevalence in older adults is second only to the 6.1% prevalence in children.

found in those under age 18, the second highest, 5.2%, occurred in adults age 65 and above. More recently, Enright et al. reported an asthma prevalence of 6% among more than five thousand elderly participants in the Cardiovascular Health Study (61).

In summary, it would appear that among both children and young adults, there has been an increase in asthma prevalence in many parts of the world. This increase has generally been attributed to an increase in both the amount and intensity of environmental and occupational allergen exposure. Among older adults, a similar increase in asthma prevalence has been described, either because the possibility of reversible airway obstruction in this age group had previously been overlooked or because of an increasing tendency among physicians to add an asthma diagnosis in older patients with chronic airflow obstruction. It must also be considered that at least a portion of the increase in all age groups is secondary to changes in disease labeling practices.

V. Morbidity and Mortality

Many of the factors that serve to confound the validity of asthma prevalence data also affect the determination of morbidity and mortality. In practical terms, morbidity is usually defined by the effect of the disease on quality of life. This may be measured by days lost from school or work or, most commonly, by hospitalization rates. In turn, this is often translated into the direct and indirect dollar costs of a disease. As noted earlier in the discussion of asthma prevalence, changes in the diagnostic labeling of hospital discharge summaries could significantly affect asthma morbidity trends. Similarly, changes in the diagnostic labels used on death certificates would have a major effect on asthma mortality statistics. Such a labeling change occurred in 1979, when the ninth revision of the *International Classification of Diseases* (ICD-9) manual was changed to include chronic bronchitis under the asthma code (asthmatic bronchitis). Prior to that time (ICD-8), chronic bronchitis had been given a separate code. The immediate effect of this change was to increase both asthma morbidity and mortality at least transiently (62,63). However, well beyond the time when trends in morbidity and mortality could be explained on this basis alone, increases in both areas have continued. Unfortunately, other confounding variables, including changes in medical practice patterns, may also have contributed to changes in the disease labels that are listed in hospital discharge summaries. As a result, studies that have attempted to assess trends in asthma morbidity have not all reached the same conclusions.

A. Morbidity

A large part of the asthma morbidity data deal with hospitalization rates for younger patients, with less information available for the elderly. Both Anderson (64) and Strachan and Anderson (65) have examined those rates over time in young people and reached somewhat different conclusions. Strachan and Anderson attributed the near doubling of asthma admissions to hospital in the United Kingdom to changes in medical practice. Specifically, they emphasized the increased use of hospital emergency rooms as a major contributing factor. Anderson, on the other hand, found that the increases are real and not related to changes in medical practice alone. He concluded that there was an increase in the number of children experiencing more severe acute attacks, possibly due to greater exposure to pollution and airborne allergens. In 1993, a report from Finland (66) noted an almost 80% increase in asthma hospitalizations between 1972 and 1986, with the largest increase in those over age 65. Much of this increase, which occurred in the absence of an ICD coding change, was attributed to frequent hospitalization of the same severely ill patients, most of whom were in the older age groups. Of interest was the fact that an excess of hospital beds in Finland was also included as a possible cause of increased asthma hospitalizations.

Hospitalization data for children in the United States were reported by Gergen and Weiss (67). Using data from the National Hospital Discharge Survey, they traced asthma hospitalization trends in children from 1979 through 1987. They reported an increase of 4.5% per year, with the youngest children having the largest increase. Although they felt that some of that increase was real, they included changes in diagnostic disease labeling from bronchitis to asthma as an important additional factor. In 1987, Evans et al. utilized National Health Interview data in the United States from 1965 to 1983 to document a significant increase in hospitalizations for asthma. The increase, although greater in children (200%), was also seen in adults (50%) (63). The financial impact of this increase in hospitalization rates was reported by Weiss et al. in 1992 (68). When direct and indirect costs were combined for 1990, the total cost was $6.2 billion. The largest single direct expenditure, $1.6 billion was for inpatient hospital services. When combined with the estimated $1 billion attributed to loss of school and work days, almost 43% of the total economic impact of asthma was accounted for by these two areas.

B. Mortality

Prior to the 1960s, reports of asthma mortality were rare, largely because asthma deaths were uncommon. This was emphasized by Osler at the turn of the century, when he taught that acute attacks of asthma never caused death (69). In 1953, Williams reviewed his own experience with 41 asthma deaths and added 140 more from the literature (70). Over 80% of the deaths were in patients over age 30. In most countries, asthma death rates were low and were declining yearly. Speizer estimated that on a worldwide basis, a diagnosis of asthma as a cause of death in most age groups was less than 2 per million (21).

Since that time, two rather abrupt increases in mortality have been reported, one in England and the other in New Zealand. Factors related to both have been thoroughly examined and demonstrate the problems inherent in determining asthma death rates, especially in the older patient. Studies of the English experience initially placed a major portion of the responsibility on the introduction of aerosolized beta-agonist bronchodilators and their misuse by patients (71,72). Subsequent analysis of the data has cast doubt on the bronchodilator relationship. In the New Zealand epidemic, it was again thought that the increased mortality was related to the introduction of a new asthma therapy, in this case, theophylline, used in combination with beta-agonist bronchodilators (73). However, when the details of the deaths were more closely examined, a different picture emerged (74): 22% of the deaths were felt to have been miscoded—all except one in individuals over age 50. Not only was there strong suspicion that those deaths were related to nonreversible obstructive lung disease (COPD), but in the majority of instances undertreatment and poor patient compliance, not overmedication, were felt to be contributing factors.

In the years since these two epidemics, considerable attention has been focused on the apparent increase in asthma mortality that has been observed in many countries. If, as noted previously, both asthma prevalence and morbidity have increased, it should be expected that mortality would also increase. The question is whether the reported mortality increases are greater than can be accounted for by prevalence and morbidity increases alone. Most reports of asthma mortality have focused on two areas. The first is related to the disease itself: how it is managed, whether overall asthma severity has increased, and whether social factors such as patient access to medical care impacts mortality. The second area deals with the identification of asthma deaths and the accuracy of the diagnostic codes extracted from death certificates.

In addressing the first area, Whitelaw has suggested that the increasing effectiveness of bronchodilators may indirectly contribute to asthma mortality by giving patients a false sense of security and, as a result, exposing them to more life-threatening allergic triggers. Instead of helping them to avoid provocative antigens, bronchodilators allow patients to continue exposures that ultimately produce severe, acute exacerbations (75). A review of asthma mortality in France by Bousquet et al. suggests a number of possible explanations for the increased death rate in that country (76). Although they were not able to document whether the increase was due to a change in the severity of the disease or an increase in prevalence, the investigators' review of the data suggested that asthma was no less severe and, in fact, could be worsening. Among the factors they felt were related to mortality was the tendency of patients to underestimate the severity of their disease. As a result, between 60 and 80% of patients died at home rather than in an acute care facility. Sulfite sensitivity, anaphylactic reactions to allergen injections, and penicillin allergy were cited as examples of preventable causes of asthma mortality. An analysis of asthma mortality in the United States by Weiss and Wagener (77) at least indirectly addressed the question of access to medical care as a factor in asthma mortality. In their review, they confirmed the increase in overall mortality from a low of 1.6 deaths per million population in 1977 to 4.2 per million in 1987. While the increased death rates in white males and females were small, increases in nonwhite deaths for both sexes were much higher. Nonwhite males experienced a mortality rate of 13.5 deaths per million, almost five times as high as the rate among white males. Detailed analyses of these data strongly suggest that the relative lack of access to health care among the economically disadvantaged may play a major role in the increase in asthma mortality among minorities in this country.

Of particular importance in the assessment of asthma mortality among older adults is the accuracy of death certificate diagnoses. Weiss and Wagener (77) estimated that under age 35, death certificate diagnoses of asthma are 95% accurate. Over age 75, accuracy decreases to less than 35%. Sutherland et al., in their examination of 84 asthma deaths in New Zealand, reported excellent agreement with the death certificate diagnosis under age 50, but beyond that age they found a 22% rate of false reporting of asthma deaths (74). As others have, they blamed the inaccuracy of the death certificate on the confusion caused by the coexistence of chronic nonreversible airways obstruction in the older age group. Because of this confusion, many studies have focused on an examination of deaths in the 5-to-35 age range (78). However, few asthma deaths occur in that age range. Evans et al. estimated that there are fewer than 110 asthma deaths per year in the United States under age 15 (63).

If death certificates are unreliable diagnostic instruments in the older individual, it is critical to know whether studies based upon their analysis overestimate or underestimate asthma mortality. Again, there is no consensus. Sears et al. (79) and others (80,81) have reported overestimates of asthma deaths of 26 and 13% respectively when dependent on certificate data alone as compared with either autopsy or expert review panel diagnoses. Conversely, Hunt et al. reached the opposite conclusion (82). In their review of 339 deaths among patients who at one time or another had been treated for asthma, death certificates listed asthma as an immediate or underlying cause in only 22 (6%). When an expert review panel examined the medical records, it concluded that asthma should have been listed in 53 deaths, almost 2½ times the number listed on the death certificates. The investigators concluded that death certificates significantly underestimate asthma death rates rather than inflating them.

Despite the apparent lack of reliability of death certificate diagnoses and disagreement over whether they over- or underestimate asthma mortality, there appears to be no doubt that in most countries asthma deaths have increased in the past 10 to 15 years. From 1980 to 1987, total deaths from asthma in the United States increased from 2891 to 4360 (83). Female deaths increased more rapidly than male deaths, and deaths among older asthmatics increased at a faster rate than those among younger asthmatics. As noted earlier, the death rate in African Americans was significantly higher than in whites. According to the NHLBI Data Fact Sheet in 1995 (84), the greatest increase was in patients over age 85. Buist and Vollmer have reviewed a number of factors that might be responsible for this increase (85). Among those listed was the effect of the ICD code change, by which asthmatic bronchitis was coded as asthma rather than bronchitis; changes in physician diagnostic patterns; an increase in the prevalence and severity of asthma; better use of diagnostic methods to detect asthma; and the possibility— raised earlier—that the availability of new asthma drugs had the unfortunate effect of increasing mortality. There is no consensus as to the relative importance of any single factor, but the overall pattern is one of significant concern.

VI. The Semantics and Diagnostic Labeling of Chronic Airflow Obstruction

At several points in this review reference has been made to the effect that disease labeling may have on asthma prevalence, morbidity, and mortality. In no age group is the potential for diagnostic confusion greater than among the elderly. For that reason, a major focus of this discussion of the epidemiology and natural history is on the diagnostic labels applied to elderly patients with chronic airflow obstruction and the historical background that provides the basis for those labels.

In 1989, Pride et al. described a study in which the case histories of four model patients with airways obstructive disease were reviewed by over a hundred pulmonary physicians from 11 North American and western European countries (86). A major objective of the study was to determine what diagnostic label or labels the physicians would attach to each of the four model patients. Analysis of the results made it clear that there were major differences among the surveyed physicians in the labels that they would attach to each patient. The authors concluded that much of this confusion was related to the redundancy of the available diagnostic terms. For example: "COPD with considerable variability and reversibility probably means exactly the same as asthma without complete reversibility." In order to place this apparent diagnostic confusion in the context of asthma in the elderly, it is appropriate to briefly review some of the attempts that have been made to clarify the diagnostic terminology in chronic airflow obstruction.

With the development of routine physiological testing of lung function in the 1950s, it became necessary to develop more precise definitions of the three major entities associated with airflow obstruction: emphysema, asthma, and chronic bronchitis. The Ciba Symposium of 1958 was organized with that goal in mind. The symposium report (87) revealed that only partial success was achieved. Although emphysema was clearly defined as a parenchymal disease of the lung, chronic bronchitis was described in nonphysiological terms, and there was no agreement among the experts on a definition of asthma. However, an attempt was made to coin two new diagnostic labels that would incorporate two or more of the specific diseases under one umbrella term. The first, *chronic nonspecific lung disease* (CNSLD), included asthma with chronic bronchitis and emphysema and was adopted primarily by the Dutch. The second, *generalized obstructive lung disease* (GOLD), separated asthma from the other two. Not long thereafter, GOLD was replaced by the term or terms in widespread use today, *chronic obstructive lung disease* (COLD), and *chronic obstructive pulmonary disease* (COPD). Both were used to define chronic airways obstruction of uncertain etiology (88), although it was recognized that patients with this syndrome varied considerably in their clinical features.

While none of these terms fully resolved the diagnostic labeling problem, there was general consensus that patients with COPD experienced a progressive downhill course with little reversibility in response to therapy. Longitudinal studies of patients with chronic bronchitis by Fletcher et al. (89) and of those with emphysema by Burrows (90) came to be regarded as prototypical of smoking-related COPD, despite the fact that chronic bronchitis had been previously defined as chronic cough and sputum without mention of airflow obstruction. A major point in the separation of COPD from asthma was the airways hyperresponsiveness and reversibility of airflow obstruction which characterize the latter. These features were emphasized by the American Thoracic Society in its 1962 definition of asthma (91). Somewhat arbitrarily, as these various terms evolved, a 15% or greater improvement in forced expiratory volume during the first second (FEV_1) following administration of an aerosolized bronchodilator became the physiological measure of reversibility required for a diagnosis of asthma (91). Later, a minimum improvement of 200 ml was added to clarify the reversibility requirement for patients with small lung volumes.

Year by year, as the diagnostic terms for chronic airflow obstruction have evolved, increasing confusion has become apparent. Authors speak of COPD with an "asthmatic component" and asthma with limited reversibility. Amid this confusion, the label *chronic bronchitis* has never been adequately defined in terms of obstruction. As a result, it has been attached to asthma either as an adjective—chronic asthmatic bronchitis—or as a separate diagnosis in addition to asthma. In 1986, Dodge et al. described this diagnostic dilemma as it existed in the Tucson epidemiological study population. Among subjects over age 40 who were given an asthma diagnosis by their physicians, 71% were also given either a prior or concomitant diagnosis of chronic bronchitis, emphysema, or both (92). Conversely, less than 30% of those with an asthma diagnosis did not also have a second or third airways obstructive diagnostic label. Contributing to this multiplicity of diagnoses was the fact that the clinical and laboratory characteristics of the older asthmatics in this study differed little from those of patients with either of the other diagnoses.

If the variable response to inhaled bronchodilators creates diagnostic confusion in defining asthma in the elderly, it may be equally confusing in patients with COPD. In a large population of COPD patients, Anthonisen reported that on any single test of bronchodilator response, significant reversibility may occur, even when little change was noted on a previous test (93). Some 30% of his study subjects who had shown little prior reversibility subsequently showed increases of greater than 15%. During the several years of this longitudinal study, 68% of his COPD subjects demonstrated reversibility, with a 15% or greater increase in FEV_1 on at least one occasion. He concluded that using only a single test was inadequate to make a determination of airflow reversibility in patients with COPD. A similar conclusion was reached by Chang et al. (94). In this pulmonary function study of elderly patients with COPD, 31% of those who were given a bronchodilator had significant reversibility. The improvement occurred equally across all age groups, and the percentage of patients responding increased as the degree of obstruction increased. Those who had never smoked were twice as likely to respond as were current or former smokers. Others have made similar observations and found that the spontaneous day-to-day variation in FEV_1 is just as great in COPD as it is in asthma (95). As a result, differentiation between asthma and COPD in the elderly on the basis of physiological reversibility in response to an inhaled bronchodilator may be difficult if not impossible for a significant percentage of patients—a problem that Pride et al. found in their study (86).

Despite the fact that asthma diagnoses in the elderly are increasingly common, very few studies have systematically assessed the clinical features accompanying this diagnosis. In the course of a longitudinal study of airways obstructive disease in Tucson, Arizona, Burrows et al. were able to identify 40 subjects who initially denied asthma but were given that diagnosis by their doctors at some time during an 8-year follow-up period (96). The average age at which asthma was first reported was 70.8 years. The most striking prediagnosis symptom was the presence of at least intermittent wheezing, found in over 62% of subjects. A history of childhood respiratory trouble was also a highly significant predictor of future asthma. Some 20% reported that they had previously consulted a doctor for chronic bronchitis. The smoking history in these elderly asthma subjects was not different from that of patients with chronic bronchitis but no asthma diagnosis. At the time of their initial evaluation, prior to their asthma diagnosis, these subjects also had significantly lower lung volumes, a higher percentage of allergen skin-test reactivity, higher IgE levels, and more eosinophilia than age-matched controls who were not subsequently given an asthma label. The major symptom difference between those with and those without asthma was a history of wheezing. Sparrow et al. (97) described the factors that predict the onset of wheezing among middle-aged and older men. In this longitudinal study, allergen skin-test reactivity, serum IgE levels, pulmonary function testing, and methacholine challenge tests were performed on several hundred males who denied a history of wheezing. Three years later the presence of wheezing was determined by questionnaire and related to the test results obtained earlier. Among smokers, cigarette consumption was the dominant predictor of future wheezing. In nonsmokers, bronchial hyperresponsiveness was the most closely related factor. None of the usual clinical markers of allergy—skin test reactivity, serum IgE levels, or blood eosinophilia—were significantly related. Conversely, other authors have emphasized the importance of those same allergic factors, especially in nonsmokers, as predictors of future wheezing and/or accelerated declines in lung function. In a study by Annesi et al., the longitudinal decline in FEV_1 during a 5-year period was related to IgE levels (98). Ohman et al. found that total IgE levels had no predictive value but that there was a relationship with specific IgE antibody levels to mite antigen (99). In their cohort study, Vollmer et al. reported that FEV_1 was inversely related to IgE on a cross-sectional basis but was not predictive of rate of decline of lung function (100). The most recent report in this area was by Tracey et al. (101). A 4-year prospective survey was done to assess the association of allergen skin-test positivity, total serum IgE, and bronchial responsiveness to methacholine with an accelerated decline in FEV_1 in subjects over 65 years of age. In nonsmokers, age was the only factor significantly associated with an accelerated decline. However, in current and former smokers, both allergy and bronchial responsiveness were significant predictive factors.

For over forty years, Dutch investigators have suggested that host allergic factors are associated with the development of chronic airflow obstruction. In 1969, Van der Lende reported that blood eosinophilia was related to a lower level of FEV_1 (102). Two more recent studies have provided some evidence in support of this "Dutch" hypothesis. Kauffmann and colleagues reported that, in nonsmokers, there was an association between eosinophilia and level of FEV_1 among both asthmatics and those who denied such a history. She suggested that eosinophilia might be a risk factor for chronic airflow obstruction in nonsmokers (103). The same investigators reported that when this population was surveyed 5 years later, a relationship between the initial eosinophilia and subsequent longitudinal decline in FEV_1 could not be confirmed (104). One might best summarize these reports and those described previously as reflective of the difficulty encountered in attempting to tease out isolated stimuli from the myriad of potential risk factors that may be involved in the development of chronic airflow obstruction. Among smokers, that factor is clearly dominant. In nonsmokers, the interactions of a number of factors, from allergy to heredity, appear to play a role. The relative importance of each and the precise nature of these interactions are uncertain and require further study.

VII. The Clinical Characteristics and Natural History of Asthma in the Elderly

A. Clinical Characteristics

With all the studies that have attempted to define risk factors for airways obstruction in adult populations, very few reports have described the clinical and physiological findings in elderly patients with asthma.

Four such reports are summarized on Table 1. Meaningful comparisons of the data are hampered by the small number of subjects in each study and the different methods which were employed in assembling their series. Braman et al. (27), and Lee and Stretton (105) described clinic patients, while Burrows et al. (106) and Burr et al. (60) identified subjects with asthma through epidemiological survey studies. Also, in an attempt to avoid confusion between asthma and COPD, Braman et al. excluded those with a smoking history. When smokers were not excluded, a high percentage of subjects had concurrent diagnoses of both chronic bronchitis and asthma. In accord with the earlier reports of Ford (6) and Derrick (57), only a minority of the older asthmatics demonstrated the allergic markers typically found in younger patients. This difference between early- and late-onset asthma is emphasized in the data of Braman et al., although their early-onset group is quite heterogeneous in terms of age at disease onset and duration of disease.

Table 1 Characteristics of Elderly Patients with Asthma in Reported Series

Author	Subject source	N	Mean age	Age at onset	Symptoms	Other AOD diagnosis	Smoke history, %	Male, %	Atopy and/or allergy history	Serum IgE, %	EOS	FEV_1 % change, mean (range)
Burrows et al. (106)	Random community	46	73	<40 (48%) >40 (52%)	Cough, sputum, wheeze, DOE	46% (CB)	63	28	28	?	37%	ND
Braman et al. (27)	Clinic	25	>70	<43 (13) >70 (12)	SOB, cough, wheeze	0	0[a] 0[a]	23	62 0	WNL — WNL	57%	18% (0–21) 10% (0–16)
Lee and Stretton (105)	Clinic	15	>60	40	Wheeze, cough, DOE	40% (CB)	73[b] curr. or ex	NA	27	—	50%	<10%
Burr (60)	Random community	14	>70	<40	Wheeze, DOE	33% (CB)	11	41	26	ND	15%	>15%

[a]Smokers were excluded.
[b]Current and ex-smokers combined.
AOD, airways obstructive disease; CB, chronic bronchitis; DOE, dyspnea on exertion; EOS, eosinophils; ND, not done; SOB, shortness of breath; WNL, within normal limits; FEV_1, percent increase in forced expiratory volume during the first second after bronchodilator.

Among their subjects with mean onset of disease prior to age 43, 62% had a history of atopy. None of the older-onset group had such a history. In the other three studies, which did not separate subjects by duration of disease, between 26 and 37% had some evidence of allergen skin-test reactivity. Depending upon the specific criteria, eosinophilia was not uncommon.

Braman et al. (27), Lee and Stretton (105), and Burr et al. (60) have provided spirometric data, including responses to inhaled bronchodilators in their reports. In the study of Braman et al., patients with long-standing disease were more severely obstructed than those with more recent onset, with a mean FEV_1 of 49.5% compared to 68.4%. In both groups the variability in baseline FEV_1 among individual patients was great, between 24 and 80% of predicted in the early-onset group, and 42 to 94% in the other. Similarly, the degree of reversibility was also variable, with as little as zero and as much as 21%, despite the fact that at some time in the past all had demonstrated at least a 15% increase. In the entire series of 25 patients, only 3 of the late-onset patients achieved a normal FEV_1 after a bronchodilator. Also, only 5 of Lee and Stretton's subjects had as much as a 10% increase in FEV_1 following bronchodilator administration. By contrast, Burr et al. (57) utilized FEV_1 response as a criterion for a diagnosis of asthma. As a result, all of their subjects had FEV_1 increases of at least 15%.

From the review of these studies, it is clear that there is no "typical" elderly patient with asthma. Statistically, he or she is someone with respiratory complaints that, in addition to cough and dyspnea, also include wheezing. Not uncommonly, the cough and dyspnea have been present for some time, leading to a diagnosis of chronic bronchitis. Asthma enters the picture when wheezing, often episodic in nature, appears. There may be a remote history of some respiratory symptoms during childhood and at least seasonal allergies during early adulthood. A mild to moderate increase in blood eosinophils is quite common, even in the absence of atopy or elevations in IgE levels. If there is a smoking history, it is usually relatively mild, with less than a total of one pack per day over 20 years. The physiological response to inhaled bronchodilators is extremely variable. Even among those who have a recent onset of disease, the 15% or greater increase in FEV_1 that is typically found in the younger patient may not be possible. For those patients with long asthma histories, only a history of prior reversibility may provide the physiological basis for an asthma diagnosis.

B. Natural History and Clinical Course

A number of factors make studies of the natural history of asthma extremely difficult. Among these is the fact that it is a disease of remissions and relapses, many of which are of short duration and only partial. Also, to determine the natural history of any chronic disease, one must perform longitudinal studies with the maintenance of a significant percentage of the initial study cohort. Such studies are extremely time-consuming and expensive. Finally, in none of such studies is it possible to assess the effect that therapeutic intervention has on the natural course of the disease. Despite these problems, a number of well-designed investigations have been reported, both in young and older asthma populations. Several of the childhood studies have been carried out over periods of many years, providing data concerning the effect of disease duration and severity on long-term prognosis. Because such studies provide insight into the status of the elderly patient with long-standing disease, they are reviewed below, in addition to studies of adult asthma patients.

Most of the early studies of the natural history of asthma were concerned with the extent to which childhood asthma remitted during the teenage years. Utilizing the childhood asthma cohort of Williams and McNicol (24), Martin et al. reported their disease status at age 21 (107). Later, Kelly et al. provided follow-up data on this same population at age 28, over twenty years after the onset of their disease (108). More than half of the patients with mild asthma as children who were wheeze-free at age 14 continued to be asymptomatic at age 21. Unfortunately, almost one-third of those who were asymptomatic at age 21 relapsed and were again wheezing 7 years later. Because their childhood asthma had been quite trivial and had been in remission for many years, the authors suggested that many of these subjects might be mislabeled as having adult-onset rather than recurrent or relapsed childhood disease. Perhaps most disturbing in the Kelly report was the fact that 95% of those with persistent asthma in childhood continued to have asthma at ages 21 and 28. Many of those with persistent disease were not under treatment, and over 40% continued to smoke. In a similar report, Roorda et al. (109) confirmed the poor prognosis of severe childhood asthma. During a 15-year follow-up study of asthmatic children aged 8 to 12, only 19% were still under a physician's care, although 76% had either continuing or recurrent respiratory symptoms. Among these young adults, women were more likely to be symptomatic than men. Factors during childhood that related to active asthma in adulthood included symptom severity, degree of bronchial hyperresponsiveness, and a low FEV_1. In perhaps the most extensive follow-up of children with asthma, Ryssing (110) suggested that no more than 30% achieve permanent remission. Taken together, these studies make it clear that among children with asthma, those with frequent symptoms are likely to have continuing disease in early adulthood, much of which is untreated. It is reasonable to project that many of these individuals will have chronic airflow obstruction in later life, with either a COPD label, an asthma label, or both. Even those who achieve remission during their teenage years have a significant likelihood of relapse during early adulthood, with less chance of subsequent remission as they enter middle age.

Utilizing the full age range of the Tucson Epidemiologic Study population, Burrows et al. described the remission and relapse rate of asthmatics from early childhood to old age during 9 years of follow-up (111). They confirmed the Martin conclusion that the likelihood of remission of childhood asthma during adolescence is directly related to the frequency and severity of symptoms.

Remissions among adults with active disease were much less common. When they did occur, they were also related to the severity of the disease. Less than 5% of older adults with frequent symptoms experienced remissions during this 9-year period. Conversely, relapse rates among adults between ages 30 and 69 approached 50% and tended to be associated with cigarette smoking. Burrows et al. concluded that the presence of even mild continuing respiratory symptoms among patients who had experienced remissions was associated with a high incidence of disease relapse (111).

Turning to the older adult with airways obstructive disease, Burrows et al. used a variety of factors to separate this population into two groups (112). In the first group were those with a high percentage of atopy, limited smoking histories, and physician-confirmed diagnoses of asthma (100%), with additional diagnoses of chronic bronchitis (56%) and/or emphysema (33%). The second group consisted of nonatopic smokers with or without a prior diagnosis of airways obstructive disease. Both groups had similar degrees of airflow obstruction at the time of entrance into the study (FEV$_1$ less than 65% of predicted) and were followed for a period of 10 years. The yearly decline in FEV$_1$ in group 1 was less than 5 ml, compared to 70 ml in the second group. Mortality in group 1 during the 10-year follow-up period was 15%, less than expected for age, with no death attributed to a pulmonary cause. The death rate in the second group was almost 60%; four-fifths of these decedents had airways obstructive disease listed on their death certificates. The investigators concluded that, on clinical grounds, one could separate obstructive lung disease into two major types, an asthmatic bronchitic form, which progressed very slowly, and an emphysematous form, which carried a very ominous prognosis. A characteristic of many patients in the second group was the insidious nature of the obstruction, such that over one-third of those with significantly abnormal spirometry at the start of the study had no pulmonary diagnosis at the time of the test. Clearly, a variety of factors were related to the differences in outcome, the most important of which may have been the difference in smoking history and the fact that subjects in group 2 had structural changes of emphysema at the start of the study, which contributed to a progressive fall in FEV$_1$.

In addition to the Burrows report, a number of investigators have conducted longitudinal follow-up studies comparing the course and prognosis of adults with asthma to that of normal controls. A summary of the data from those studies is shown in Table 2. For comparison purposes, the data of Burrows et al. are also included, although their comparison was with COPD, not normal controls. In each instance, the yearly decline in pulmonary function as reflected in the FEV$_1$ was greater in asthmatics than in age-matched normal controls. Although each study tended to emphasize a different factor, there was general agreement that disease severity and the presence of chronic bronchitis in addition to asthma were related to accelerated declines in lung function and increased morbidity. Since all of the studies included smokers, it is not possible to draw conclusions about the outcome

Table 2 Longitudinal Studies of Adult Asthma Patients

Author	Year	N	Years of follow-up	Age range	Smoke %	Factors associated with an accelerated decline in lung function						
						FEV_1 $\downarrow$/year	Age	Severity	Atopy	Smoke	BHR	CB
Peat et al. (113)	1987	92	18	22–69	28	↑	−	+	−	?	+	?
Schachter et al. (114)	1984	73	7	7–17[a]							?	+
				18+	55	↑	−	+	−	?		
Almind et al. (115)	1992	211	7	13–61	15	↑	+	?	−	+	?	+
Ulrik et al. (116)	1995	1075	19	13–70+	27	int ↑ ext −	+	+	+	+	?	+
Burrows et al. (112)	1987	27	9	62+8	44	−	?	?	+	−	?	+

[a]Seventy-three subjects with asthma were followed, but the precise number aged 18 and older is not provided. Follow-up data for the adults are listed.
FEV_1 $\downarrow$/year, decline greater than normal and/or control group; BHR, bronchial hyperresponsiveness; CB, chronic bronchitis; int, intrinsic; ext, extrinsic.

in nonsmoking adults with asthma. Also, it would not be unusual for cough and sputum to be a risk factor in accelerating the course of adult asthmatics with a smoking history. When the asthma populations were divided into groups with allergic (extrinsic) and nonallergic (intrinsic) disease, the latter group was associated with a more rapid functional decline, and increased mortality. In part, this was secondary to the increased age of the nonallergic subjects, and, as alluded to above, the higher incidence of associated chronic bronchitis. In their study, Peat et al. (113) included a measure of nonspecific bronchial responsiveness, which was correlated with a more rapid decline in FEV_1. Schacter et al. noted that a high percentage of adults with asthma in their series had concomitant chronic bronchitis (114). Finally, two of the authors reported an increased mortality in patients with adult asthma as compared with nonasthmatic controls (115,116)—a finding that was also evident in a British study by Markowe et al. (117). Almind et al. (115) also commented on the decrease in reversibility of airway obstruction with time, an observation that has been made by others (118). In none of these studies is mention made of the manner in which the asthma patients were managed. As a result, it is difficult to know how much of the data is confounded by that unknown variable. Despite these limitations, there appears little question that in the absence of disease remission, adult asthmatics with continuing symptoms have an accelerated decline in pulmonary function, and most likely, an increase in premature mortality as well, at least when compared with normals.

VIII. Summary

Within the universe of chronic airways obstructive disease, the place of asthma in general and, specifically, asthma in the elderly is illustrated in Fig. 2. The Venn diagram on the left (2a) represents the spectrum of the common airways obstructive diseases in the general population. Asthma is represented as a largely pure disease, as one would expect to find it in children and young adults. Smaller areas reflect the mixed picture found with chronic bronchitis in the very young and in combination with both emphysema and bronchitis, as is often seen in the older patient. On the right (2b) the diagram has been modified to represent the differences between the asthmatic population in general and asthma as it exists in the elderly. In this latter population, a much smaller proportion of asthma is pure and a greater proportion is combined with other airways obstructive diagnoses— primarily, chronic bronchitis. The term *chronic bronchitis* is used here as it has classically been defined: the presence of chronic cough and phlegm without the requirement of an obstructive component. The term *asthmatic bronchitis* has been used to identify this combination, and the heavy border encompassing the generic term *COPD* has been redrawn to exclude this entity.

Included in this diagnostic mix of elderly patients with an asthma label are a variety of clinical patterns. For some, the traditional features of significant revers-

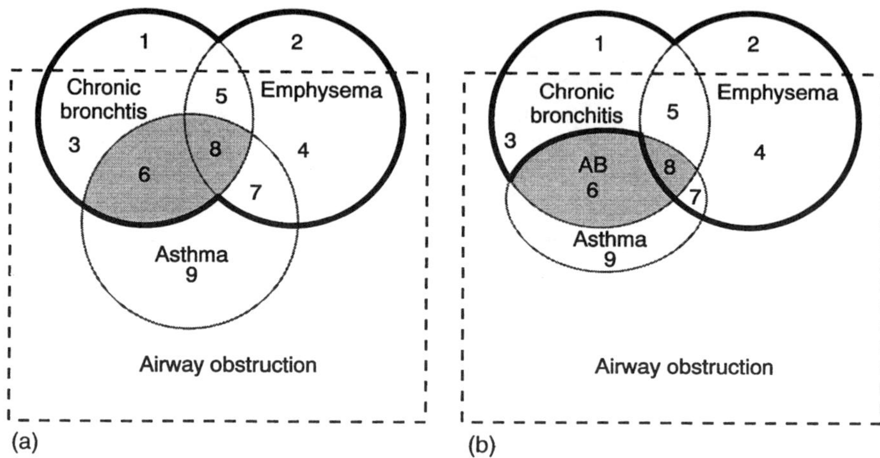

Figure 2   Venn diagrams illustrating the spectrum of chronic airways obstructive diseases are shown. (a) Chronic obstructive pulmonary disease in the overall population. Pure asthma, without a concomitent obstructive diagnosis (area 9), represents a large proportion of patients with asthma. Area 6 includes a combination of chronic bronchitis and asthma (asthmatic bronchitis). (b) Chronic airflow obstruction in the elderly. The diagram has been modified (119) to reflect the clinical differences in asthma as it occurs in the elderly. A majority of asthma diagnoses are accompanied by a second or third chronic obstructive disease. The most common combination, asthma plus chronic bronchitis (*asthmatic bronchitis*), is reflected by the greater size of area 6. The heavy borders, which encompass chronic obstructive pulmonary disease, have been redrawn to exclude this area, although many would include it. (From Ref. 119.)

ibility and airway hyperresponsiveness are clearly present, and an asthma label seems entirely appropriate. Usually these are patients with a relatively recent onset of wheezing and a negative smoking history. Not infrequently, cough and wheeze appear or are made worse by a viral lower respiratory infection, leading to an asthma diagnosis. There are virtually no biopsy data that would allow one to know the nature of the airway pathology. For others, the asthma label appears to be one that may have been quite appropriate at onset but can be more difficult to justify by the traditional asthma criteria after a period of twenty or thirty years. Often in these patients, baseline pulmonary function is grossly abnormal and is only marginally improved by bronchodilators. Any signs of an allergic component that may have been present previously, are no longer evident.

Perhaps the most difficult patients diagnostically are those with chronic airflow obstruction who have significant reversibility of airflow obstruction only intermittently. Most often, they are labeled COPD with an asthmatic component. The COPD label is usually predicated on the presence of a significant smoking history with persistent cough and sputum. Without the smoking history, the same patients might well be given an asthma diagnosis.

Given this widely divergent clinical population with the same diagnostic label and the lack of an epidemiological gold standard for the diagnosis of asthma, it is not possible to know with any certainty if the prevalence of asthma in the elderly has changed in recent years. While the word *asthma* is more commonly used in describing elderly individuals with chronic airflow obstruction, it is not at all clear that the clinical features and pathological changes in many of those individuals are the same or even similar to those of younger patients with the same diagnostic label. If airway remodeling, with the laying down of collagen in the lamina propria is a feature of long-standing asthma, then many elderly patients with asthma may have an entirely different disease pathologically than younger asthma patients with the same diagnosis.

Similarly, it is difficult to know the natural history of asthma in this age group. Most studies which have concluded that there is an accelerated decline in lung function and an increase in premature mortality have included both smokers and nonsmokers. Longitudinal studies of nonsmoking elderly asthma patients have not been carried out. As a result, the independent effect of asthma on FEV_1 and mortality has not been determined. In addition, mortality data have been dependent primarily upon death certificate diagnoses, which may either over- or underestimate actual cause of death.

Until more precise definitions become available to characterize COPD, a significant percentage of elderly patients with chronic airflow obstruction will continue to be provided with multiple diagnostic labels. Whether these labels are important clinically is uncertain. It has been argued that the importance of using the asthma label for older patients lies in the increased effort that will be made to induce reversibility when the word *asthma* is included. Others would argue that inducing reversibility is a primary clinical objective, irrespective of the label employed. At present, it seems appropriate to continue to use the asthma label in this population with or without a second or third COPD diagnosis.

Abbreviations

COPD	chronic obstructive pulmonary disease
COLD	chronic obstructive lung disease
CNSLD	chronic nonspecific lung disease
GOLD	generalized obstructive lung disease
IgE	immunoglobulin E
ICD 8 and 9	International Code of Diagnoses, volumes 8 and 9

References

1. Barbee R, Kaltenborn W, Lebowitz M. Longitudinal changes in allergen skin test reactivity in a community population sample. J Allergy Clin Immunol 1987; 79: 16–24.
2. Barbee RA, Halonen M, Lebowitz MD, Burrows B. Distribution of IgE in a community population sample: Correlations with age, sex, and allergen skin test reactivity. J Allergy Clin Immunol 1981; 68:106–111.
3. Barbee R, Lebowitz M, Thompson H, et al. Immediate skin-test reactivity in a general population sample. Ann Intern Med 1976; 84:129–133.
4. Armstrong X. Practice of Medicine. London: 1837.
5. Rackemann F. A working classification of asthma. Am J Med 1947; 3: 601–606.
6. Ford RM. Aetiology of asthma: A review of 11,551 cases (1958 to 1968). Med J Aust 1969; 1:628–631.
7. American Thoracic Society. Definitions and classification of chronic bronchitis, asthma, and pulmonary emphysema. Am Rev Respir Dis 1962; 85:762–768.
8. Dunnill MS. The pathology of asthma. In: Porter R, Birch J, eds. Identification of Asthma. Edinburgh: Churchill Livingstone, 1971:35–46.
9. Laitinen LA, Heino M, Laitinen A, et al. Damage of the airway epithelium and bronchial reactivity in patients with asthma. Am Rev Respir Dis 1985; 131: 599–606.
10. Bousquet J, Chanez P, Lacoste JY, et al. Eosinophilic inflammation in asthma. N Engl J Med 1990; 33:1033–1039.
11. Djukanovic R, Roche WR, Wilson JW, et al. Mucosal inflammation in asthma. Am Rev Respir Dis 1990; 142:434–457.
12. Foresi A, Bertorelli G, Pesci A, et al. Inflammatory markers in bronchoalveolar lavage and in bronchial biopsy in asthma during remission. Chest 1990; 98:528–535.
13. Laitinen LA, Laitinen A, Haahtela T. Airway mucosal inflammation even in patients with newly diagnosed asthma. Am Rev Respir Dis 1993; 147:697–704.
14. Lozewicz S, Gomez E, Ferguson H, Davies RJ. Inflammatory cells in the airways in mild asthma. Br Med J 1988; 297:1515–1516.
15. Beasley R, Roche WR, Roberts JA, Holgate ST. Cellular events in the bronchi in mild asthma and after bronchial provocation. Am Rev Respir Dis 1989; 139: 806–817.
16. Jeffery PK, Wardlaw AJ, Nelson FC, et al. Bronchial biopsies in asthma. Am Rev Respir Dis 1989; 140:1745–1753.
17. Macklem PT. A hypothesis linking bronchial hyperreactivity and airway inflammation: Implications for therapy. Ann Allergy 1990; 64:113–116.
18. Chetta A, Foresi A, Del Donno M, et al. Bronchial responsiveness to distilled water and methacholine and its relationship to inflammation and remodeling of the airways in asthma. Am J Respir Crit Care Med 1996; 153:910–917.
19. NHLBI/WHO workshop. Global strategy for asthma management and prevention. March 1993.
20. Toren K, Brisman J, Järvholm B. Asthma and asthma-like symptoms in adults assessed by questionnaires. Chest 1993; 104:600–608.

21. Speizer FE. Epidemiological aspects of asthma. Triangle 1978; 17:117–123.
22. Dodge R, Burrows B. The prevalence and incidence of asthma and asthma-like symptoms in a general population sample. Am Rev Respir Dis 1980; 122:567–575.
23. Vergnenegre A, Antonini MT, Bonnaud F, et al. Comparison between late onset and childhood asthma. Allergol Immunopathol 1992; 20:190–196.
24. Williams H, McNicol K. Prevalence, natural history, and relationship of wheezy bronchitis and asthma in children: An epidemiological study. Br Med J 1969; 8: 321–325.
25. Tollerud DJ, O'Connor GT, Sparrow D, Weiss ST. Asthma, hay fever, and phlegm production associated with distinct patterns of allergy skin-test reactivity, eosinophilia, and serum IgE levels. Am Rev Respir Dis 1991; 144:776–781.
26. Burrows B, Martinez F, Halonen M, et al. Association of asthma with serum IgE levels and skin test reactivity to allergens. N Engl J Med 1989; 20:271–277.
27. Braman SS, Kaemmerlen JT, Davis SM. Asthma in the elderly: A comparison between patients with recently acquired and long standing disease. Am Rev Respir Dis 1991; 143:336–340.
28. Woolcock AJ, Peat JK, Salome CM, et al. Prevalence of bronchial hyperresponsiveness and asthma in a rural adult population. Thorax 1987; 42:316–368.
29. Peat JK, Woolcock AJ. Sensitivity to common allergens: Relation to respiratory symptoms and bronchial hyperresponsiveness in children from three different climatic areas of Australia. Clin Exp Allergy 1991; 21:573–581.
30. Brand PLP, Postma DS, Kerstjens HAM, et al. Relationship of airway hyperresponsiveness to respiratory symptoms and diurnal peak flow variations in patients with obstructive lung disease. Am Rev Respir Dis 1991; 143:916–921.
31. Peat JK, Salome CM, Berry G, Woolcock AJ. Relation of dose-response slope to respiratory symptoms in a population of Australian schoolchildren. Am Rev Respir Dis 1991; 144:663–667.
32. Burney PG, Britton JR, Chinn S, et al. Descriptive epidemiology of bronchial reactivity in an adult population: Results from a community study. Thorax 1987; 42:38–44.
33. Cockcroft DW, Murdock KY, Berscheid BA. Relationship between atopy and bronchial responsiveness to histamine in a random population. Ann Allergy 1984; 53: 26–29.
34. Sears MR, Burrows B, Flannery EM, et al. Relation between airway responsiveness and serum IgE in children with asthma and in apparently normal children. N Engl J Med 1991; 325:1067–1071.
35. Townley R, Ryo U, Kolotkin B, Kang B. Bronchial sensitivity to methacholine in current and formal asthmatic and allergic patients and control subjects. J Allergy Clin Immunol 1975; 56:429–442.
36. Townley R. Mechanisms and management of bronchial asthma. In: Tices, ed. Practice of Medicine. Vol. 1. Hagerstown, MD: Harper & Row, 1972, chap 40.
37. Townley R, McGeady S, Bewtra A. The effect of beta adrenergic blockade bronchial sensitivity to acetyl-beta-methacholine in normal and allergic rhinitis subjects. J Allergy Clin Immunol 1976; 57:358–366.
38. Reed C, Townley R. Asthma: Classification and pathogenesis. In: Middleton, Reed, Ellis, eds. Allergy—Principles and Practice. St. Louis: Mosby, 1978:659–677.
39. Juniper E, Frith P, Hargreave F. Airway responsiveness to histamine and metha-

choline: Relationship to minimum treatment to control symptoms of asthma. Thorax 1981; 36:575–579.

40. Pratter MR, Hingston DM, Irwin RS. Diagnosis of bronchial asthma by clinical evaluation: An unreliable method. Chest 1983; 84:42–47.

41. Woolcock AJ, Dowse GK, Temple K, et al. The prevalence of asthma in the South-Fore people of Papua New Guinea: A method for field studies of bronchial reactivity. Eur J Respir Dis 1983; 64:571–581.

42. Enarson DA, Vedal S, Schulzer M, et al. Asthma, asthmalike symptoms, chronic bronchitis, and the degree of bronchial hyperresponsiveness in epidemiologic surveys. Am Rev Respir Dis 1987; 136:613–617.

43. Smith AJ. A five-year prospective survey of rural children with asthma and hay fever. J Allergy 1971; 47:23–30.

44. Speight A, Lee D, Hey E. Underdiagnosis and undertreatment of asthma in childhood. Br Med J 1983; 286:1253–1256.

45. Skarpass I, Gulsvik A. Prevalence of bronchial asthma and respiratory symptoms in school children in Oslo. Allergy 1985; 40:295–299.

46. Auerbach H, Springer C, Godfrey S. Total population survey of the frequency and severity of asthma in 17 year old boys in an urban area in Isreal. Thorax 1993; 48:139–141.

47. Haahtela T, et al. Prevalence of asthma in Finnish young men. Br Med J 1990; 301:266–268.

48. Turner KJ, Dowse GK, Stewart GA, et al. Prevalence of asthma in the South Fore people of the Okapa District of Papua New Guinea. Int Arch Allergy Appl Immunol 1985; 77:158–162.

49. Manfreda J, Becker AB, Wang PZ, et al. Trends in physician-diagnosed asthma prevalence in Manitoba between 1980 and 1990. Chest 1993; 103:151–157.

50. Burney PGJ, Chinn S, Rona RJ. Has the prevalence of asthma increased in children? Evidence from the national study of health and growth 1973–86. Br Med J 1990; 300:1306–1310.

51. Gerstman BB, Bosco LA, Tomita DK, et al. Prevalence and treatment of asthma in the Michigan Medicaid patient population younger than 45 years, 1980–1986. J Allergy Clin Immunol 1989; 83:1032–1039.

52. Cuthbert OD. The incidence and causative factors of atopic asthma and rhinitis in an Orkney farming community. Clin Allergy 1981; 11:217–225.

53. Ross I. Bronchial asthma in Malaysia. Chest 1984; 78:369–375.

54. Peat JK, Tovey ER, Mellis CM, et al. Importance of house dust mite and alternaria allergens in childhood asthma: An epidemiologic study in two climatic regions of Australia. Clin Exp Allergy 1993; 23:812–820.

55. National Center for Health Statistics. National Health Interview Survey. 1989.

56. Broder I, Higgins MW, Mathews KP, et al. Epidemiology of asthma and allergic rhinitis in a total community, Tecumseh, Michigan: III. Second survey of the community. J Allergy Clin Immunol 1974; 53:127–138.

57. Derrick EH. The significance of the age of onset of asthma. Med J Aust 1971; 1: 1317–1319.

58. Bannerjee DK, Lee GS, Malik SK. Underdiagnosis of asthma in the elderly. Br J Dis Chest 1987; 81:23–29.

59. Allen SC. Missed asthma: A study of 13 old people. Br J Clin Pract 1988; 42: 158–160.
60. Burr M, Charles T, Roy KL, et al. Asthma in the elderly: An epidemiologic survey. Br Med J 1979; 1:1041–1044.
61. Enright PL, Kronmal RA, Higgins MW, et al. Prevalence and correlates of respiratory symptoms and disease in the elderly. Chest 1994; 106:827–834.
62. Sly RM. Increases in deaths from asthma. Ann Allergy 1984; 53:20–25.
63. Evans R, Mullally DI, Wilson RW, et al. National trends in the morbidity and mortality of asthma in the U.S. Chest 1987; 91:65S–74S.
64. Anderson HR. Increase in hospital admissions for childhood asthma: Trends in referral, severity, and readmissions from 1970 to 1985 in a health region of the United Kingdom. Thorax 1989; 44:614–619.
65. Strachan DP, Anderson HR. Trends in hospital admission rates for asthma in children. Br Med J 1992; 304:819–820.
66. Keistinen T, Tuuponen T, Kivelä SL. Asthma related hospital treatment in Finland: 1972–86. Thorax 1993; 48:44–47.
67. Gergen PJ, Weiss KB. Changing patterns of asthma hospitalization among children: 1979–87. JAMA 1990; 264:1689–1693.
68. Weiss KB, Gergen PJ, Hodgson TA. An economic evaluation of asthma in the United States. N Engl J Med 1992; 326:862–866.
69. Osler W. The Principles and Practice of Medicine. 4th ed. Edinburgh:Pentland, 1901.
70. Williams DA. Deaths from asthma in England and Wales. Thorax 1953; 8:137–140.
71. Speizer F, Doll R, Heaf P. Observations on recent increase in mortality from asthma. Br Med J 1968; 1:335–339.
72. Stolley P, Schinnar R. Association between asthma mortality and isoproterenol aerosols: A review. Prev Med 1978; 7:319–338.
73. Wilson J, Sutherland D, Thomas A. Has the change to beta-agonist combined with oral theophylline increased cases of fatal asthma? Lancet 1981; 1:1235–1237.
74. Sutherland D, Beaglehole R, Fenwike J, et al. Death from asthma in Auckland. NZ Med J 1984; 97:845–848.
75. Whitelaw WA. Asthma deaths. Chest 1991; 99:1507–1510.
76. Bousquet J, Hatton F, Godard P, Michel FB. Asthma mortality in France. J Allergy Clin Immunol 1987; 80:389–394.
77. Weiss KB, Wagener DK. Changing patterns of asthma mortality: Identifying target populations at high risk. JAMA 1990; 264:1683–1687.
78. Arrighi HM. U.S. Asthma mortality 1941–1989. J Allergy Clin Immunol 1994; 93:247.
79. Sears MR, Rea HH, deBoar G, et al. Accuracy of certification of deaths due to asthma: A national study. Am J Epidemiol 1986; 124:1004–1011.
80. Subcommittee of the BTA Research Committee. Accuracy of death certificates in bronchial asthma: Accuracy of certification procedures during the confidential inquiry by the British Thoracic Association. Thorax 1984; 39:505–509.
81. Kircher T, Nelson J, Burdo H. The autopsy as a measure of accuracy of the death certificate. N Engl J Med 1985; 313:1263–1269.
82. Hunt LW, Silverstein MD, Reed CE, et al. Accuracy of the death certificate in a population-based study of asthmatic patients. JAMA 1993; 269:1947–1952.

83. Centers for Disease Control. Asthma—United States, 1980–1987. MMWR 1990; 39:493–497.
84. NHLBI Data Fact Sheet 10, 1995. U.S. Department of Health and Human Services. Public Health Service, NIH - 10/95 (NHIS-1988).
85. Buist AS, Vollmer WM. Reflections on the rise in asthma morbidity and mortality. JAMA 1990; 264:1719–1720.
86. Pride NB, Vermeire P, Allegra L. Diagnostic labels applied to model case histories of chronic air flow obstruction: Responses to questionnaire in 11 North American and western European countries. Eur Respir J 1989; 2:702–709.
87. Ciba Guest Symposium-Terminology, definitions, and classifications of chronic pulmonary emphysema and related conditions. Thorax 1959; 14:286–299.
88. Burrows B, Niden AH, Fletcher CM, Jones NL. Clinical types of chronic obstructive lung disease in London and Chicago. Am Rev Respir Dis 1964; 90:14–27.
89. Fletcher C, Peto R, Tinker C, Speizer FE. The natural history of chronic bronchitis and emphysema: An eight-year study of early chronic obstructive lung disease in working men in London. Oxford, England: Oxford University Press: 1976.
90. Burrows B. Course and prognosis in advanced disease. In: Perry TL, ed. Chronic Obstructive Pulmonary Disease. Vol. 28. Lung Biology in Health and Disease. New York: Marcel Dekker, 1985;31–42.
91. American Thoracic Society. Chronic bronchitis, asthma, and pulmonary emphysema: A statement by the committee on diagnostic standards for nontuberculous respiratory disease. Am Rev Respir Dis 1962; 85:762–768.
92. Dodge R, Cline MG, Burrows B. Comparisons of asthma, emphysema, and chronic bronchitis diagnoses in a general population sample. Am Rev Respir Dis 1986; 133:981–986.
93. Anthonisen NR, Wright EC, IPPB Trial Group. Bronchodilator response in chronic obstructive pulmonary disease. Am Rev Respir Dis 1986; 133:814–819.
94. Chang JT, Moran MB, Cugell DW, Webster JR. COPD in the elderly: A reversible cause of functional impairment. Chest 1995; 108:736–740.
95. Eliasson O, DeGraff AC. The use of criteria for reversibility and obstruction to define patient groups for bronchodilator trials: Influence of clinical diagnosis, spirometric, and anthropometric variables. Am Rev Respir Dis 1985; 132:858–864.
96. Burrows B, Lebowitz M, Barbee R, Cline M. Findings before diagnosis of asthma among the elderly in a longitudinal study of a general population sample. J Allergy Clin Immunol 1991; 88:870–877.
97. Sparrow D, O'Connor GT, Basner RC, et al. Predictors of new onset of wheezing in middle-aged and older men: The normative aging study. Am Rev Respir Dis 1993; 147:367–371.
98. Annesi I, Oryszezyn MP, Frette C, Neukirch F, et al. Total circulating IgE and FEV_1 in adult men: An epidemiologic longitudinal study. Chest 1992; 101:642–648.
99. Ohman JL, Sparrow D, MacDonald MR. New onset wheezing in an older male population: Evidence of allergen sensitization in a longitudinal study. J Allergy Clin Immunol 1993; 91:752–757.
100. Vollmer WM, Buist AS, Johnson LR, et al. Relationship between serum IgE and cross-sectional and longitudinal FEV_1 in two cohort studies. Chest 1986; 90:416–423.

101. Tracey M, Villar A, Dow L, et al. The influence of increased bronchial responsiveness, atopy, and serum IgE on decline in FEV_1. Am J Respir Care Med 1995; 151: 656–662.

102. Van der Lende R. Epidemiology of chronic nonspecific lung disease (chronic bronchitis): A critical analysis of three field surveys of CNSLD carried out in the Netherlands. Thesis. Assen, The Netherlands: van Gorcum, 1969.

103. Kaufmann F, Neukirch F, Korobaeff M, et al. Eosinophils, smoking, and lung function. Am Rev Respir Dis 1986; 134:1172–1175.

104. Frette C, Annesi I, Korobaeff M, et al. Blood eosinophilia and FEV_1. Am Rev Respir Dis 1991; 143:987–992.

105. Lee HY, Stretton TB. Asthma in the elderly. Br Med J 1972; 4:93–95.

106. Burrows B, Barbee R, Cline M, et al. Characteristics of asthma among elderly adults in a sample of the general population. Chest 1991; 100:935–942.

107. Martin AJ, McLennan LA, Landau LI, Phelan PD. The natural history of childhood asthma in adult life. Br Med J 1980; 14:1397–1400.

108. Kelly WJW, Hudson I, Phelan PD, et al. Childhood asthma in adult life: A further study at 28 years of age. Br Med J 1987; 294:1059–1062.

109. Roorda RJ, Gerritsen J, Van Aalderen WMC, et al. Risk factors for the persistence of respiratory symptoms in childhood asthma. Am Rev Respir Dis 1993; 148:1490–1495.

110. Ryssing E. Continued follow-up investigation concerning the fate of 298 asthmatic children. Acta Paediatr 1959; 48:255–260.

111. Burrows B. The natural history of asthma. J Allergy Clin Immunol 1987; 80:373–377.

112. Burrows B, Bloow JW, Traver GA, Cline MG. The course and prognosis of different forms of chronic airways obstruction in a sample from the general population. N Engl J Med 1987; 317:1309–1314.

113. Peat JK, Woolcock AJ, Cullen K. Rate of decline of lung function in subjects with asthma. Eur J Respir Dis 1987; 70:171–179.

114. Schachter EN, Doyle CA, Beck GJ. A prospective study of asthma in a rural community. Chest 1984; 85:623–630.

115. Almind M, Viskum K, Evald T, et al. Seven year follow-up study of 343 adults with bronchial asthma. Dan Med Bull 1992; 39:561–565.

116. Ulrik CS, Frederiksen J. Mortality and markers of risk of asthma death among 1,075 outpatients with asthma. Chest 1995; 108:10–15.

117. Markowe HLJ, Bulpitt CJ, Shipley MJ, et al. Prognosis in adult asthma: A national study. Br Med J 1987; 295:949–952.

118. Brown PJ, Greville HW, Finucane KE. Asthma and irreversible airway obstruction. Thorax 1984; 39:131–136.

119. Snider GL, Faling J, Rennard S. Chronic bronchitis and emphysema. In: Murray JF, Hadel JA, eds. Textbook of Respiratory Medicine. Orlando, FL: Saunders, 1994: 1331–1397.

2

The Role of Allergy and Airway Inflammation

CHARLES E. REED

Mayo Medical School
Rochester, Minnesota

I. Introduction

The word *allergy* carries a dual meaning in the context of this topic. One of its meanings is asthma provoked by acute or chronic exposure to a specific environmental allergen, such as *Alternaria*, pollen, cat dander, or house dust mites. In its second, more general meaning, *allergy* can be understood as the special type of allergic inflammation that is the histopathological basis of asthma and that can be summarized by the phrase "chronic desquamating eosinophilic bronchitis." Since the first meaning applies to only some patients while the second applies to them all, it is appropriate to discuss these two meanings separately.

II. Asthma from Environmental Allergens

In such cases the allergen (or, more often, allergens) is quite specific and varies from patient to patient as well as from place to place. Conventional wisdom has generally considered elderly asthmatic patients in two categories: those whose disease persisted from childhood and those whose disease began late in life. IgE-mediated allergy to specific allergens has often been considered to persist from childhood but to begin late in life only rarely. Data about the role of environmental allergens in asthma in the elderly are quite scarce. Braman and colleagues reported that none of their 25 elderly asthmatic patients had positive skin tests to common allergens, whether or not the disease began in old age (1). Those patients whose disease began in early life were, however, more likely to have a history of other allergic diseases. The Tucson epidemiology study found that both the concentration of IgE in the serum and the frequency and size of positive allergy skin tests decline with age, but that many elderly asthmatics had positive skin tests (2) (see Chap. 1). A population-based study of the incidence of asthma in Rochester, Minnesota, confirmed that the disease most often begins in early childhood (3). However, asthma may have its onset at any age, and the incidence rate continues to be about 100 per 100,000 throughout adult life into the eighth decade. The prevalence of asthma in patients 65 years of age and older was 4.5%, a value greater than the 3.4% prevalence in adults aged 30–64 but less than the 6.8% prevalence in children aged 1–19. The relationship of allergy to environmental agents was not examined in these elderly Rochester patients.

In order to obtain additional information about skin tests in the elderly, I reviewed a random sample of a quarter of the approximately 1200 patients with a physician's diagnosis of asthma 65 years of age or older who were referred to the Mayo Clinic, a tertiary care center, in 1993. Of 228 patients who met our epidemiological criteria for a diagnosis of asthma, 63 (27%) had skin tests performed. The indications for skin testing were not specified, so it is possible, even likely, that patients with a history suggesting an allergen exposure were overrepresented. Among these 63 patients, the results were positive in 18 (28%). When considered by age to onset of asthma, 56% of tests in patients whose disease began before age 40 were positive, compared to 21% in patients whose disease began after the age of 41. Skin tests were positive in about 20% of patients whose disease began after the age of 65. These positive tests reflected allergy to the usual things: *Alternaria*; tree, grass, and weed pollens; animal danders; and mites. Because patients referred to a tertiary care center are likely to have more severe disease than the population as a whole, I reviewed the records of 51 similarly selected local patients who received primary care at Mayo. Fifteen (29%) of these patients had skin tests performed at some time during their disease. The results were similar to those of the referred patients, although, as judged by spirometry, the cases were milder.

Occupational allergy has been estimated to account for about 5% of the cases of asthma in working-age adults, and active disease often persists after exposure ceases (4). Thus, it is somewhat unexpected that residual impairment from occupational asthma was not mentioned in any of these patient records. Nor is it considered in publications on asthma in the elderly. Because recognition and control of exposure to allergens is an important component of effective asthma treatment, recognition of environmental allergens—whether they be occupational, domestic, or communitywide—deserves more attention that it customarily receives. Environmental control might help in the management of as many as one-fifth of cases of asthma in the elderly, even for those whose disease has only recently begun. Obviously, prospective studies of this often overlooked issue are needed.

III. Allergic Inflammation

In the majority of elderly patients (the "intrinsic" cases), no environmental allergen can be identified. Some other stimulus or stimuli, as yet unidentified, must initiate and perpetuate the eosinophilic bronchial inflammation. Allergic inflammation of the airway has two outcomes. The first and best understood is obstruction from swelling of the airway wall, mucous plugging, and desquamation of the ciliated epithelium that responds to glucocorticoids but not to bronchodilators. This inflammation exaggerates airway hyperresponsiveness. The other outcome is permanent airway remodeling causing obstruction that does not reverse with any treatment. This second outcome is the source of considerable difficulty both for the differential diagnosis of asthma and for its management.

The past 10 years have seen remarkable successes in the application of cellular and molecular biology to understanding the role of cytokines in the pathogenesis of allergic inflammation. These results are beginning to resolve the long-standing clinical paradox arising from the consideration that the physiology, pathology, and pharmacology are the same for all asthmatic patients, yet the factors that provoke the disease are often very different. The old controversy about whether asthma is a single disease or a complex of different diseases is becoming irrelevant. Different stimuli can evoke key proinflammatory cytokines from different cells, but the final result is similar. A cytokine is a regulatory protein secreted by one cell that controls growth, differentiation, survival, and the functions of another cell. Unlike neurotransmitters and mast cell mediators of allergic disease that act on membrane and cytoplasmic functions to cause bronchospasm, cytokines act on the nucleus to induce DNA transcription and protein synthesis to cause airway inflammation.

A. Asthma, Eosinophils, and Cytokines

A review of eosinophil function provides the most direct introduction to an understanding of the role of cytokines in the pathogenesis of allergic inflammation, because eosinophils play one of the leading roles in the inflammation of bronchial asthma (5–7). The numbers of eosinophils in peripheral blood, broncho-alveolar lavage (BAL) fluid, and bronchial biopsies from patients with asthma are elevated compared to normal controls and patients with chronic bronchitis from smoking. Also, in asthma, the degree of eosinophilia can be correlated with disease severity and bronchial hyperreactivity (5,8,9). In a monkey model of asthma, inhibition of eosinophil migration into the airway by administration of monoclonal antibody to intracellular adhesion molecule-1 (ICAM-1) or vascular cell adhesion molecule-1 (VCAM-1) suppresses the development of airway hyperresponsiveness in vivo (10–12). Eosinophils from patients with asthma or allergy are activated compared with those of control subjects. For example, peripheral blood eosinophils from patients with asthma are "hypodense," a putative marker of cell activation, and have a prolonged survival (13,14). Activated circulating eosinophils express the adhesion molecule CD11b/CD18 (15). This integrin molecule binds to ICAM-1 and is important in cell-cell interaction, particularly adhesion to endothelium (16). Activated eosinophils also express receptors for immunoglobulins, which are important in degranulation, the final stage of eosinophil function (17). Even more striking activation is present in eosinophils in the airway tissue and lumen. After bronchial allergen challenge of patients with hay fever, eosinophils collected from BAL fluids, as compared with blood eosinophils, show increased superoxide production, increased adherence to collagen, and sustained elevation of intracellular calcium after N-formyl-methionyl-leucyl-phenylalanine (FMLP) stimulation (18). Furthermore, eosinophils in sputum or BAL fluids from patients with asthma express even more of the integrin CD11b/CD18 than activated circulating cells (19). These eosinophils from BAL also express ICAM-1, CD69, and human histocompatibility leukocyte antigen (HLA-DR), all of which are not expressed on blood eosinophils (13). Thus, eosinophils from patients with asthma, especially those derived from the lungs, show an activated phenotype associated with functional changes, increased intercellular adhesion, increased viability, and increased sensitivity to degranulation.

Eosinophil functions are regulated by cytokines, specifically granulocyte-macrophage colony-stimulating factor (GM-CSF), interleukin-3 and interleukin-5 (IL-3, IL-5), tumor necrosis factor alpha (TNF-α), and interferon gamma (IFN-γ) (20) (Fig. 1). These cytokines promote the growth and differentiation of eosinophils in the bone marrow and activate mature circulating eosinophils to express surface receptors, including CD11b/CD18, ICAM-1, HLA-DR, and CD69. They also promote eosinophil survival and ultimate degranulation (21,22). In allergic inflammation, IL-5 seems to be the most important cytokine because it is detected in various biological fluids from patients with allergy (23) and pulmonary eosinophilia (24). In animals, administration of neutralizing anti–IL-5 abolishes eosinophil infiltration into the tissues as well as blocking antigen-induced hyperresponsiveness (25,26). In contrast, transgenic mice overexpressing IL-5 have no pathological abnormalities apart from marked eosinophilia, suggesting a requirement for an additional factor besides IL-5 for initiation of disease (27). Eosinophil degranulation with release of toxic proteins in vitro follows engagement of their IgG and IgA receptors or stimulation with soluble mediators, such as platelet-activating factor (PAF) (28,29).

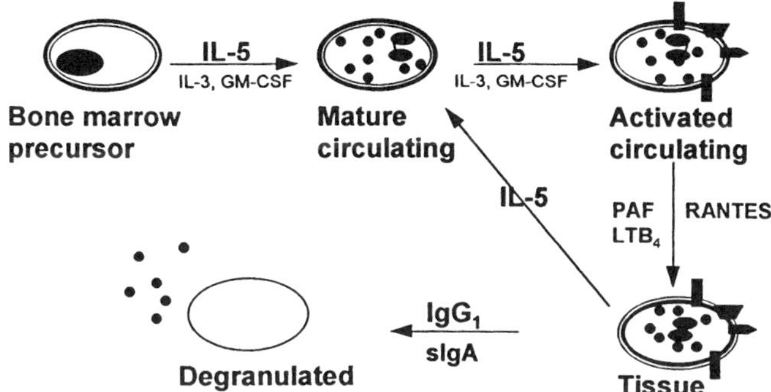

Figure 1 Locally produced cytokines, particularly IL-5, stimulate granulocyte precursors in the bone marrow to proliferate and differentiate into eosinophils. A second exposure to circulating cytokines leads to activation and expression of surface proteins, particularly adhesion molecules LFA(CD11b/CD18) and VLA. After adhesion to endothelial cells, eosinophils are drawn into the tissues by chemotactic factors, particularly the chemokines RANTES and eotaxin, and by platelet activating factor. Activated eosinophils themselves produce leukotrienes and cytokines, IL-5, and GM-CSF. Also, eosinophils activated by IL-3, IL-5, or GM-CSF are long-lived, surviving up to 7 days longer than normal mature eosinophils in tissue culture. IgG₁ or secretory IgA provides the stimulus for the final step, degranulation, and release of toxic granule proteins, particularly eosinophil major basic protein (MBP), which cause tissue damage and contribute to airway hyperresponsiveness.

Although several cytokines including IL-3, IL-5, and GM-CSF activate eosinophils, only IL-5 specifically causes eosinophilia (30). Analyses of specimens from patients with asthma have provided evidence for the presence of IL-5 in secretions and tissues. The levels of IL-5 in these fluids correlate with the degree of eosinophilia and the quantities of eosinophil granule proteins, suggesting that IL-5 causes the eosinophilia and also is related to eosinophil activation and release of granule proteins into tissues. Thus, IL-5 plays a central role in the pathophysiology of asthma. Presently, five cells are recognized as able to produce IL-5, including T cells of both the CD4[+] and CD8[+] subtypes (29), mast cells (31,32), eosinophils themselves (33,34), and, finally, natural killer (NK) cells (35).

Thus, considerable evidence suggests that eosinophils from patients with asthma, especially those derived from the lungs, are activated in vivo, and eosinophils in vitro can be activated by using immunoglobulins, lipid mediators, and cytokines. However, many connections between the in vivo and in vitro findings are still incomplete. We do not know the in vivo trigger(s) of eosinophil degranulation and subsequent epithelial damage. Furthermore, little is known about the mechanism(s) of eosinophil activation during the natural course of asthma. The above information has been obtained in vitro or in animal or human models.

B. Cytokines and Cell-Cell Interactions—Atopic Asthma— CD4[+] TH2-like Lymphocytes

Investigators at the Brompton Hospital in London under Barry Kay's direction have pioneered studies on the role of lymphocytes and their cytokines. T cells in BAL fluids and bronchial biopsies from patients with asthma are activated, especially CD4[+] T-helper cells producing IL-4 and IL-5. Because of the similarity of these human T cells to well-characterized mouse cells, they are called TH2-like cells (36). Numerous experiments have analyzed specimens from patients with atopic asthma comparing them with those from patients with atopy but without asthma and to normal control subjects (36,37). In patients with allergic asthma, lymphocytes are activated and eosinophils increased. Analyses of circulating peripheral blood CD4[+] and CD8[+] T-lymphocyte subsets in patients with acute, severe asthma indicates that CD4[+] cells are activated as compared with those in normal control subjects, whereas CD8[+] cells are not (38). In contrast, bronchial biopsies from patients with stable atopic asthma show increases in activated eosinophils and T lymphocytes of both CD4[+] and CD8[+] types (39). Analyses of T cells in BAL fluid from patients with atopic asthma show increased numbers of cells positive for mRNA for IL-2, IL-3, IL-4, IL-5, and GM-CSF but no difference in the number of cells expressing mRNA for INF-γ. The mRNA for IL-4 and IL-5 is expressed predominantly by T lymphocytes (40). Overall, comparisons of atopic subjects with normal control subjects support the hypothesis that CD4[+] TH2 cells producing IL-4 and IL-5 are characteristic of atopic asthma (38). A recent publication from the Brompton group reports analyses of bronchial biopsies from seven mild atopic patients and nine nonasthmatic controls by immunocytochemistry and in situ hybridization (34). They report that the asthmatics had significant increases in the percentages of cells expressing mRNA for IL-2, IL-4, and IL-5. Greater than 70% of the cells expressing mRNA for IL-4 and IL-5 are activated T cells (CD3[+]). The remaining IL-4 and IL-5 signals colocalize to tryptase+ mast cells and activated eosinophils. IL-4 promotes IgE antibody production, and IL-5 promotes eosinophilia and eosinophil degranulation. Stimulated peripheral blood mononuclear cells from all asthmatic patients produce IL-5, but only cells from atopic asthmatics produce IL-4 (41) (Figs. 2 and 3).

C. Cytokines and Nonatopic Asthma—CD8[+] Lymphocytes— Toluene Diisocyanate and Viruses

What about the allergic inflammation that is present in the majority of elderly patients who are not atopic? A somewhat expanded view of the role of T cells in

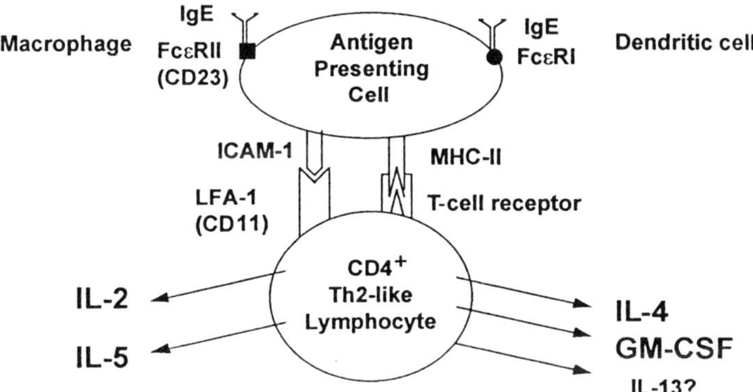

Figure 2 CD4+ TH2-like lymphocytes. Allergen reacting with IgE bound to either low-affinity FcεRII on macrophages or perhaps to high-affinity FcεRI on dendritic cells in the airway is presented to CD4+ helper T cells through the MHC class II (HLA-DR) molecule. This leads to production of the cytokines IL-2 (growth factor for the lymphocytes themselves), IL-4, and IL-5. Possibly other cytokines are formed as well.

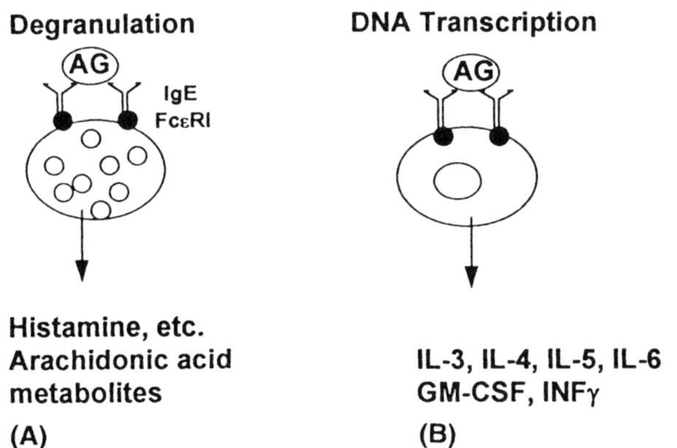

Figure 3 Mast cells: (A) immediate; (B) late. Allergen binding to IgE on mast cells cross-links the high-affinity receptor for IgE (FcεRI). This stimulus immediately leads to release of mast cell granules and preformed mediators. It also leads to activation of phospholipase A2 and production of products of arachidonic acid metabolism. This stimulus also leads to transcription of the genes coding for eosinophil-activating cytokines. This synthesis of new protein requires several hours and presumably is an important component of the "late phase" of the response to an allergen.

asthma emerges to help clarify this question. The Davos group compared atopic and nonatopic asthmatics (42). They confirm that BAL fluid from atopic asthmatics contain activated CD4$^+$ lymphocytes. In contrast, the BAL fluid of nonallergic asthmatics contains both CD4$^+$ and CD8$^+$ cells. The cytokine profile of the allergic patients is IL-5 and IL-4 (with associated increase in IgE), contrasting to the cytokine profile of the nonallergic patients, which is IL-5 and IL-2 (without IL-4 and no increase in IgE). The group studying toluene diisocyanate (TDI)–induced asthma in Italy, led by Leo Fabbri, isolated T-cell clones from bronchial biopsies of two patients with atopic asthma 48 hr after provocation with grass pollen extract. Of the 111 T-cell clones, 70% exhibited a clear-cut TH2-helper profile, and these included IgE synthesis in autologuous peripheral blood B cells in the presence of grass allergens. In contrast, the majority of T-cell clones derived from the bronchial mucosa of two nonatopic patients with TDI-induced asthma under the same experimental conditions were CD8$^+$. In response to stimulation, most of these cells produced IFN-γ or IFN-γ and IL-5, but not IL-4 (43). Analysis of peripheral blood lymphocytes from patients with TDI-induced asthma showed that the percentage of CD8$^+$ lymphocytes increases significantly 8 hr after TDI exposure, again in keeping with a role for CD8$^+$ cells (44) (Fig. 4).

Respiratory infections are a common cause of asthma at all ages, but the mechanisms of the virus-induced episode remain obscure (45). Many indirect

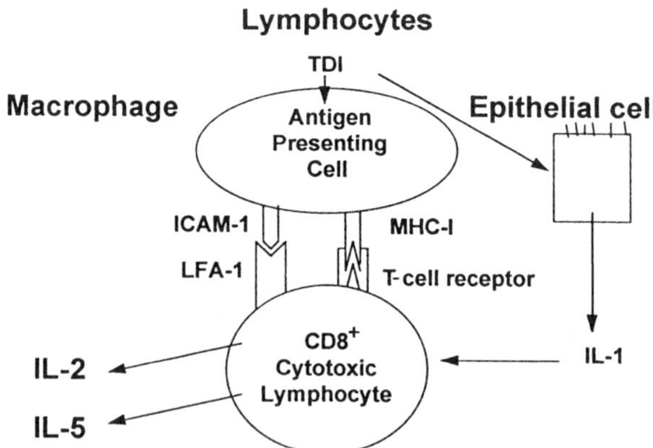

Figure 4 Toluene diisocyanate can stimulate both epithelial cells and macrophages to activate lymphocytes by unknown molecular mechanisms. It is not clear which one (or both) of these pathways accounts for the activation of CD8$^+$ cells and production of IL-5. Nor is it at all clear why only some individuals exposed to diisocyanates develop asthma. A similar pathway seems to operate in western red cedar asthma.

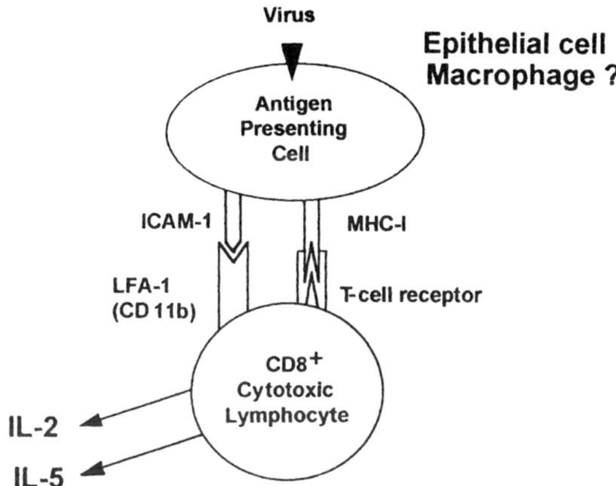

Figure 5 Much remains to be learned about the details of virus-induced asthma. All respiratory viruses may not activate the same pathways. This schema is only a first approximation of the role of CD8+ cells in virus-induced asthma and, by extension, other forms of intrinsic asthma. As with the non-IgE–mediated occupational asthmas, there are no clues about why only some persons respond to rhinovirus infections with asthma.

arguments point to the involvement of cytokines induced by viral antigens. Experimental evidence that this hypothesis may be true is beginning to be reported. An analysis of virus-specific CD8+ cells in a transgenic mouse model of asthma reveals that the virus-specific CD8+ cells can switch to IL-5 production and induce airway eosinophilia (46). Furthermore, BAL cells from virus-infected guinea pigs transfer bronchial hyperresponsiveness, implying a cytokine-mediated event (47). And antibody to IL-5 inhibits virus-induced airway hyperresponsiveness (48). Rhinovirus induces TNF-α production by macrophages; whether this activation of antigen-presenting cells leads to lymphocyte cytokine production remains to be seen. Another respiratory virus, influenza virus, does increase CD8+ cells producing IL-5, IL-10, and INF-γ (49). Considered as a whole, these results suggest that IL-5 may be the link between virus infection and acute exacerbations of asthma (Fig. 5).

Although the above studies indicating a central role for eosinophils and IL-5 produced by a variety of cells in generating the inflammation of asthma have been conducted in young or middle-aged adults, there is no reason to suspect that these immunological pathways differ with age. The results are surely relevant to asthma in the elderly. These cellular events in atopic and nonatopic asthma not only emphasize the critical role of T cells and their cytokines but also stress a heterogeneity of pathways that can lead to differentiation of progenitor cells into cells with different phenotypes but similar responses (Tables 1 and 2). It is important to emphasize that these intercellular pathways intersect and interact (50). The complex relationship between CD4$^+$ and CD8$^+$ cells, including pathways for their activation and their interdependence, is still incompletely defined. And in the clinical context of this issue, atopic and nonatopic asthma are by no means mutually exclusive. The same patient may be allergic to cats and also have asthma provoked by colds, and, more seriously, may have progressive chronic asthma of unknown cause. These exciting studies about cytokines clarify the cellular mechanisms of the disease but do not even begin to address the question of why a few people develop asthma and most do not.

D. Relationship of Inflammation to Airways Hyperresponsiveness

Airways hyperresponsiveness is as characteristic of asthma as eosinophilia, and these two characteristics correlate with each other (9). Airways hyperresponsiveness has a complex multifactorial basis that includes both inherited and acquired components. Although an important part of airways hyperresponsiveness can be explained by the geometrical and mechanical effects of submucosal thickening from inflammation, eosinophil granule proteins can be related to bronchial hyperreactivity in additional ways (51). Studies in animal models have been especially informative. Application of human eosinophil major basic protein (MBP) to guinea pig tracheal rings with intact epithelium causes a significant augmentation of acetylcholine responses. Intraepithelial injection of MBP substantially augments the response of canine tracheal smooth muscle to intra-arterial acetyl-

Table 1 Cytokines that Can Be Expressed by Various Cells

Cell	Cytokine
CD4 TH1-like lymphocyte	IL-2, INF-γ
CD4 TH2-like lymphocyte	IL-2, IL-4, IL-5
CD8 lymphocyte	IL-2, IL-5
NK lymphocyte	IL-5
Mast cell	IL-3, IL-4, IL-5
Macrophage	IL-1, IL-6, TNF-α, GM-CSF, IL-8, IL-10, IL-12
Eosinophil	IL-5, IL-8
Epithelial cell	IL-1 IL-6, TNF-α, GM-CSF
Neutrophil	IL-1, IL-8
Endothelial cell	GM-CSF, IL-8, SCF

This list is surely only partial.

Table 2 Cells and Cytokines in the Bronchoalveolar Lavage Fluid of Asthmatics

Allergic asthma	Intrinsic asthma
Eosinophils	Eosinophils
Epithelial cells	Epithelial cells
Neutrophils	Neutrophils
Mast cells	Mast cells
Macrophages	Macrophages
Activated CD4$^+$ Th2-like cells	Activated CD8$^+$ cells (decreased in blood)
IL-1 (from macrophages)	Not done
TNF-α (from macrophages)	Not done
IL-6 (from macrophages)	Not done
IL-8 (from eosinophils)	Not done
GM-CSF (from several cells)	Not done
IL-4[a]	IL-2
IL-5[a]	IL-5

[a]Some 70% of cells producing IL-4 and IL-5 are CD4$^+$ lymphocytes; 30% are mast cells.

choline. MBP injection directly into the subepithelial tracheal smooth muscle does not, suggesting that MBP stimulates the respiratory epithelium and thereby alters the contractility of underlying tracheal smooth muscle (52). Therefore, MBP affects respiratory epithelium, which, in turn, alters respiratory smooth muscle contractility, possibly by way of nitric oxide.

Repeated inhalation of *Ascaris suum* antigens in sensitized cynomolgus monkeys results in a prolonged inflammatory reaction characterized by an increase in airway eosinophils (53). This airway eosinophilia is associated with an increase in airway responsiveness. The number of BAL eosinophils and the MBP levels in the BAL fluids correlate significantly with methacholine response. The ability of eosinophil granule proteins to directly alter pulmonary function was also analyzed in cynomolgus monkeys (54). Instillation of MBP into the trachea of the monkeys causes a significant dose-related increase in airways responsiveness to inhaled methacholine. Furthermore, MBP and eosinophil peroxidase (EPO) induce a transient bronchoconstriction immediately after instillation, which requires an hour to resolve (53).

Cholinergic reflexes have long been recognized to be an important part of bronchospasm. In the lung, acetylcholine release from the vagus is under the control of inhibitory muscarinic receptors on the postganglionic nerves. These inhibitory receptors are classified as M_2 muscarinic receptors, whereas the muscarinic receptors on airway smooth muscle are classified as M_3 receptors. Acetylcholine released from the vagus nerve stimulates both M_3 muscarinic receptors on airway smooth muscle, causing contraction, and M_2 muscarinic receptors on nerves, decreasing further release of acetylcholine. Antigen inhalation in guinea pigs is associated with increased release of acetylcholine from the vagus nerves. Because positively charged proteins—including polyarginine, polylysine, basic histones, and protamine—are antagonists for the M_2 receptor, the possibility that a cationic eosinophil granule protein—such as MBP, EPO, ECP, or EDN—might be responsible for an antigen-induced pulmonary M_2 receptor abnormality was tested by analyzing the binding of purified eosinophil granule proteins to cholinergic receptors isolated from guinea pig heart (M_2 receptors) and guinea pig submandibular gland membrane (M_3 receptors) (55). MBP inhibited the specific binding of N-[^{3}H]methylscopolamine (^{3}HNMS) to M_2 receptors but not to M_3 receptors. MBP also inhibited the atropine-induced dissociation of ^{3}HNMS-receptor complexes in a dose-dependent fashion, showing that interaction of MBP with the M_2 receptor is allosteric. Therefore, MBP may function as an endogenous allosteric inhibitor of agonist binding to the M_2 muscarinic receptor. EPO also inhibited binding, but on a molar basis, EPO was less potent than MBP. These proteins may be important causes of M_2 receptor dysfunction, and they may enhance vagally induced bronchospasm in asthma.

MBP also activates kallikrein, thereby generating bradykinin. Animal studies suggest that this is the major pathway of eosinophil-induced bronchial hyperresponsiveness in guinea pigs (56). It's not yet clear how important bradykinin may be in the pathogenesis of hyperresponsiveness in asthma.

E. Relationship of Inflammation to Irreversible Obstruction

An important outcome of studies of the natural history of asthma in the elderly has been the observation that in many cases, particularly in the more severe ones, pulmonary function slowly declines and the obstruction becomes no longer fully reversible (57–60). In 1993, about 20% of patients aged 65 and older seen at the Mayo Clinic for asthma had a postbronchodilator FEV_1 of less than 50% of the normal predicted value for their age, sex, and race. Fortunately, though, about 20% of them had mild reversible disease with a normal postbronchodilator FEV_1 (Fig. 6). The factors responsible for the decline are not clear. Braman et al. reported that incomplete restoration of normal FEV_1 after treatment occurred more often in patients whose disease began early in life (1). In contrast, we found no correlation between the duration of the disease and the FEV_1 in the elderly patients at Mayo. Other factors, particularly severity and continuous activity of the disease, are likely to be more important. A variety of considerations lead to the conclusion that this irreversible obstruction is the result of "airway remodeling," predominantly in peripheral airways (61,62). The conclusion that obstruction of the peripheral airways is particularly important is supported by the spirometric findings of the patients described in Fig. 6. In these patients, the $FEF_{25-75\%}$ was

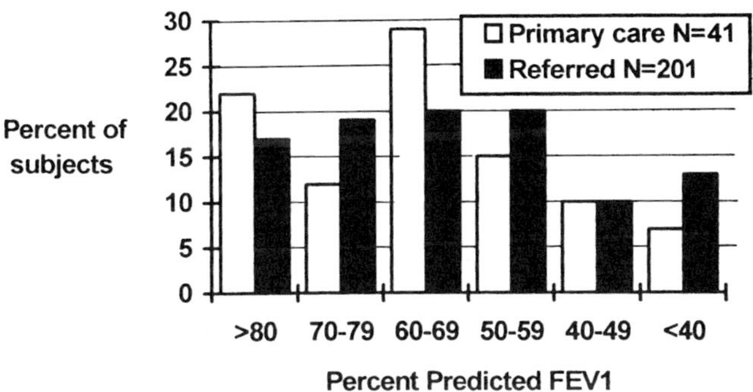

Figure 6 Spirometry in elderly asthmatics. These patients are a random selection of a quarter of the total of about 1200 patients 65 years of age and older who were diagnosed as having asthma (from a study at the Mayo Clinic in Rochester, Minnesota, in 1993). The plotted values are those measured after inhalation of adrenergic bronchodilator. For the patients referred to the Mayo Clinic from other cities, spirometry was performed at the time of the outpatient visit when the patients were in their usual state of health, but the results do not necessarily represent the maximal values that could be obtained with optimum doses of prednisone. However, if spirometry had been done on several visits, the highest value would be plotted. In this setting, about 20% of the patients had FEV_1 of less than 50% of their age-, sex-, and race-adjusted predicted value. The primary care patients lived in the Rochester area. Many of them had been followed for many years. The most recent result is plotted. The patients referred from other areas were somewhat more severely affected than the local patients. In neither group was there a correlation between the duration of asthma and the FEV_1 (data not shown).

substantially more impaired than the FEV_1. The pathology of asthma is fully discussed in Chap. 3 by Dr. Sobonya. The two main histopathological changes that account for this fixed obstruction are hypertrophy of bronchial smooth muscle and collagen deposition beneath the basement membrane. This subepithelial fibrosis may permanently narrow the airway by circular cicatricial contracture (62). Inspection of thin-section computed tomography of the lung in these irreversible asthmatics indicates that the pathology may be still more complex. Bronchiectasis, emphysema, and linear fibrosis are common (63).

In any event, presumably this remodeling occurs through the action of inflammatory cytokines. Information on this important subject is just beginning to accumulate (64–66). In the lung, one of the candidate cytokines, platelet-derived growth factor (PDGF), comes from activated macrophages (despite its name) (67). PDGF stimulates the growth of smooth muscle and of fibroblasts. One study reported modestly increased amounts of PDGF mRNA in macrophages of asthmatics as compared with normal controls and patients with COPD (68). Another center failed to confirm this finding (69). Eosinophils producing large amounts of PDGF are present in nasal polyps and in the airways of asthmatics (70). Other candidate cytokine growth factors for fibroblasts and smooth muscle include epidermal growth factor from epithelial cells, transforming growth factors α and β, insulin-like growth factors, and fibroblast growth factor. They have not yet been studied in relation to the airway remodeling of elderly asthmatics.

IV. Summary and Conclusions

In the narrow meaning of the word, *allergy* to environmental agents is relatively uncommon in elderly patients with asthma. Epidemiologically reliable information on its prevalence is lacking, but the upper limit of the frequency of IgE antibody to environmental allergens in elderly patients can be estimated to be about 20%. Positive tests are more common in patients whose disease began before the age of 40, but they may occur in patients with onset after age 65. Because continued exposure to environmental agents often leads to progressive and irreversible disease, recognition of preventable exposure for patients who do have IgE antibody to allergens encountered in domestic or occupational exposures is worthwhile, even though the frequency is low.

In the broad sense of the word, *allergic inflammation* underlies all cases of asthma. It is now clear that many of the clinical, physiological, and histopathological manifestations of asthma are mediated through cytokines produced by activated lymphocytes and other cells. Among the cytokines the most important and specific seems to be IL-5, acting on eosinophils. Generation of IL-5 can occur through several pathways, such as activation of CD4$^+$ Th2-like helper lymphocytes, CD8$^+$ cytotoxic lymphocytes, mast cells, and eosinophils themselves. Not all of these pathways operate in all patients or after all stimuli. For example, formation of IgE antibody occurs only when CD4$^+$ Th2-like cells producing IL-4 are involved. CD8$^+$ lymphocytes may be more important in virus-induced episodes and in non-IgE–mediated occupational exposures. The source of chronic eosinophilic inflammation in the absence of obvious provoking causes is still unknown. And the cellular mechanisms that leads to airway remodeling and fixed airway obstruction can only be speculated upon.

Inasmuch as eosinophilic allergic inflammation with asthma often coexists in the elderly with COPD from other causes such as smoking, some better means of identifying the allergic component is needed. Despite all the recent advances in understanding the biology of allergic inflammation, there is as yet no satisfactory clinical laboratory test to confirm its presence or determine its severity. Enumeration of eosinophils (or eosinophil granule proteins) in the sputum is helpful, but the reliability, sensitivity, and specificity of this test remain to be established. Its value is compromised by the fact that many patients with chronic airways obstruction are under treatment with glucocorticoids, which reduces cytokine production and obscures the eosinophilia.

Abbreviations

BAL	bronchoalveolar lavage
EPO	eosinophil peroxidase
FMLP	N-formyl-methionyl-leucyl-phenylalanine
GM-CSF	granulocyte-macrophage colony-stimulating factor
^{3}HNMS	tritiated methyl scopoloamine
ICAM-1	intercellular adhesion molecule-1
IgA, IgE, IgG	immunoglobilins A, E, and G
IL-1 to IL-12	interleukin-1 to interleukin-12
INF-γ	interferon gamma
LFA	leukocyte factor antigen (CD11b/CD18), an integrin
MBP	eosinophil major basic protein
MHC	major histocompatibility complex
mRNA	messenger ribonucleic acid
PAF	platelet activating factor
PDGF	platelet-derived growth factor
SCF	stem cell factor (a growth and activating factor for mast cells)
TDI	toluene diisocyanate
TNFα	tumor necrosis factor alpha
VCAM-1	vascular cell adhesion molecule-1
VLA	very late antigen (CD49/CD29), an integrin

References

1. Braman SS, Kaemmerlen JT, Davis SM. Asthma in the elderly: A comparison between patients with recently acquired and long-standing disease. Am Rev Respir Dis 1991; 143:336–340.
2. Burrows B, Lebowitz MD, Barbee RA, Cline MG. Findings before diagnoses of asthma among the elderly in a longitudinal study of a general population sample. J Allergy Clin Immunol 1991; 88:870–877.
3. Yunginger JW, Reed CE, OConnell EJ, et al. A community-based study of the epidemiology of asthma: Incidence rates, 1964–1983. Am Rev Respir Dis 1992; 146:888–894.
4. Bernstein DI, Bernstein IL. Occupational asthma. In: Middleton E Jr, Reed CE, Ellis EF, et al, eds. Allergy: Principles and Practice, 4th ed. St. Louis: Mosby, 1993:1369–1394.
5. Bousquet J, Chanez P, Lacoste JY, et al. Eosinophilic inflammation in asthma. N Engl J Med 1990; 323:1033–1039.

6.   Seminario MC, Gleich GJ. The role of eosinophils in the pathogenesis of asthma. Curr Opin Immunol 1994; 6:860–864.

7.   Martin LB, Kita H, Leiferman KM, Gleich GJ. Eosinophils in allergy—Role in disease, degranulation, and cytokines. Int Arch Allergy Immunol 1996; 109:207–215.

8.   Walker C, Kaegi MK, Braun P, Blaser K. Activated T cells and eosinophilia in bronchoalveolar lavages from subjects with asthma correlated with disease severity. J Allergy Clin Immunol 1991; 88:935–942.

9.   Wardlaw AJ, Dunnette S, Gleich GJ, et al. Eosinophils and mast cells in bronchoalveolar lavage in subjects with mild asthma: Relationship to bronchial hyperreactivity. Am Rev Respir Dis 1988; 137:62–69.

10. Gundel RH, Wegner CD, Torcellini CA, Letts LG. The role of intercellular adhesion molecule-1 in chronic airway inflammation. Clin Exp Allergy 1992; 22:569–575.

11. Wegner CD, Gundel RH, Reilly P, et al. Intercellular adhesion molecules 1 (ICAM-1) in the pathogenesis of asthma. Science 1990; 247:456–459.

12. Pretolani M, Ruffie C, Lapa, et al. Antibody to very late activation antigen 4 prevents antigen-induced bronchial hyperreactivity and cellular infiltration in the guinea pig airway. J Exp Med 1994; 180:795–805.

13. Hartnell A, Robinson DS, Kay AB, Wardlaw AJ. CD69 is expressed by human eosinophils activated *in vivo* in asthma and *in vitro* by cytokines. Immunology 1993; 80:281–286.

14. Virchow JC Jr, Oehling A, Boer L, et al. Pulmonary function, activated T cells, peripheral blood eosinophilia, and serum activity for eosinophil survival *in vitro*: A longitudinal study in bronchial asthma. J Allergy Clin Immunol 1994; 94:240–249.

15. Hartnell A, Moqbel R, Walsh GM, et al. Fc gamma and CD11/CD18 receptor expression on normal density and low density human eosinophils. Immunology 1990; 69:264–270.

16. Bochner BS, Schleimer RP. The role of adhesion molecules in human eosinophil and basophil recruitment. J Allergy Clin Immunol 1994; 94:427–438.

17. Kaneko M, Swanson MC, Gleich GJ, Kita H. Allergen-specific IgG1 and IgG3 through Fc gamma RII induce eosinophil degranulation. J Clin Invest 1995; 95:2813–2821.

18. Calhoun WJ, Bates ME, Schrader L, et al. Characteristics of peripheral blood eosinophils in patients with nocturnal asthma. Am Rev Respir Dis 1992; 145:577–581.

19. Kroegel C, Liu MC, Hubbard WC, et al. Blood and bronchoalveolar eosinophils in allergic subjects after segmental antigen challenge: Surface phenotype, density heterogeneity, and prostanoid production. J Allergy Clin Immunol 1994; 93:725–734.

20. Walker C, Braun RK, Boer C, et al. Cytokine control of eosinophils in pulmonary diseases. J Allergy Clin Immunol 1994; 94:1262–1271.

21. Fujisawa T, Abu-Ghazaleh R, Kita H, et al. Regulatory effect of cytokines on eosinophil degranulation. J Immunol 1990; 144:642–646.

22. Kita H, Weiler DA, Abu-Ghazaleh R, et al. Release of granule proteins from eosinophils cultured with IL-5. J Immunol 1992; 149:629–635.

23. Sedgwick JB, Calhoun WJ, Gleich GJ, et al. Immediate and late airway response of allergic rhinitis patients to segmental antigen challenge: Characterization of eosinophil and mast cell mediators. Am Rev Respir Dis 1991; 144:1274–1281.

24. Walker C, Bauer W, Braun RK, et al. Activated T cells and cytokines in bronchoalveo-

lar lavages from patients with various lung diseases associated with eosinophilia. Am J Respir Crit Care Med 1994; 150:1038–1048.

25. Nakajima H, Iwamoto I, Tomoe S, et al. CD4+ T-lymphocytes and interleukin-5 mediate antigen-induced eosinophil infiltration into the mouse trachea. Am Rev Respir Dis 1992; 146:374–377.

26. Van Oosterhout AJ, Ladenius AR, Savelkoul HF, et al. Effect of anti-IL-5 and IL-5 on airway hyperreactivity and eosinophils in guinea pigs. Am Rev Respir Dis 1993; 147: 548–552.

27. Dent LA, Mellor AL, Strath M, Sanderson CJ. Eosinophilia in transgenic mice expressing interleukin 5. J Exp Med 1990; 172:1425–1433.

28. Abu-Ghazaleh RI, Fujisawa T, Mestecky J, et al. IgA-induced eosinophil degranulation. J Immunol 1989; 142:2393–2399.

29. Kroegel C, Chilvers ER, Giembycz MA, et al. Platelet-activating factor stimulates a rapid accumulation of inositol (1,4,5) trisphosphate in guinea pig eosinophils: Relationship to calcium mobilization and degranulation. J Allergy Clin Immunol 1991; 88:114–124.

30. Howard MC, Miyajima A, Coffman RL. T-cell-derived cytokines and their receptors. In: Paul WE, ed. Fundamental Immunology, 3d ed. New York: Raven Press, 1996:763.

31. Okayama Y, Semper A, Holgate ST, Church MK. Multiple cytokine mRNA expression in human mast cells stimulated via Fc epsilon RI. Int Arch Allergy Immunol 1995; 107:158–159.

32. Okayama Y, Petit-Frere C, Kassel O, et al. IgE-dependent expression of mRNA for IL-4 and IL-5 in human lung mast cells. J Immunol 1995; 155:1796–1808.

33. Dubucquoi S, Desreumaux P, Janin A, et al. Interleukin 5 synthesis by eosinophils: Association with granules and immunoglobulin-dependent secretion. J Exp Med 1994; 179:703–708.

34. Ying S, Durham SR, Corrigan CJ, et al. Phenotype of cells expressing mRNA for TH2-type (interleukin 4 and interleukin 5) and TH1-type (interleukin 2 and interferon gamma) cytokines in bronchoalveolar lavage and bronchial biopsies from atopic asthmatic and normal control subjects. Am J Resp Cell Mol Biol 1995; 12:477–487.

35. Warren HS, Kinnear BF, Phillips JH, Lanier LL. Production of IL-5 by human NK-cells and regulation of secretion by IL-4, IL-10 and IL12. J Immunol 1995; 154:5144–5152.

36. Corrigan CJ, Kay AB. T cells and eosinophils in the pathogenesis of asthma. Immunol Today 1992; 13:501–507.

37. Bradley BL, Azzawi M, Jacobson M, et al. Eosinophils, T-lymphocytes, mast cells, neutrophils, and macrophages in bronchial biopsy specimens from atopic subjects with asthma: Comparison with biopsy specimens from atopic subjects without asthma and normal control subjects and relationship to bronchial hyperresponsiveness. J Allergy Clin Immunol 1991; 88:661–674.

38. Corrigan CJ, Kay AB. CD4 T-lymphocyte activation in acute severe asthma: Relationship to disease severity and atopic status. Am Rev Respir Dis 1990; 141:970–977.

39. Azzawi M, Bradley B, Jeffery PK, et al. Identification of activated T lymphocytes and eosinophils in bronchial biopsies in stable atopic asthma. Am Rev Respir Dis 1990; 142:1407–1413.

40. Robinson DR, Hamid Q, Ying S, et al. Evidence for a predominant "Th2-type" bronchoalveolar lavage T-lymphocyte population in atopic asthma. N Engl J Med 1992; 326:298–304.

41. Doi S, Gemou-Engesaeth V, Kay AB, Corrigan CJ. Polymerase chain reaction quantification of cytokine messenger RNA expression in peripheral blood mononuclear cells of patients with acute exacerbations of asthma: Effect of glucocorticoid therapy. Clin Exp Allergy 1994; 24:854–867.

42. Walker C, Bode E, Boer L, et al. Allergic and nonallergic asthmatics have distinct patterns of T-cell activation and cytokine production in peripheral blood and bronchoalveolar lavage. Am Rev Respir Dis 1992; 146:109–115.

43. Maestrelli P, Del Prete GF, De Carli M, et al. CD8 T-cell clones producing interleukin-5 and interferon-gamma in bronchial mucosa of patients with asthma induced by toluene diisocyanate. Scand J Work Environ Health 1994; 20:376–381.

44. Finotto S, Fabbri L, Rado V, et al. Increase in numbers of CD8+ lymphocytes and eosinophils in peripheral blood of subjects with alte asthmatics reactions induced by toluene diisocyanate. Br J Ind Med 1991; 48:116–121.

45. Busse WW. The role of respiratory infections in airway hyperresponsiveness and asthma. Am J Respir Crit Care Med 1994; 150:S77–S79.

46. Coyle AJ, Erard F, Bertrand C, et al. Virus-specific CD8+ cells can switch to interleukin 5 production and induce airway eosinophilia. J Exp Med 1995; 181:1229–1233.

47. Folkerts G, Verheyen A, Janssen M, Nijkamp FP. Virus-induced airway hyperresponsiveness in the guinea pig can be transferred by bronchoalveolar cells. J Allergy Clin Immunol 1992; 90:364–372.

48. Van Oosterhout AJ, van Ark I, Folkerts G, et al. Antibody to interleukin-5 inhibits virus-induced airway hyperresponsiveness to histamine in guinea pigs. Am J Respir Crit Care Med 1995; 151:177–183.

49. Baumgarth N, Brown L, Jackson D, Kelso A. Novel features of the respiratory tract T-cell response to influenza virus infection: Lung T cells increase expression of gamma interferon mRNA in vivo and maintain high levels of mRNA expression for interleukin-5 (IL-5) and IL-10. J Virol 1994; 68:7575–7581.

50. Le Gros G, Erard F. Non-cytotoxic, IL-4, IL-5, IL-10 producing CD8+ T cells: Their activation and effector functions. Curr Opin Immunol 1994; 6:453–457.

51. Gleich GJ, Adolphson C. Bronchial hyperreactivity and eosinophil granule proteins. Agents Actions Suppl 1993; 43:223–230.

52. White SR, Ohno S, Munoz NM, et al. Epithelium-dependent contraction of airway smooth muscle caused by eosinophil MBP. Am J Physiol 1990; 259:L294–L303.

53. Grundel RH, Gerritsen ME, Gleich GJ, Wegner CD. Repeated antigen inhalation results in a prolonged airway eosinophilia and airway hyperresponsiveness in primates. J Appl Physiol 1990; 68:779–786.

54. Gundel RH, Letts LG, Gleich GJ. Human eosinophil major basic protein induces airway constriction and airway hyperresponsiveness in primates. J Clin Invest 1991; 87:1470–1473.

55. Jacoby DB, Gleich GJ, Fryer AD. Human eosinophil major basic protein is an endogenous allosteric antagonist at the inhibitory muscarinic M2 receptor. J Clin Invest 1993; 91:1314–1318.

56. Coyle AJ, Ackerman SJ, Burch R, et al. Human eosinophil-granule major basic protein and synthetic polycations induce airway hyperresponsiveness in vivo dependent on bradykinin generation. J Clin Invest 1995; 95:1735–1740.

57. Buske Kirschbaum A, Kirschbaum C, Stierle H, et al. Conditioned increase of natural killer cell activity (NKCA) in humans. Psychosom Med 1992; 54:123–132.

58. Ulrik CS, Backer V, Dirksen A. Mortality and decline in lung function in 213 adults with bronchial asthma: A ten-year follow up. J Asthma 1992; 29:29–38.

59. van Schayck CP, Dompeling E, van Herwaarden CL, et al. Interacting effects of atopy and bronchial hyperresponsiveness on the annual decline in lung function and the exacerbation rate in asthma. Am Rev Respir Dis 1991; 144:1297–1301.

60. Ulrik CS, Backer V, Dirksen A. A 10 year follow up of 180 adults with bronchial asthma: Factors important for the decline in lung function. Thorax 1992; 47:14–18.

61. Jeffery PK. Histological features of the airways in asthma and COPD. Respiration 1992; 59(Suppl 1):13–16.

62. Kuwano K, Bosken CH, Pare PD, et al. Small airways dimensions in asthma and in chronic obstructive pulmonary disease. Am Rev Respir Dis 1993; 148:1220–1225.

63. Paganin F, Seneterre E, Chanez P, et al. Computed tomography of the lungs in asthma—Influence of disease severity and etiology. Am J Respir Crit Care Med 1996; 153:110–114.

64. Brody AR. Control of lung fibroblast proliferation by macrophage-derived platelet-derived growth factor. Ann NY Acad Sci 1994; 725:193–199.

65. Reidy MA. Factors controlling smooth-muscle cell proliferation. Arch Pathol Lab Med 1992; 116:1276–1280.

66. Casscells W. Smooth muscle cell growth factors. Prog Growth Factor Res 1991; 3: 177–206.

67. Bonner JC. Regulation of platelet-derived growth factor (PDGF) and alveolar macrophage-derived PDGF by alpha 2-macroglobulin. Ann NY Acad Sci 1994; 737: 324–338.

68. Aubert JD, Hayashi S, Hards J, et al. Platelet-derived growth factor and its receptor in lungs from patients with asthma and chronic airflow obstruction. Am J Physiol 1994; 266:L655–L663.

69. Chanez P, Vignola M, Stenger R, et al. Platelet-derived growth factor in asthma. Allergy 1995; 50:878–883.

70. Ohno I, Nitta Y, Yamauchi K, et al. Eosinophils as a potential source of platelet-derived growth factor B-chain (PDGF-B) in nasal polyposis and bronchial asthma. Am J Respir Cell Mol Biol 1995; 13:639–647.

3

Pathology of Asthma in the Elderly

RICHARD E. SOBONYA

University of Arizona Health Sciences Center
Tucson, Arizona

Many pathologists have thought they had absolute criteria of bronchial or allergic asthma. We clinicians felt that they did not.

—Robert W. Lanson, M.D., 1937

I. Introduction

The structural changes associated with clinical asthma occur particularly in bronchi—that is, those airways having seromucinous glands and cartilage plates in their walls and measuring greater than 2 mm in luminal diameter. However, changes reflecting asthma also involve small airways, those nonalveolated airways without cartilage measuring 2 mm or less. Changes in the alveolar parenchyma—such as hyperinflation, atelectasis, or transient eosinophilic infiltrates—are of less importance and are secondary to the airways disease. True destructive emphysema does not occur as a consequence of asthma (1).

The pathology of asthma has been well documented in younger patients with relatively untreated disease who die in status asthmaticus (2–4). This pathology is described below and compared with that of simple chronic bronchitis (without airflow obstruction) and chronic obstructive bronchitis (small airways disease). However, the nature and severity of pathological changes seen in asthma often do not reflect clinical or pathophysiological findings: structural alterations do not provide a complete basis for clinical asthma. A recent study of bronchial biopsies in asthmatics points out that the degree of inflammation does not correlate with the patient's symptoms or bronchial hyperresponsiveness (5). The pathology of fatal asthma, including status asthmaticus, shows wide variation in the degree of common pathological findings, such as bronchial mucous plugging, increased smooth muscle, and increased bronchial glands (see below). Basement membrane thickening (now known to be subepithelial fibrosis) is almost universally present in asthmatics (6), but does not indicate the degree of symptomatology or physiologic derangement. When the effects of age, chronicity of disease, therapy, and the coexistence of other diseases are added to the pathology of asthma, a complex morphologic picture emerges (1). The pathology of asthma will be examined in the elderly asthmatic, whether a patient with newly diagnosed asthma or one with asthma stretching over decades. But even now, as was the case 60 years ago, the pathologic criteria for this clinically complex disease falls short of absolute.

II. Comparative Pathology of Asthma, Simple Chronic Bronchitis, and Chronic Obstructive Bronchitis (Small Airways Disease) as Part of Chronic Obstructive Pulmonary Disease

Asthma is a chronic inflammatory disease (7). While the histologic evidence for this fact has been with us since the 1920's (2), only in the last few decades has that concept increased our understanding of asthma. The older definition of asthma (8), a clinical one, referred to a chronic disease with productive cough and dyspnea due to clinical airflow obstruction from episodic, reversible airways narrowing. The addition of the role of inflammation has produced this updated definition: "Asthma is a chronic inflammatory disorder of the airways.... In susceptible individuals this inflammation causes recurrent episodes of wheezing, breathlessness, chest tightness, and cough ..." (7). This paradigm shift from the mechanical aspects of bronchospasm and mucous plugging to the inflammatory events that underlie them has allowed much progress in elucidating the pathogenesis and drug therapy of asthma.

The meaning of the clinical entity called chronic obstructive pulmonary disease (COPD) has recently been clarified and refined in a statement from the American Thoracic Society (9). This condition is defined as "a disease state characterized by the presence of airflow obstruction due to chronic bronchitis or emphysema." The majority of patients with COPD have both emphysema and chronic bronchitis. Various types of chronic bronchitis have been described. Simple chronic bronchitis is defined clinically as chronic productive cough unexplained by an underlying disease (8). Pathological alterations are confined to the larger airways, and clinically significant expiratory airflow limitation is not present. Chronic obstructive bronchitis is a disease of small airways and produces airflow obstruction. The chronic bronchitis that is part of COPD is chronic obstructive bronchitis. In reality, this disease is more of a bronchiolitis than a bronchitis, hence the alternative term *small airways disease*. A third form of chronic bronchitis, asthmatic bronchitis, is seen in asthmatics whose airflow obstruction is no longer fully reversible; it can be thought of as a combination of asthma and chronic obstructive bronchitis. This entity is discussed further on in the chapter. The final thrust of this revised definition of COPD is the exclusion of patients with asthma, as much as possible, from being classified as having COPD.

A comparison of the large airways in asthma and simple chronic bronchitis shows many similarities and a few striking differences (10–12). A striking feature of asthma is epithelial shedding or sloughing into the airway lumen, leaving only a layer of basal cells or no epithelium at all on the basement membrane (5,10,13), as seen in Fig. 1. This finding is emphasized in descriptions of the pathology of

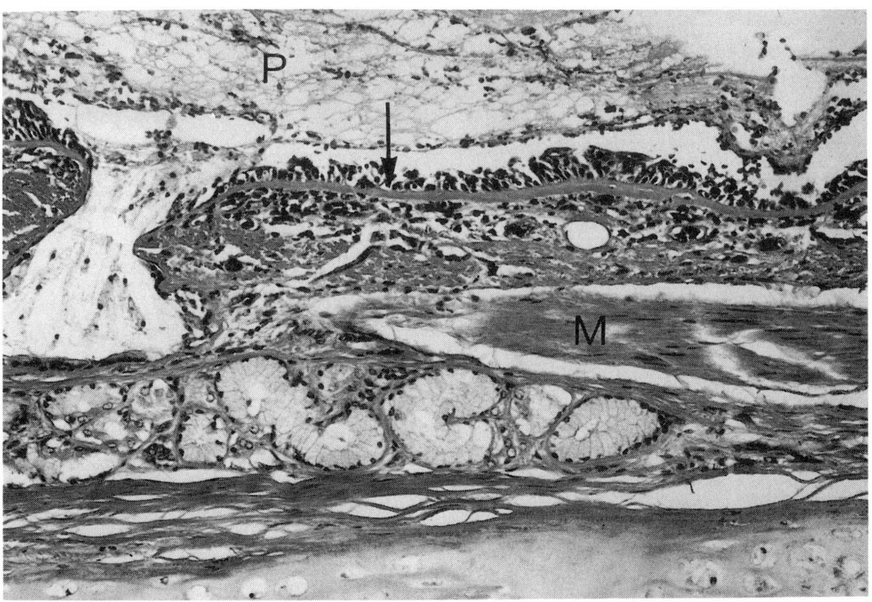

Figure 1   Low-power view of the bronchial wall in active asthma in an elderly patient with corticosteroid-treated, long-standing disease. Mucous plugging (P), a thick basement membrane (arrow), and prominent muscle (M) are seen; eosinophils are absent. Focal epithelial denudation is seen in the area of the gland duct on the left side of the picture. (H&E, ×195.)

asthma but not those of simple chronic bronchitis. However, a comparison of bronchial biopsies from asthmatics and patients with COPD, presumably having some degree of simple chronic bronchitis as well, showed a similar degree of epithelial loss in the two groups (5). Artifactual loss of epithelium during biopsy and the sampling error inherent in small biopsies may account for the degree of epithelial loss in larger airways in COPD. Still, in resected or autopsy lungs, the degree of epithelial loss in asthmatics is much more striking than that in simple chronic bronchitis occurring with COPD. The epithelium of large airways in asthma also typically shows goblet-cell hyperplasia; instead of the ratio of one goblet cell for approximately each three to five ciliated columnar cells (14), the ratio becomes 1:1 or greater (15). Squamous metaplasia occasionally occurs. Similar goblet cell hyperplasia occurs in simple chronic bronchitis (16,17), and squamous metaplasia is common.

Both simple chronic bronchitis and asthma are characterized by the production of mucoid sputum as well as mucous plugs in airways lumens (15). The plugging in asthma is related to active disease, and the plugs are described as more dense and more tenacious. Cytologically, the plugs in asthma usually contain Curschmann's spirals, which are curlicues of inspissated mucus from bronchial gland ducts (18). Creola bodies, aggregates of detached epithelium that occasionally simulate neoplasia, are also more common in asthma (19). If they have systematic eosinophilia, the mucus of asthmatics may contain many eosinophils as well as acicular eosinophilic crystals known as Charcot-Leyden crystals (18). These crystals are composed primarily of lysophopholipase (20). Mucous plugging in patients with simple chronic bronchitis or COPD is far less extensive and the plugs are not as tenacious. Curschmann's spirals, Creola bodies, and Charcot-Leyden crystals are usually absent.

By morphometric analysis, both asthmatics and simple chronic bronchitics typically have enlarged bronchial glands (16,17,21,22) with a tendency for more mucinous acini than normal (Fig. 1). However, occasionally there is overlap with the normal range in both entities. Bronchial gland duct ectasia is common in asthmatics, and rupture of one of these dilated ducts may be the mechanism of interstitial emphysema (air) in status asthmaticus (23). Bronchial muscle is increased in asthmatics (24,25) (Fig. 1), and this increase entails a significant degree of smooth muscle cell hyperplasia as well as hypertrophy (24,25). There typically is no increase in smooth muscle in bronchitics (21,22).

The basement membrane has long been a focus of interest in asthma because it is clearly thickened in nearly all cases (3,6) (Fig. 1). The original concept, based on light microscopy, was that the membrane itself was thickened, perhaps by deposition of immunoglobulins. Now it is clear from electron microscopic studies (26–29) that subepithelial collagen deposition (fibrosis) accounts for the appearance of thickening. Immunohistochemical studies showed that the true basement membrane, which is largely collagen IV, was no thicker than in controls, but collagen III and fibronectin were deposited in the reticular layer beneath. Immuno-globulins (IgM and G but not E) have been localized to the region of the basement membrane in some asthmatics and occasionally in nonasthmatics (30,31). However, these deposits do not explain the apparent thickening seen. Bronchitics and patients with other chronic respiratory infections may have a modest degree of basement membrane thickening, but this rarely approaches that seen in asthma. Thus, basement membrane alteration remains the most reliable histological finding suggesting clinical asthma (32).

Elastic fibers in the lamina propria of the airways are altered in asthma; fragmentation, tangling, and thickening are seen (33). It is not known if similar changes occur in bronchitis. The volume percent of interstitial tissue is not significant different in asthma and simple chronic bronchitis (21), though vascular dilatation is more commonly described in the latter. The striking feature of the interstitial connective tissue in asthma is the type and extent of inflammation (34), as discussed in detail in Chap. 4. Aggregates of lymphocytes and plasma cells are common in asthmatic airways, even between attacks. CD3$^+$ T lymphocytes are present in the epithelium of asthmatic airways, but their numbers are reduced in fatal asthma (35). Eosinophils appear during attacks and are abundant in connective tissue and between epithelial cells (35–38). Their presence is correlated with the severity of asthma in some studies but not in others (36,37). The bronchitic airways similarly have lymphoplasmacytic infiltrates, but eosinophils are not common (5). Acute infections result in infiltrates of neutrophils. Mast cells in asthma have been regarded as apparently reduced with degranulation (12). They are increased in smokers (39) and are increased and not degranulated in simple chronic bronchitis (12). The difficulties of identifying degranulated mast cells in tissue by histological methods rather than electron microscopy or immunohisto-chemistry are apparent.

Histological changes in the small airways in asthma were noted in earlier descriptions of the pathology of asthma, but the gross findings in large and medium-sized bronchi were emphasized. Changes seen in small airways include mucous plugging, a mixed inflammatory infiltrate with many eosinophils, and basement membrane thickening. These were variably present but were less severe than bronchial changes (2,3). More recent studies have emphasized morphometric techniques in evaluating small airways in asthma and have shown increased wall thickness, increased area of smooth muscle, mucous plugging, and eosinophilic inflammation (40–42), as seen in Fig. 2. Wall thickening in asthmatics is due to increased epithelium, muscle, and submucosa and occurs in large and small airways (43). This thickening may be as important as muscle shortening (contraction) in determining airways responsiveness.

The small airways changes in asthma can be compared to chronic obstructive bronchitis (small airways disease), as seen in COPD, in which the injury is largely attributed to cigarette smoking. A recent review summarizes small airways

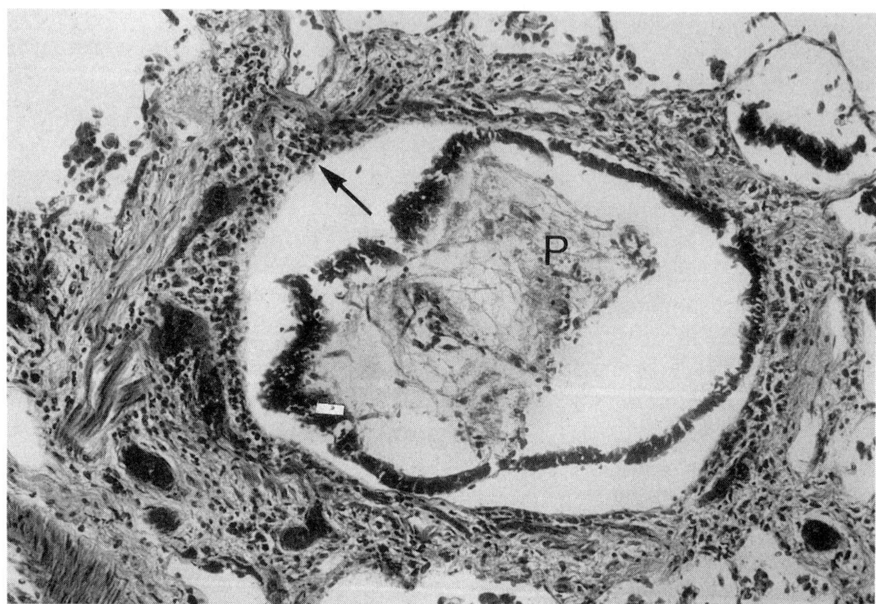

Figure 2 A small airway from an elderly asthmatic showing mucous plugging (P) and diffuse lymphocytic inflammation (arrow) of the wall. These changes are the same as those in chronic obstructive bronchitis (small airways disease). (H&E, ×150.)

disease in COPD (44): inflammation without many eosinophils, wall thickening, and fibrosis are typical features. Wall thickening is important because a small airway with a thick wall, though it may have a normal luminal area during maximal dilatation, will have a reduced luminal area with muscle contraction (shortening) compared to airways of normal wall thickness (45). The wall area of small airways was greater in asthmatics than in controls, and small airways muscle was increased in asthmatics more than in COPD patients, but both showed increases over controls (42). This wall thickening may contribute to airways hyperresponsiveness in COPD (46). Loss of epithelium and squamous metaplasia of bronchiolar epithelium are seen in the chronic obstructive bronchitis of COPD, but the most noted lesion is goblet cell metaplasia (47). Loss of alveolar attachments to small airways influences small airways function in COPD (48), since this process is a reflection of emphysema. This finding is not seen in asthma. In summary, small airways in asthma may show wall thickening, increased muscle area, and mucous plugs; these features are similar to small airways disease in COPD but quantitatively are more severe. Inflammation is seen in both conditions but shows a predominance of eosinophils in asthma. Fibrosis seems to be more evident in the chronic obstructive bronchitis of COPD.

The pathology of fatal asthma is more varied than might be expected. Early reports, such as that by Cardell and Pearson in 1959 (3), stressed the findings of mucous plugging, infiltration of eosinophils, and a thickened basement membrane. They concluded that "these features are diagnostic of severe active asthma" (3). All their cases except one infant who did not have basement membrane thickening showed these three features. However, more recent studies have noted cases of fatal asthma without bronchial mucous plugging (49). Similarly, sudden-onset fatal asthma has been described to have relatively few eosinophils and more neutrophils (50). Cluroe et al. (23) reviewed the histology of 72 cases of clinical fatal asthma. Asthma was diagnosed pathologically if at least four of five of the following histological criteria were present: mucous plugging, basement membrane thickening, epithelial shedding, eosinophilic infiltrates, and smooth muscle enlargement. Only 53 of the 72 cases (74%) could be called asthma histologically. The reasons for this lack of concordance probably include a more expanded definition of asthma as well as modification of the disease by drug therapy, especially systemic corticosteroids (see below).

A comparison of histological changes in asthma compared to simple chronic bronchitis is seen in Table 1. In many instances the range of abnormality of a

Table 1 Pathology of Untreated Asthma Compared to Simple Chronic Bronchitis

Airways pathology	Asthma	Simple chronic bronchitis
Mucous plugging	Usually widespread during attacks	Occasional
Epithelial sloughing	Continuous process, major finding	Occurs but not prominent
Basement membrane thickening	Nearly always present, striking	Mild degrees seen
Thickened bronchial wall	Major finding	Occurs
Lymphocytic inflammation	Prominent	Present, moderate
Eosinophilia	Major finding	Not seen
Increased muscle	Major finding	Uncommon[a]
Increased glands	Major finding	Major finding, often striking
Small airways disease	Variable	May occur[b]

[a]Increased smooth muscle suggests asthma with or instead of simple chronic bronchitis.
[b]Small airways disease with airflow limitation indicates chronic obstructive bronchitis.

particular histological alteration (bronchial gland enlargement, epithelial sloughing, inflammation) overlaps significantly between the two diseases. On the other
hand, widespread mucous plugging, greatly increased smooth muscle, and eosinophilic inflammation each strongly correlate with asthma. Greatly enlarged bronchial glands strongly suggest chronic bronchitis (17,51,52), especially in the
absence of features suggesting asthma. Subepithelial fibrosis is the single best
histological feature correlating with asthma. The looseness of these correlations
should not be surprising, as the definitions of both diseases are predominantly
clinical. Finally, the clinical precipitating factors for acute asthma do not influence
the pathology of this disease. Intrinsic and extrinsic types of asthma do not differ
in gross or microscopic histological features.

III. Effects of Aging: Asthmatic Bronchitis

The pathology of asthmatic airways is likely to be influenced by the subject's age,
the duration and intensity of disease, exposure to injurious agents, sampling
variation inherent in bronchoscopic biopsies, and therapy. The extent of this
variation is not known, however, because no study to date has analyzed the
pathology of asthmatic airways in a group of cases controlled for all the above
factors. However, we can examine each of these factors and speculate how they
might affect the morphology of asthma in the elderly.

Several age-related changes have been described in human airways. Squamous metaplasia of the epithelium can occur in adults of any age (53) but is most
prevalent in adults of age 41 to 50 years, decreasing as age advances. Exposure to
cigarette smoke increases the likelihood of squamous metaplasia (53,54). Bronchial gland mass is increased in aged nonsmokers (55) and oncocytes are more
frequent in the bronchial glands of older persons (56). An oncocyte is mitochon-
dria-rich but relatively nonfunctional type of glandular cell, and oncocytes are
more frequent with age in other organs in the body as well, such as parathyroids
and salivary glands. Adipose tissue in the lamina propria of airways likewise is a
change seen more in older persons. Because of exposure to atmospheric irritants,
one would assume that the extent of lymphoplasmacytic infiltrate normally seen in
the airways would be increased. Bronchial cartilage may become ossified in the
elderly and may even acquire bone marrow cells. Large airways diameter does not
change with age once the adult size has been reached (57). None of these changes
would appear to modify the appearance of asthma in an older person (2–4).

One cannot distinguish untreated asthma in a 70-year-old from that in a 20-
year-old by routine histopathology of the airways (2–3). Perhaps by morphometric analysis, one could discern differences in type and extent of inflammation,
but there is striking intrasubject variability in airway inflammation in asthma (58),
making such comparisons difficult. Similarly, the range of variation of typical

findings in asthma—such as bronchial gland or smooth muscle area (20,21,23,24), airway area, and basement membrane thickness (3)—hampers detection of any morphological differences in asthma in older compared to younger patients.

Changes in small airways due to age alone are not easily separated from other factors. The accumulation of atmospheric pigment has been shown (59), and one would assume that inflammation and fibrosis may be increased, reflecting chronic low-grade inhalation of atmospheric irritants. Small airways diameters increase from early adulthood till approximately age 40, and then they decline (57). The small airways of an elderly asthmatic thus will reflect effects of aging, atmospheric irritants, and particularly any cigarette use.

Some elderly asthmatics have relatively new disease, while others may have been asthmatic from childhood or adolescence (60,61). Asthma presenting as a new disease in the elderly may appear to be more in the nature of chronic bronchitis with episodic bronchospasm or bronchitis with bronchospasm during acute infections (62,63). This entity has been termed *asthmatic bronchitis* and is more frequently seen in elderly women. The limited pathological evaluation of such patients has shown changes of simple chronic bronchitis but with increased smooth muscle (22). Thus, they would resemble asthma morphologically and could be considered such. In terms of ICD-9 coding, the point is moot, as both simple chronic bronchitis and asthma can be combined and coded as asthmatic bronchitis. Asthmatic bronchitis, because of the component of airflow obstruction, thus becomes a type of COPD, while asthma by itself is not subsumed under this mantle (9). The difficulties in classification of various forms of asthma and COPD are discussed further in Chap. 1.

IV. Remodeling of Asthmatic Airways

With chronic asthma, airflow obstruction (limitation) may become relatively irreversible; these changes reflect both the duration and severity of the disease (64). The structural changes causing resistance to airflow during acute asthma are twofold: (1) mucous plugging and airways wall thickening by edema and inflammation, producing airway narrowing, and (2) smooth muscle shortening (15,45). These changes are reversible spontaneously or with therapy. The changes that account for the irreversible component to chronic asthma are less well understood. The concept of airways remodeling has been introduced to explain the structural lesions of irreversible asthma (65).

The subepithelial fibrosis of asthmatic bronchi creating the "thickened basement membrane" is a change that is not influenced by therapy (1,29) and persists between attacks (26,38) and with advancing age. The occasional report of an infant dying of asthma with a bronchial basement membranes of normal thickness (3) indicate that this change results from disease activity over time. This thickened membrane is an irreversible fibrosing process that indicates airway remodeling (66–68). Such remodeling may lead to decreased responsiveness to bronchodilator and anti-inflammatory drugs such as corticosteroids. Injury to bronchial elastic fibers may decrease lung elastic recoil and interfere with airway stability and distensibility (33). Airway remodeling in asthma is the subject of a monograph scheduled for release at about the time of this writing (69).

Small airways disease of the type seen in COPD has been suggested as a cause for lack of reversibility in long-standing asthma (70,71) and has been seen in some elderly asthmatics with long-standing disease (1). Fibrosis in small airways of asthmatics may occur as shown in Fig. 3, producing irreversible airflow obstruction, as in COPD. However, some elderly asthmatics with irreversible disease seem to have flow limitation due to thickened airway walls (45,65); perhaps glandular and smooth muscle enlargement fails to regress with therapy (67). The epithelial denudation commonly seen in asthma may be the stimulus for release of cytokines and other mediators that stimulates smooth muscle proliferation (67). The extent of reversibility of smooth muscle proliferation in asthma is still to be determined.

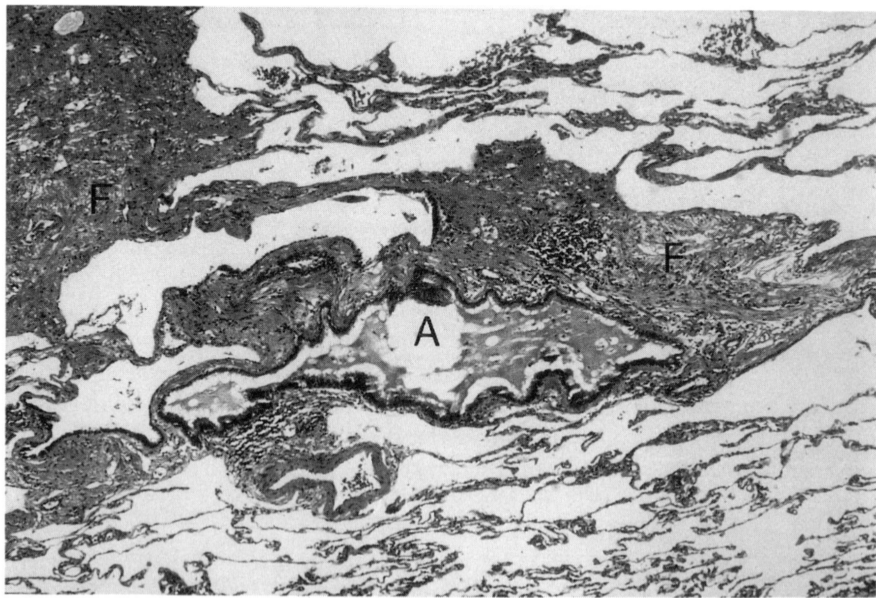

Figure 3 A small airway (A) distorted by fibrosis (F) in an elderly asthmatic. Such an irreversible change is rare in a normal lung but may be seen in chronic obstructive bronchitis as well. (H&E, ×150.)

The presence of eosinophils is evidently not necessary for the onset of fixed airflow limitation in asthma, as systemic corticosteroid therapy eliminates nearly all blood and lung tissue eosinophilia (1,29,38). Thus an elderly asthmatic on prolonged systemic corticosteroid therapy with symptoms for decades may have airways showing differences from those of a recently diagnosed, largely untreated asthmatic. Airways in the former individual may show little lymphocytic inflammation and no eosinophilia. Smooth muscle will be prominent, as will the basement membrane. Bronchial glands may be normal or modestly increased in size. Nonetheless, the symptomatology and physiological impairment will not differ from that of the young asthmatic.

V. Summary

The triad of pathological changes identified in early descriptions of fatal asthma—namely, mucous plugs in airways, eosinophilic infiltrates, and a thickened basement membrane—distinguish asthma from simple chronic bronchitis and the obstructive chronic bronchitis (small airways disease) seen in COPD. These changes may be modified in chronic asthma as seen in the elderly. Mucous plugs are a variable component of acute disease, and eosinophilic infiltrates may disappear with aerosolized or systemic corticosteroids or similar drug therapy. The subepithelial fibrosis that gives the appearance of thickened basement membrane, elastic tissue injury, small airways disease, and fixed thickening of airway walls may produce irreversible airflow obstruction. Detailed study of the bronchial tree in asthma of various durations in patients with varying therapies at all ages have not yet been done. This is a promising area for research to further our understanding of asthma as it changes clinically with time.

Abbreviations

COPD   chronic obstructive pulmonary disease
IgE   immunoglobulin E
IgG   immunoglobulin G
IgM   immunoglobulin M

References

1. Sobonya RE. Concise clinical study: Quantitative structural alterations in long-standing allergic asthma. Am Rev Respir Dis 1984; 130:289–292.
2. Huber HL, Koessler KK. The pathology of bronchial asthma. Arch Intern Med 1922; 30:689–760

3. Cardell BS, Pearson RSB. Death in asthmatics. Thorax 1959; 14:341–352.
4. Dunnill MS. The pathology of asthma, with special reference to changes in the bronchial mucosa. J Clin Pathol 1960; 13:27–33.
5. Ollerenshaw SL, Woolcock AJ. Characteristics of the inflammation in biopsies from large airways of subjects with asthma and subjects with chronic airflow limitation. Am Rev Respir Dis 1992; 145:922–927.
6. Crepea SB, Harman JW. The pathology of bronchial asthma: I. The significance of membrane changes in asthma and nonallergic pulmonary disease. J Allergy 1955; 26:453–460.
7. Global Initiative for Asthma, National Institutes of Health, Pub. No. 95-3659, 1995.
8. American Thoracic Society. Chronic bronchitis, asthma, and pulmonary emphysema: A statement by the committee on diagnostic standards for non-tuberculous respiratory diseases. Am Rev Respir Dis 1962; 85:762–764.
9. American Thoracic Society. Standards for the diagnosis and care of patients with chronic obstructive pulmonary disease. Am J Respir Crit Care Med 1995; 152:S77–S120.
10. Jeffery PK. Comparative morphology of the airways in asthma and chronic obstructive pulmonary disease. Am J Respir Crit Care Med 1994; 150:S6–S13.
11. Glynn AA, Michaels L. Bronchial biopsy in chronic bronchitis and asthma. Thorax 1960; 15:142–153.
12. Salvato G. Some histological changes in chronic bronchitis and asthma. Thorax 1968; 23:168–172.
13. Djukanovic R, Roche WR, Wilson JW, et al. State of the art: Mucosal inflammation in asthma. Am Rev Respir Dis 1990; 142:434–457.
14. McDowell EM, Barett LA, Glavin F, et al. The respiratory epithelium: 1. human bronchus. J Natl Cancer Inst 1978; 61:539–549.
15. Aikawa T, Shimura S, Sasaki H, et al. Marked goblet cell hyperplasia with mucus accumulation in the airways of patients who died of severe acute asthma attack. Chest 1992; 101:916–921.
16. Reid L. Pathology of chronic bronchitis. Lancet 1954; 1:275–279.
17. Reid L. Measurement of the bronchial mucous gland layer: A diagnostic yardstick in chronic bronchitis. Thorax 1960; 15:132–141.
18. Sakula A. Charcot-Leyden crystals and Curschmann spirals in asthmatic sputum. Thorax 1986; 41:503–507.
19. Naylor B. The shedding of the mucosa of the bronchial tree in asthma. Thorax 1962; 17:69–72.
20. Weller PF, Bach D, Austen KF. Human eosinophil lysophospholipase: The sole protein content of Charcot-Leyden crystals. Proc Natl Acad Sci USA 1980; 77:7440–7443.
21. Dunnill MS, Massarella GR, Anderson JA. A comparison of the quantitative anatomy of the bronchi in normal subjects, in status asthmaticus, in chronic bronchitis, and in emphysema. Thorax 1969; 24:176–179.
22. Takizawa T, Thurlbeck WM. Muscle and mucous gland size in the major bronchi of patients with chronic bronchitis, asthma, and asthmatic bronchitis. Am Rev Respir Dis 1971; 104:331–336.

23. Cluroe A, Holloway L, Thomson K, et al. Bronchial gland duct ectasia in fatal bronchial asthma: Association with interstitial emphysema. J Clin Pathol 1989; 42: 1026–1031.

24. Hossain S. Quantitative morphometry of bronchial muscle in females. Pakistan Med Rev 1970; 5:411–422.

25. Hossain S. Quantitative measurement of bronchial muscle in men with asthma. Am Rev Respir Dis 1973; 107:99–109.

26. Cutz E, Levison H, Cooper DM. Ultrastructure of airways in children with asthma. Histopathology 1978; 2:407–421.

27. Roche WR, Beasley R, Williams JH, Holgate ST. Subepithelial fibrosis in the bronchi of asthmatics. Lancet 1969; 1:520–523.

28. Brewster CEP, Howarth PH, Djukanovic R, et al. Myofibroblasts and subepithelial fibrosis in bronchial asthma. Am J Respir Cell Mol Biol 1990; 3:507–511.

29. Jeffery PK, Godfrey RW, Adelroth E, et al. Effects of treatment on airway inflammation and thickening of basement membrane reticular collagen in asthma. Am Rev Respir Dis 1992; 145:890–899.

30. Callerame ML, Condemi JJ, Bohrod MG, Vaughn JH. Immunologic reactions of bronchial tissues in asthma. N Engl J Med 1971; 183:459–464.

31. Gerber MA, Paronetto F, Kochwa S. Immunohistochemical localization of IgE in asthmatic lungs. Am J Pathol 1971; 62:339–351.

32. Thieme ET, Sheldon JM. A correlation of the clinical and pathologic findings in bronchial asthma. J Allergy 1938; 9:246–269.

33. Bousquet J, Lacoste J-Y, Chanez P, et al. Bronchial elastic fibers in normal subjects and asthmatic patients. Am J Respir Crit Care Med 1996; 153:1648–1654.

34. Gross NJ. Airway inflammation in COPD: Reality or myth? Chest 1995; 107:210S–213S.

35. Bosquet J, Chanez P, Lacoste J-Y, et al. Eosinophilic infiltration in asthma. N Engl J Med 1990; 323:1033–1039.

36. Synek M, Beasley R, Frew AJ, et al. Cellular infiltration of the airways in asthma of varying severity. Am J Respir Crit Care Med 1996; 154:224–230.

37. McFadden ER Jr. Asthma: Morphologic-physiologic interactions. Am J Respir Crit Care Med 1994; 150:S23–S26.

38. Laitanen LA, Laitanen A, Heino M, Haahtela T. Eosinophilic airway inflammation during exacerbation of asthma and its treatment with inhaled corticosteroid. Am Rev Respir Dis 1991; 143:423–427.

39. Lamb D, Lumsden A. Intra-epithelial mast cells in human airway epithelium: Evidence for smoking-induced changes in their frequency. Thorax 1982; 37:334–342.

40. Saetta M, Di Stefano A, Rosina C, et al. Quantitative structural analysis of peripheral airways and arteries in sudden fatal asthma. Am Rev Respir Dis 1991; 143:138–143.

41. Carroll N, Elliot J, Morton A, James A. The structure of large and small airways in nonfatal and fatal asthma. Am Rev Respir Dis 1993; 147:404–410.

42. Kuwano K, Bosken CH, Pare PD, et al. Small airways dimensions in asthma and in chronic obstructive pulmonary disease. Am Rev Respir Dis 1993; 148:1220–1225.

43. James AL, Pare PD, Hogg JC. The mechanics of airway narrowing in asthma. Am Rev Respir Dis 1989; 139:242–246.

44. Wright JL, Cagle P, Churg A, et al. State of the art: Diseases of the small airways. Am Rev Respir Dis 1992; 146:240–262.

45. Moreno RH, Hogg JC, Pare PD. Mechanics of airway narrowing. Am Rev Respir Dis 1986; 133:1171–1180.

46. Wiggs BR, Bosken C, Pare PD, et al. A model of airway narrowing in asthma and in chronic obstructive pulmonary disease. Am Rev Respir Dis 1992; 145:1251–1258.

47. Karpick RJ, Pratt PC, Asmundsson T, Kilburn KH. Pathological findings in respiratory failure: Goblet cell metaplasia, alveolar damage, and myocardial infarction. Ann Intern Med 1970; 72:189–197.

48. Saetta M, Ghezzo H, Kim WD, et al. Loss of alveolar attachments in smokers: A morphometric correlate of lung function impairment. Am Rev Respir Dis 1985; 132:894–900.

49. Reid LM. The presence or absence of bronchial mucus in fatal asthma. J Allergy Clin Immunol 1987; 80(part 2):415–416.

50. Sur S, Crotty TB, Kephart GM, et al. Sudden-onset fatal asthma: A distinct entity with few eosinophils and relatively more neutrophils in the submucosa? Am Rev Respir Dis 1993; 148:713–719.

51. Field WEH, Davey EN, Reid L, Roe FJC. Bronchial mucus gland hypertrophy: Its relation to symptoms and environment. Br J Dis Chest 1966; 60:66–80.

52. Jamal K, Cooney TP, Fleetham JA, Thurlbeck WM. Chronic bronchitis: Correlation of morphologic findings to sputum production and flow rates. Am Rev Respir Dis 1984; 129:719–722.

53. Spain DM. Metaplasia of bronchial epithelium: Effect of age, sex, and smoking. JAMA 1970; 211:1331.

54. Peters EJ, Morice R, Benner SE, et al. Squamous metaplasia of the bronchial mucosa and its relationship to smoking. Chest 1993; 103:1429–1432.

55. Hernandez JA, Anderson AE Jr, Holmes WI, et al. The bronchial glands in aging. J Am Geriatr Soc 1965; 13:799–803.

56. Matsuba K, Takizawa T, Thurlbeck WM. Oncocytes in human bronchial mucous glands. Thorax 1972; 27:181–184.

57. Niewoehner DE, Kleinerman J. Morphologic basis of pulmonary resistance in the human lung and effects of aging. J Appl Physiol 1974; 36:412–418.

58. Richmond I, Booth H, Ward C, Walters EH. Intrasubject variability in airway inflammation in biopsies in mild to moderate stable asthma. Am J Respir Crit Care Med 1996; 153:899–903.

59. Sobonya RE, Anderson JR, Buseck PR, et al. Atmospheric pigment and lung structure: Morphometric correlates (abstr). Am Rev Respir Dis 191; 143:A95.

60. Braman SS, Kaemmerlen JT, Davis SM. Asthma in the elderly: A comparison between patients with recently acquired and long-standing disease. Am Rev Respir Dis 1991; 143:336–340.

61. Vergnenegre A, Antonini MT, Bonnaud F, et al. Comparison between late onset and childhood asthma. Allergol Immunopathol 1992; 20:190–196.

62. Lee HY, Stretton TB. Asthma in the elderly. Br Med J 1972; 4:93–95.

63. Burrows B, Barbee RA, Cline MG, et al. Characteristics of asthma among elderly adults in a sample of the general population. Chest 1991; 100:935–942.

64. Brown PJ, Greville HW, Finucane KE. Asthma and irreversible airflow obstruction. Thorax 1984; 39:131–136.
65. Knox AJ. Airway re-modelling in asthma: Role of airway smooth muscle. Clin Sci 1994; 86:647–652.
66. Chetta A, Foresi A, Del Donno M, et al. The remodelling of the airways is related to severity of asthma (abstr). Am Rev Respir Crit Care Med 1996; 153:A879.
67. Stewart AG, Tomlinson PR, Wilson J. Airway wall remodelling in asthma: A novel target for the development of anti-asthma drugs. Trends Pharm Sci 1993; 14:275–279.
68. Gabbrielli S, Di Lollo S, Stanflin N, Romagnoli P. Myofibroblast and elastic and collagen hyperplasia in the bronchial mucosa: A possible basis for the progressive irreversibility of airway obstruction in chronic asthma. Pathologica 1994; 86:157–160.
69. Stewart AG, ed. Airway Wall Remodelling in Asthma. Boca Raton, FL: CRC Press, 1996.
70. Partridge MR, Saunders KB. The site of airflow limitation in asthma: The effects of time, acute exacerbations of disease and clinical features. Br J Dis Chest 1981; 75:263–272.
71. Despas PJ, Leroux M, Macklem PT. Site of airway obstruction in asthma as determined by measuring maximal expiratory flow breathing air and a helium-oxygen mixture. J Clin Invest 1972; 51:3235–3243.

4

Physiology of the Aging Lung

PAUL L. ENRIGHT

University of Arizona
Tucson, Arizona

JOSEPH R. RODARTE

Baylor College of Medicine
Houston, Texas

I. Introduction

In 1955, Bates and Christie stated that "Emphysema is a gross exaggeration of what happens to the lung with advancing years" (1). Although the anatomic changes of the respiratory system with aging differ from those of emphysema, there are marked similarities in the pulmonary function changes that occur. Understanding the functional changes occurring with aging is important to understand the effects of asthma in the elderly. Differences in pulmonary function in elderly as compared with young asthmatics may result in part from differences in the aging lung rather than differences in the disease.

There are methodological difficulties inherent in any study of the effect of aging in humans. The human life span precludes longitudinal studies from adolescence to senescence. This is particularly problematic in respiratory function, which is not commonly measured in asymptomatic individuals. Cross-sectional studies presume that the contemporary elderly were previously like the contemporary young and that today's youth will, with time, become like the current elderly. However, there have been dramatic changes in environment, lifestyle, and medicine in developed countries over the last 60 years. These changes have altered the distribution of heights (stature), life expectancies, and, for many, the severity of

Table 1 Effects of Age Alone on Pulmonary Function Test Results

Lower maximal expiratory flows: FEV_1, FEV_1/FVC, $FEF_{75\%}$
Increased FRC and RV, lower VC, but stable TLC
Lower DL_{CO}
Lower Po_2 and Sao_2 due to $\dot{V}/\dot{Q}$ mismatch (no change in Pco_2)
Lower respiratory muscle strength (MIP and MEP) and endurance
Stiffer chest wall (less compliant)
Increased lung tissue compliance (loss of lung recoil)
Reduced respiratory drive (for hypoxia, hypercarbia, and resistive loads)
Increased airways reactivity

previous illness, particularly infections. Changes in lung function over a lifetime are gradual and difficult to determine accurately with short-term follow up. Small differences in the rate of change of lung function parameters extrapolate to substantially different predictions over 20 years. In general, the rate of decline of lung function in longitudinal studies is slightly less than it is in cross-sectional studies. Since a low FEV_1 is a predictor of all-cause mortality, cross-sectional studies in the elderly should reflect a survivorship and might be expected to predict a slower rate of decline than longitudinal studies. Such an effect, if it occurs, may be obscured by the confounding effect of social changes in cross-sectional studies. In spite of these methodological difficulties, there are clearly defined changes in respiratory function with aging.

In this chapter, we first review the changes in lung function that are known to occur in the healthy (normal persons who have never smoked) with aging. We include the major categories of pulmonary function (PF) tests: static lung volumes, maximal expiratory flow, lung mechanics, and gas exchange, plus bronchodilator response and nonspecific airway reactivity (Table 1). We then discuss how these PF tests may be used by a clinician to assist in the diagnosis of asthma in an elderly patient, and then how these tests may be used to objectively measure the efficacy of asthma therapy.

II. Static Lung Volumes

Total lung capacity (TLC) is the volume of air within the respiratory system when a subject makes a maximal voluntary inspiratory effort. It is determined by the balance of forces between (1) the maximally activated inspiratory muscles and (2) the elastic recoil of the lung and chest wall. In cross-sectional studies, TLC is independent of age (2), but in longitudinal studies there is a slight decrease in TLC. A nearly constant TLC with aging appears to be the fortuitous result of changes in all the factors that determine TLC. In the elderly, maximal inspiratory pressure (MIP) decreases with age (3); however, this measurement is made at residual volume (RV), which increases with age, so respiratory muscles are shorter and less efficient as RV increases. The ability of inspiratory muscles to generate pressure at high lung volumes (near TLC) may not decrease with age—this has not been studied.

The static elastic recoil of the lung clearly decreases with aging, making it easier for the lungs to expand toward TLC (4). This reduction of elastic recoil tends to increase TLC; however, the chest wall becomes stiffer with aging, and its inward elastic recoil is increased as the lungs expand, so that a maximal inspiratory effort is not able to achieve a higher lung volume even though the lungs themselves may expand more easily. In contrast to this balance of changes in lung versus chest wall elasticity seen in normal aging, the loss of lung elastic recoil due to smoking-induced emphysema is associated with large increases in TLC (hyperinflation).

Residual volume (RV) is the volume of air remaining in the respiratory system when subjects have expired as much air as possible. The RV and RV/TLC ratio increase from middle age to older age (Fig. 1).

The major determinant of RV in adults is the lung volume at which lung elastic recoil falls to zero during exhalation and maximal expiratory flow is near zero because of airway compression and closure (5). Since lung elastic recoil

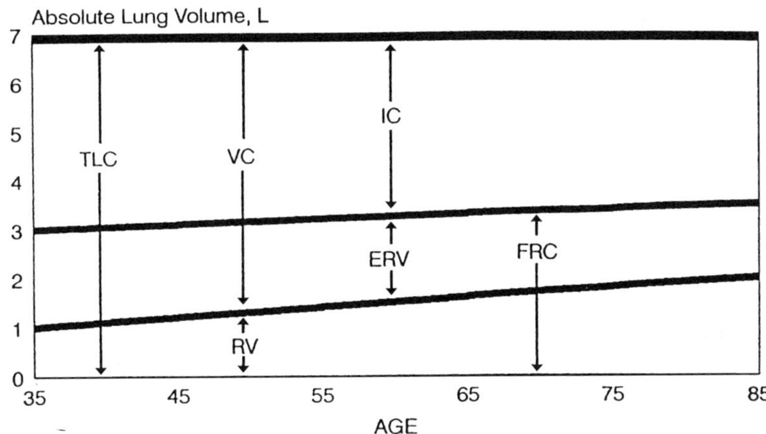

Figure 1 Total lung capacity (TLC) remains unchanged due to aging, but residual volume (RV) increases, causing vital capacity (VC) to decline steadily throughout adult life. The components of VC—the inspiratory capacity (IC), and expiratory reserve volume (ERV)—both decline due to aging, even in healthy persons.

decreases due to normal aging, the RV increases in healthy elderly persons. Vital capacity (VC) is the difference between the absolute lung volume at TLC and at RV. Since TLC is relatively constant while RV increases with age, the VC decreases with age. Vital capacity is a major measurement performed in clinical spirometry and is discussed in detail later.

Functional residual capacity (FRC) is the lung volume at the end of normal quiet respiration. It is the equilibrium volume of the respiratory system when all respiratory muscles are relaxed. The FRC volume is about half of the TLC volume when the person is sitting or standing (Fig. 1). At FRC, the elastic recoil of the lung (forcing the lungs to contract) is balanced by the elastic recoil of the chest wall (forcing the lungs to expand). The FRC is altered by body position, the shape of the spine, the position of the arms, and clothing that constrains the abdomen. The FRC increases slightly with aging ($<$100 ml per decade) as the lung elastic recoil decreases (2).

Tidal volume, the volume excursion during quiet breathing, does not change with age. Inspiratory capacity, the difference between FRC and TLC, and inspiratory reserve volume, the difference between FRC plus TV and TLC, decrease minimally with age, since FRC increases slightly while TLC remains constant. Expiratory reserve volume (ERV) is the difference between RV and FRC (Fig. 1). The increases in RV with aging are larger than changes in FRC; therefore ERV decreases with age. In the very elderly, as RV approaches half of TLC, passive expiratory flow may be so diminished that subjects cannot exhale fully during the normal expiratory time and will inspire before reaching relaxation volume (the usual FRC volume). In this situation, FRC becomes dynamically determined and is larger than the subject's relaxation volume.

III.   Maximal Expiratory Flow

Maximal expiratory flow is a function of lung volume; higher flows are always possible at a higher lung volume. For forced exhalation beginning from TLC (the usual spirometry maneuver), the initial (peak) flow is determined by the recoil of the lung and chest wall and the speed with which the respiratory muscles can generate positive pleural pressure. Once maximal flow is achieved, maximal flow throughout the remainder of the vital capacity is determined by the intrinsic properties of the lung. There are modest decreases of peak expiratory flow (PEF) with age. However, the major fractional reductions in maximal expiratory flow occur at lower lung volume as the flow-volume (F-V) curve becomes more concave to the volume axis (Fig. 2) (2). The volume at which flow falls to zero (residual volume) also increases with age, as noted above.

The determinants of maximal expiratory flow are lung elastic recoil pressure, the cross-sectional area of the airways, and airway compliance. Much of the

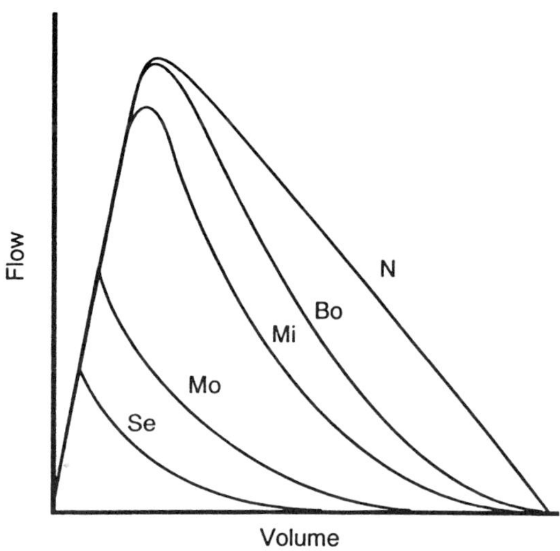

Figure 2   Flow-volume curves with increasing degrees of obstruction. N, normal (100% predicted FEV_1); Bo, borderline obstruction (85% predicted); Mi, mild obstruction (70% predicted); Mo, moderate obstruction (60% predicted); Se, severe obstruction (35% predicted).

reduction in maximal expiratory flow and the shape of the F-V curve is determined by decreases in the lung's elastic recoil with aging.

Measurements of lung elastic recoil or FVC maneuvers in a body plethysmograph (with flow as a function of absolute lung volume) are usually not used clinically due to their complexity and cost. The major index of maximal expiratory flow is the volume that can be expired during the first second of a forced expiration (FEV_1). Since the majority of the volume is expired in the first second, the FEV_1 is a global average of flow over most of the vital capacity. As a time-based average, the FEV_1 is weighted by the lower flows occurring at low lung volumes; therefore, the decreases in FEV_1 with age are somewhat greater than the decreases in FVC, in spite of the relative preservation of maximal flows at higher lung volume, and the FEV_1/FVC ratio falls with aging (6,7).

IV.   Nonuniform Regional Ventilation

At volumes below TLC, the lung is not uniformly expanded because of a vertical gradient in pleural pressure. In younger individuals, dependent lung regions (near the diaphragm in the upright position) are ventilated more than nondependent (apical) regions. There is also a vertical gradient in perfusion, with more blood flow to the dependent areas of the lung. These ventilation and perfusion gradients are generally well matched, providing optimal gas exchange. However, at low lung volumes, dependent regions reach their regional RV before nondependent regions, and the vertical gradient in ventilation may be abolished or even reversed. In younger individuals, this does not occur within tidal breathing volumes (above FRC). However, in elderly individuals, in whom RV has increased much more than FRC, during passive exhalation, airflow in dependent lung regions may cease before FRC is reached, so that the vertical gradient in ventilation is reduced or abolished during tidal breathing. This causes a mismatch of ventilation to perfusion, and an increased alveolar-to-arterial (A-a) oxygen gradient in the absence of lung disease (8).

V. Spirometry

The most common test of lung function, spirometry, is easily performed by elderly patients using an instrument found in many physicians' offices: a spirometer. Modern office spirometers use a flow sensor, which is connected to a microprocessor that calculates the results (FEV_1 and FVC), and prints the flow-volume curves from the patient's best forced expiratory breathing maneuver. Instrument accuracy and the methods for performing the test and interpreting the results have been standardized by the American Thoracic Society (ATS) (9,10).

Using spirometry, the presence of airways obstruction is determined by a low FEV_1/FVC ratio and visualized on the flow-volume (F-V) curve as concavity toward the volume axis or tail at the end of the maneuver (Fig. 2). The descending limb of the F-V curve of healthy young adults is a straight line of about 45° until the end of the maneuver, corresponding to exponential emptying of the lungs. The shape of the F-V curve becomes progressively more curvilinear as a healthy adult becomes older, corresponding to decreases in expiratory flows at low lung volumes. The reduced flows at low lung volumes, even in healthy elderly persons, is a result of a decrease in the mean diameter of membranous bronchioles (small airways) (11). Since the FEV_1 is the average flow during the first second of the maneuver, it includes flows over most of the vital capacity and is also reduced with normal aging (6).

Spirometry was measured in the Cardiovascular Health Study of 5200 elderly persons during the 1990s (7). Over 90% of the elderly persons in this sample of women and men aged 65+ were able to perform good-quality spirometry tests. Spirometry reference values were calculated from a healthy subgroup without heart or lung disease, confirming the results of previous smaller studies showing a 30-ml mean cross-sectional decline per year in FEV_1 with aging. The

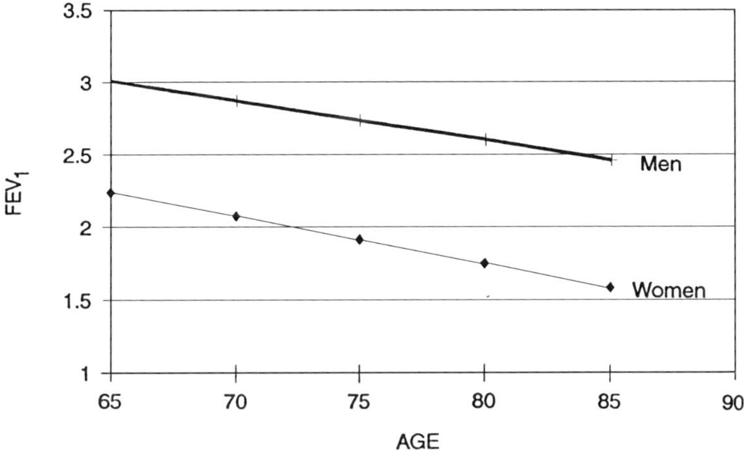

Figure 3 The FEV_1 normally declines about 30 ml per year with aging, even in healthy elderly men and women without lung disease. (Data from Ref. 7.)

decline in FVC with aging (due to increased RV, see above) is somewhat less than the decline in FEV_1, so that the ratio of FEV_1/FVC also declines with age in the elderly (Fig. 3). Many nonpulmonary factors contribute to a decline in the FEV_1 in elderly persons: in the Cardiovascular Health Study, all of the factors listed in Table 2 were significantly associated with a lower FEV_1. The strongest factors were cigarette smoking, a diagnosis of emphysema, chronic bronchitis or asthma, and wheezing symptoms—all of which are known to cause airways obstruction (a low FEV_1/FVC ratio). Several of the factors associated with a lower FEV_1 in the elderly are due to restriction of lung volumes with a normal FEV_1/FVC ratio— these include obesity, malnutrition, heart disease, and chest wall abnormalities. For a given height, gender, and age, the FVC and FEV_1 of healthy elderly black persons was about 12% lower than those for the healthy elderly white persons in this study, but there was no ethnic difference in the FEV_1/FVC ratio (12).

VI. Respiratory Muscle Strength

Another vital component of respiratory function is respiratory muscle strength and endurance. Diaphragm strength is reduced by about 25% in healthy elderly persons as compared with young adults (Fig. 4). The vital capacity will be reduced if the diaphragm is weak or if the expiratory muscles of the abdominal and thoracic wall cannot empty the lungs below the resting respiratory position (FRC).

Table 2 Factors Associated with a
Lower FEV$_1$ in Elderly Participants

Factors associated with obstruction
   Cigarette smoking
   Emphysema or chronic bronchitis
   A diagnosis of asthma
   Wheezing
Factors associated with restriction
   Dyspnea on exertion
   Obesity
   Underweight (body mass index < 20)
   Hypertension
   Hypotension
   Major ECG abnormality
   Pitting ankle edema
   Diabetes, on medication
   Prior chest surgery

Source: From Ref. 7.

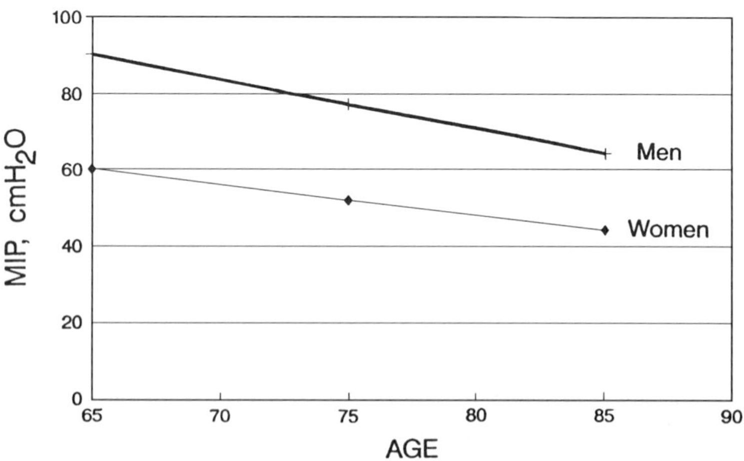

Figure 4 Maximal inspiratory pressure (MIP), a measure of the strength of the diaphragm, declines more rapidly with aging in healthy elderly men than in healthy elderly women. (Data from Ref 3.)

The load on these respiratory muscles increases with aging, since chest wall compliance decreases more than lung tissue compliance increases (13).

Diaphragm strength may be easily and inexpensively measured in the outpatient office. The patient exhales slowly, then makes a maximal attempt to inhale from a mouthpiece connected to a pressure gauge (-200 cmH_2O range, with a small leak) for 2 sec. The largest pressure from five such maneuvers (the highest two of which match within 10%) is reported as the maximal inspiratory pressure (MIP) (14).

Maximal inspiratory pressure was measured in 4400 elderly participants of the Cardiovascular Health Study (3). The results from the healthy subset of men and women confirmed that respiratory muscle strength is stronger in men (mean 57 cmH_2O for women and 83 for men) and declines with aging. The mean MIP for healthy 85-year-old men was about 28% lower than for 65-year-old men (65 versus 90 cmH_2O). A lower MIP was associated with many factors in this cohort, including decreased handgrip strength, a lower FVC, lower body mass index (malnutrition), and current smoking. The skill of the technician in coaching the patient to give maximal effort also affects the results by more than 10%.

VII. Arterial Blood Gases

Acid-base balance is tightly controlled; therefore, normal values for arterial pH and Pa_{CO_2} do not change throughout adult life in healthy persons. However, due to increased nonuniformity of ventilation with aging, mean arterial oxygen tension (Pa_{O_2}) declines during middle life even in healthy persons who have never smoked (15,16). An often quoted rule of thumb to determine the lower limit of the normal range of Pa_{O_2} at sea level for those over age 60 was to subtract 1 mmHg from 80 for every year over age 60 (17). Unfortunately, these traditional reference studies did not include adequate samples of subjects over age 60, yet they were used to extrapolate beyond age 60 the downward trend in Pa_{O_2} seen in those studied from ages 40 to 60. Recent studies of elderly persons show this assumption of a linear decline to be incorrect (18,19) (Fig. 5). Mean Pa_{O_2} remains relatively constant at 83 mmHg from age 65 to 90 in healthy elderly persons at sea level. These results suggest that oxygen saturation also does not change over this age range. This plateau may be due to a survival effect.

VIII. Diffusing Capacity

A test of the single-breath pulmonary diffusing capacity for carbon monoxide (DL_{CO}-SB) is available at most pulmonary function laboratories. The 15-min noninvasive DL_{CO} test is clinically valuable for the differential diagnosis of both airways obstruction and restriction of lung volumes. The DL_{CO} is the amount of

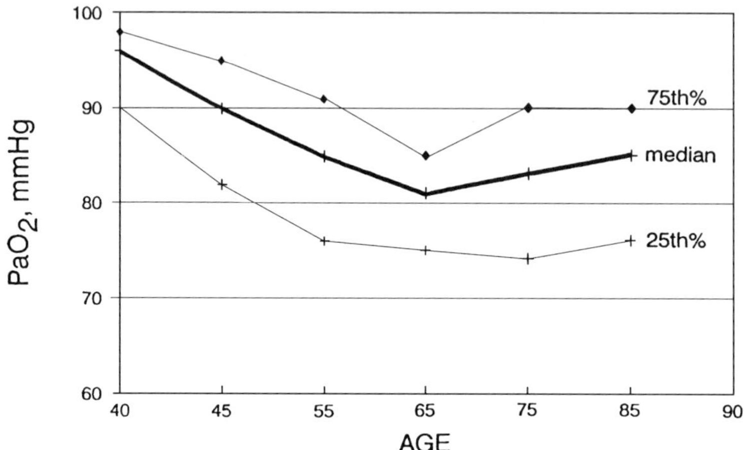

Figure 5   Arterial oxygen (Pao_2) decreases throughout middle age in healthy persons but stabilizes after about age 60, probably due to a survival effect. The median, 25th percentile, and 75th percentile ranges for each age group are graphed. (Data from Ref. 19.)

3% carbon monoxide that is absorbed into the blood (mm/min per mmHg) during a 10-sec breath-hold. Instrument accuracy and the methods for performing the test and interpreting the results have been standardized by the American Thoracic Society (20,21), but DL_{CO} results are not as reproducible as the FEV_1 or FVC (in the same patient tested twice in the same laboratory or in a different laboratory).

In smokers with airways obstruction, the DL_{CO} is an excellent index of the degree of anatomic emphysema—a low DL_{CO} correlates highly (R > 0.85) with a low mean lung tissue density on lung computed tomography (CT) scans and the degree of anatomic emphysema (22,23). Smokers with airways obstruction but normal DL_{CO} values usually have chronic "obstructive" bronchitis but not emphysema; and nonsmoking patients with asthma and borderline to moderate airways obstruction have normal or high (percent predicted) DL_{CO} values.

In healthy persons, the absolute value of DL_{CO} in adults varies with height, age, gender, and race. Reference values from large population studies are used to obtain percent predicted values for individual patients (24,25). The mean DL_{CO}s for an average-height, middle-aged, never-smoking Caucasian man and woman are 33 and 24 ml/min per mmHg, respectively. The DL_{CO} is higher in very obese persons (in the highest decile of body mass index) and lower in patients with anemia.

After age 40, the DL_{CO} declines with age in healthy, never-smoking individ-

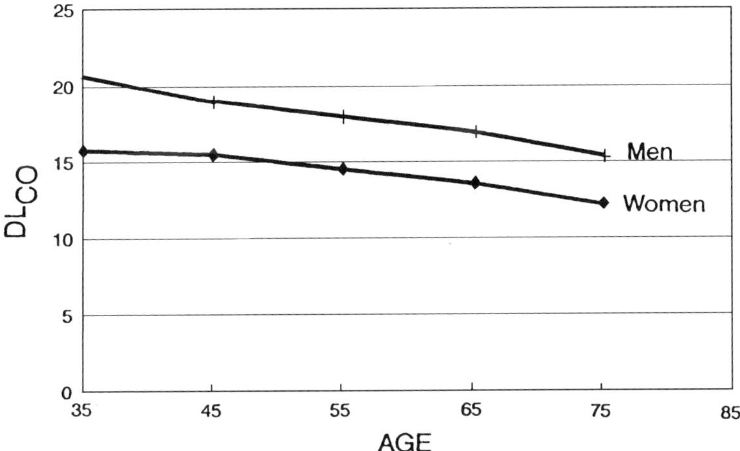

Figure 6 The mean diffusing capacity (DL_{CO}, an index of the ability of the lungs to take up oxygen at rest) declines slowly in healthy, never-smoking men and women throughout adult life. (Data from Ref. 27.)

uals at a rate of about 5% per decade—somewhat more rapidly than does the vital capacity. Older studies suggested that this decline was linear (24,26), but the recent analysis of DL_{CO} values from a cross-sectional national sample of 1635 never-smoking adults (27) found that while men experienced a linear decline of about 2 DL_{CO} units per decade, women lost only about 0.54 DL_{CO} units per decade from ages 25 to 46, but 1.47 thereafter (after adjustment for height, race, and hemoglobin levels) (Fig. 6). This finding suggests a protective hormonal effect on DL_{CO} decline for women prior to menopause (or a cohort effect). A prospective longitudinal study would be necessary to determine the etiology of the cross-sectional gender difference.

IX. Bronchodilator Response

There is evidence that airways beta receptor function in elderly patients with COPD is impaired, but this is not the case in *healthy* elderly persons, where there is a steep dose-response relationship for inhaled $beta_2$-selective bronchodilators (28). A population survey of 2609 participants aged 7 to 75 found no age effect for the FEV_1 response to inhaled terbutaline. The upper limit of the normal range of the bronchodilator (BD) response (percent change in FEV_1 from baseline) was 9% in the healthy subset of the population (29).

In patients with asthma, age was not a significant predictor of the acute response to inhaled BD drugs such as albuterol or ipratropium (up to six inhalations from a metered-dose inhaler; or MDI) when elderly patients were compared with young adults (30). The elderly patients had a slightly larger mean improvement in FVC as compared with the younger adults. The average time to peak effect of these drugs was 5 to 10 min in both the young and elderly patients with asthma. A separate study demonstrated that the mean time for maximum response to albuterol was just as short as that to isoproterenol (31). In a review of over 1000 consecutive PF tests done at three PF laboratories in Connecticut during the early 1980s, there was no systematic correlation among bronchodilator response and age, height, or weight (32).

The ATS suggests that a cutpoint of $>12\%$ and >200 mL improvement in FEV_1 be used to interpret a significant BD response (9). Results of the above studies suggest that this criterion is appropriate for the entire age range of young adults to elderly adults.

X. Nonspecific Airways Hyperreactivity

Evidence of nonspecific airways hyperreactivity is present in almost all patients with current asthma. The most commonly performed test of airways reactivity is the methacholine (or histamine) challenge test—available from most PF laboratories—safely and easily performed in the outpatient clinic setting in 30–45 min. The result is expressed as a PC-20, the interpolated concentration of methacholine at which the patient's FEV_1 falls by 20%. In a patient with normal baseline spirometry, a PC-20 of less than 8 mg/ml is evidence of bronchial hyperreactivity (BHR) (Fig. 7).

Tens of thousands of methacholine challenge tests have been performed safely in the clinical setting and during epidemiological studies of participants in community surveys (33). The correlates of BHR have been determined from nonasthmatic study participants: these include older age, cigarette smoking, respiratory symptoms, and airways obstruction at the baseline.

Several recent population-based epidemiological studies that performed methacholine or histamine challenge tests found that the prevalence of BHR was higher in elderly persons as compared with middle-aged adults, even after correcting for the baseline degree of airways obstruction, smoking status, and atopy (34–38). The Normative Aging Study (34) included only men, and an Italian study showed the age association in men but not in women (38). Two studies did not show an age association with BHR, but one did not correct for other correlates (39) and the other did not include any subjects over age 60 (40).

In an Australian study, the prevalence of BHR was about 10% for young and middle-aged adults, but it jumped to 20% for those in their 70s (36) (Fig. 8).

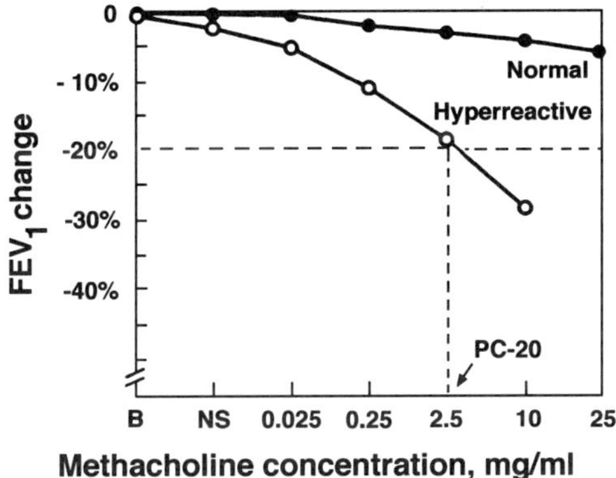

Figure 7 A graph of the results of a positive methacholine challenge test showing bronchial hyperreactivity (BHR). The PC-20 (about 2.5 mg/ml in this case) is the interpolated concentration of inhaled methacholine, which caused a 20% decrease in the patient's FEV_1 when compared to the baseline (B) value. The response to the normal saline (NS) diluent is sometimes measured before methacholine is given.

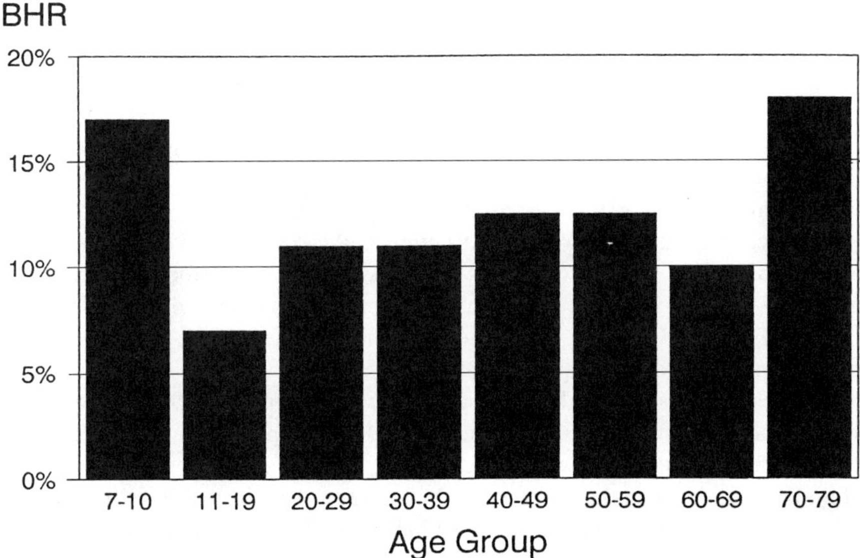

Figure 8 The prevalence rates of bronchial hyperreactivity (BHR) by age group from a population survey in Australia, showing a higher BHR rate in the 70- to 79-year-old group when compared with middle-aged groups. (From Ref. 36.)

The adjusted odds ratio for BHR in this elderly group was about 3.5 as compared with the younger subjects. However, BHR was defined in this study as a PC-15 below 50 mg/ml of histamine, giving much higher sensitivity (and prevalence) for BHR than when using the ATS and European Respiratory Society (ERS) definition of a PC-20 below 8 mg/ml of methacholine.

When using a fixed cutpoint to define BHR for all ages, the above study results show that elderly persons are more likely to have a positive methacholine challenge test than are young and middle-aged adults. The investigators suggested that perhaps the higher prevalence of BHR in the elderly was due to a combination of factors: the cumulative effects of cigarette smoking, occupational exposures, and air pollution; loss of lung elastic recoil due to the aging process (more prechallenge airways obstruction), or increased comorbidity (subclinical congestive heart failure, for instance). However, neither the ATS nor ERS guidelines suggest that the BHR threshold be adjusted upward for elderly patients (41,42).

XI. Pulmonary Function Tests to Assist in the Diagnosis of Asthma

The diagnosis of asthma in the elderly in many cases is more difficult than in younger adults due to the higher prevalence of comorbidity (see Chap. 6). The elderly are much more likely than middle-aged adults to have COPD and cardiovascular disease, both often due to cigarette smoking, and both with symptoms that may mimic asthma. Elderly persons with asthma are also less likely to have highly positive skin tests for allergens or high IgE levels, making these tests less useful in helping to confirm a diagnosis of asthma than in younger persons (see Chap. 4). The above factors increase the value of objective PF tests in the differential diagnosis of asthma in the elderly patient (43).

Since intermittent airways obstruction is the primary physiological manifestation of asthma, the first (and least expensive) PF test to perform is spirometry, especially if the patient is experiencing symptoms at the time of presentation (Fig. 9). If the FEV_1/FVC ratio is below the lower limit of the normal range (assuming that appropriate reference equations for elderly patients are used and the quality of the test session was good), the patient has airways obstruction (9). The degree of severity of the obstruction is then determined by the percent predicted FEV_1.

If the patient has airways obstruction, then repeat spirometry following administration of an inhaled bronchodilator (pre- and post-BD spirometry) is indicated. The technician or nurse should administer two inhalations of albuterol from an MDI, 1 min apart, followed by a 15-min delay to allow near maximal bronchodilator action before spirometry is repeated. Inhaled albuterol in this dose in elderly patients does not increase the pulse rate or blood pressure or cause cardiac arrhythmias (30).

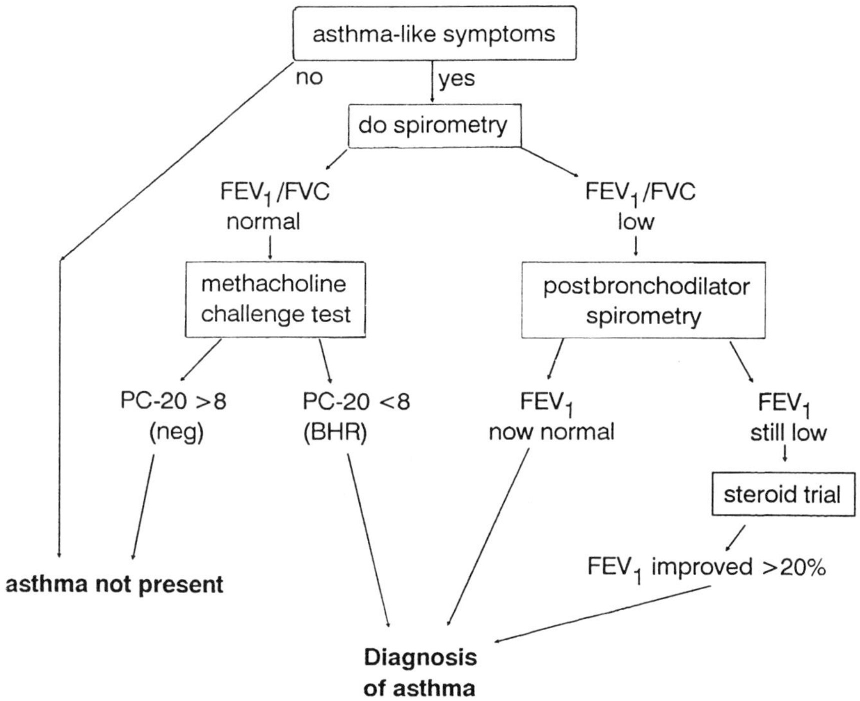

Figure 9   The role of PF tests in making a diagnosis of asthma in a patient with symptoms suggesting asthma. (Data from Ref. 41.)

The pre-post BD spirometry results are useful *only* if there is a significant improvement in the FEV$_1$. A positive (significant) BD response is defined as an FEV$_1$ increase of both 12% and 200 ml or greater (9). Smaller changes in FEV$_1$ are within the short-term FEV$_1$ repeatability (noise of measurement). The quality of the spirometry test sessions—both pre- and post-BD—must be good, otherwise the change in FEV$_1$ should not be interpreted. Changes in spirometry parameters other than the FEV$_1$ should be interpreted with caution: the use of body plethysmography or changes in the forced or slow vital capacity are no more sensitive than the change in FEV$_1$ for detecting bronchodilation (44,45). If the patient cannot perform satisfactory FVC maneuvers, a >40% improvement in airways conductance, using a body plethysmograph, may be substituted for a significant improvement in FEV$_1$.

With good test quality, baseline airways obstruction followed by a BD response resulting in an FEV$_1$ in the normal range, is consistent with asthma in a patient with a history suggesting asthma. However, the lack of a positive BD response is of no help in making the diagnosis (it does not rule out asthma), since chronic asthma often leads to airways inflammation, which is not acutely reversible. Furthermore, many elderly patients with a history of smoking, current symptoms suggesting asthma, baseline airways obstruction, and a "positive" BD response still have obstruction (a low FEV_1) following aggressive therapy for asthma. Unfortunately, the BD response is frequently not helpful in attempts to separate asthma from COPD (46,47) and is not a good predictor of objective improvement with subsequent chronic bronchodilator or inhaled corticosteroid therapy (48,49), nor does it predict survival (50).

The method of calculating a BD response by using percent change from baseline, which is used by almost all PF laboratories in the United States, makes it difficult to separate asthma from emphysema: for a given absolute FEV_1 increase (300 ml, for instance), patients who have a very low baseline FEV_1 (as commonly seen in COPD) have a large percentage change as compared with patients who have a relatively high baseline FEV_1 (as commonly seen in patients with asthma). In other words, small absolute changes become large percentage changes in patients with a low baseline FEV_1, so that the patients with the greatest impairment of lung function (COPD) may appear to have the greatest reversibility (51).

All methods of calculating the BD response are somewhat affected by the degree of baseline airways obstruction and poor short-term reproducibility as evidenced by a large (35–60%) coefficient of variation (48,51,52). However, the "percent possible" method (change as a percentage of predicted minus baseline) has a lower coefficient of variation and less dependence on baseline FEV_1 than does the traditional percent change calculation method and has been recommended for use in Europe (2).

Baseline and pre-post BD spirometry may be normal in patients with a history suggesting asthma. Commonly, the patient is asked to return for retesting when symptoms occur; however, this delays the diagnosis and may be impractical. Inhalation challenge testing will usually confirm the diagnosis in this situation and may be performed in the office or hospital PF laboratory in less than an hour. A negative test rules out asthma with a high degree of confidence (41), but a positive test is seen with hay fever, COPD, congestive heart failure, and some other lung diseases. An alternative to an inhalation challenge test for the detection of airways hyperreactivity (with less sensitivity and specificity, however) is to measure airway lability for 2 weeks in the patient's own environment, using ambulatory monitoring of PEF or FEV_1. The patient should not be using asthma medication during this time. Adults with active asthma usually have PEF lability $>20\%$, but this pattern may also be seen in patients with COPD or congestive heart failure (40).

Measurement of the diffusing capacity (DL_{CO}) is quick and safe, and it helps to distinguish between emphysema and other causes of chronic airway obstruction. Emphysema lowers the DL_{CO}, obstructive chronic bronchitis does not affect the DL_{CO}, and asthma frequently increases the DL_{CO}. The DL_{CO} instrument, however, is expensive, difficult to maintain, and rarely available outside of the pulmonary function laboratory of a hospital. An even more expensive alternative to DL_{CO} testing to clearly differentiate asthma from emphysema in a cigarette smoker is the lung CT scan (23). Of course, both diseases may coexist in a smoker.

XII. Pulmonary Function Tests to Assess Asthma Therapy in the Elderly

A. The Need for Objective Measurements

The inhaled corticosteroids and beta-selective bronchodilators used to treat asthma in elderly persons should be adjusted upward and downward (step treatment) according to changes in asthma severity. When oral corticosteroids are used, the side effects can cause serious morbidity in the elderly; therefore, objective measurements of the effectiveness of the prescribed therapy are highly desirable.

Two lung function tests are used as asthma therapy outcome measures in the outpatient clinic setting: (1) the pre- or post-BD FEV_1 during a clinic visit and (2) PEF lability measured at home over 2–3 weeks (53) (see Table 3).

B. Spirometry

The FEV_1 is the most reproducible PF parameter and is linearly related to the severity of asthma symptoms in groups of elderly patients (54) (Fig. 10). However, the wide variability of FEV_1 for a given set of respiratory symptoms makes prediction of the degree of obstruction for an individual patient very risky—hence the need for objective measurements.

Table 3 Advantages, Disadvantages, and Applicable Settings for Pulmonary Function Tests Used to Measure Asthma Outcomes

Test	Setting	Advantages	Disadvantages
Spirometry (clinic visit)	C,H,S,	Most reliable, reproducible	Snapshot, expense
Ambulatory PEF or FEV_1 (lability index)	A,C S	Sensitive, no side effects, very low cost	Patient compliance, 2-week wait
Airway responsiveness (methacholine)	A C?	Sensitive, results in 1 hr, index of inflammation	Contraindications, expense, time and skill

A, asymptomatic (normal FEV_1); C, clinically symptomatic; S, severe asthma; H, hospitalized, recovering.
Source: From Ref. 3.

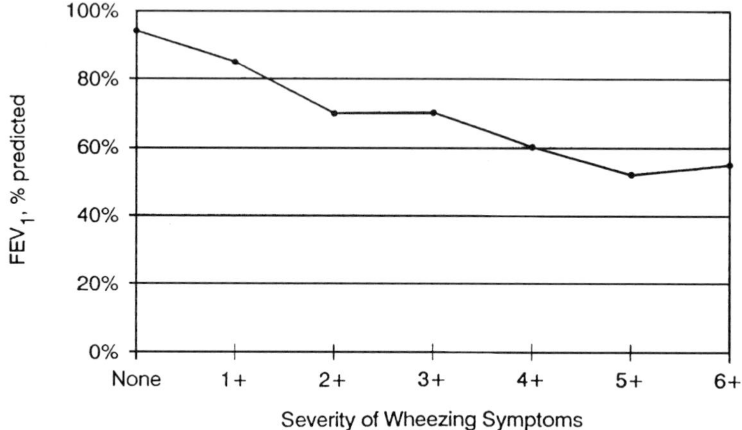

Figure 10 The degree of airways obstruction is correlated with the severity of self-reported wheezing in persons aged 55 and older with a history of asthma from a community survey. Many subjects also reported chronic bronchitis or COPD. (From Ref. 54.)

An accurate FEV_1 may be obtained in less than 5 min from over 90% of elderly persons in the outpatient setting, and there are no contraindications. In the Lung Health Study, in 5000 middle-aged subjects who had borderline to moderate airways obstruction due to cigarette smoking (not treated asthma), investigators could be 95% confident that a change of FEV_1 of more than 9% (180 ml in women or 280 ml in men) was a significant change over a 1-month interval (55). However, other studies without a strict quality-assurance program have noted up to twice that variability in patients with asthma. In a patient with asthma in the outpatient setting, an FEV_1 improvement of more than 20% and 200 ml is necessary to let one conclude with reasonable confidence that improvement from visit to visit was not due merely to measurement noise.

The post-BD FEV_1 measures the best lung function that can be achieved by inhaled BD therapy at the day of the visit; therefore, it is a more stable measure in asthmatics than a comparison of visit-to-visit *baseline* FEV_1s. Although a positive acute response to a BD helps to confirm the diagnosis of asthma, the *degree* of bronchodilator reversibility from visit to visit is *not* a useful index of asthma outcome.

The relationship between the degree of baseline obstruction and the increase in FEV_1—when expressed as the percentage change from baseline—is bell-shaped, with the largest mean response seen in asthmatics with moderate obstruction, where the FEV_1 may sometimes double following a bronchodilator. Those with severe baseline obstruction are more likely to have airway edema and secretions blocking airways, neither of which conditions responds within minutes to inhaled BDs. Those with only mildly reduced baseline FEV_1 "don't have far to go" before they become maximally bronchodilated and reach their personal best FEV_1 or *ceiling*. Paradoxical reductions in FEV_1 following a BD may also be seen and are often due to the effect of variable initial effort on intrathoracic gas compression (56).

C. Ambulatory Monitoring

Using peak flow meters or the new inexpensive hand-held spirometers (which provide both PEF and FEV_1) provides multiple measurements of the degree of obstruction for days to weeks in the patients' natural setting. The often asymptomatic obstruction of an asthmatic has both short-term (within a day and day-to-day) and longer-term variations, which are triggered by naturally occurring stimuli. This variability is best measured by PF lability but not by spirometry during clinic visits (53). Home monitoring of changes in FEV_1 is more sensitive and specific for bronchoconstriction than is PEF monitoring (57).

The $FEF_{25-75}\%$ and the FEV_1/FVC ratio should not be used to determine bronchodilator response, for challenge testing, or for trend analysis over longer periods of time, since paradoxical changes are frequent. When the FVC improves more than flows, the $FEF_{25-75}\%$ and the FEV_1/FVC decrease. The FVC increases due to a reduction in the RV (less air trapping and airways closure)—the $FEF_{25-75}\%$ is then measured over a lower absolute lung volume, where flows are reduced. Measurement of changes in the "isovolume" $FEF_{25-75}\%$ partially corrects for this problem, but this measurement is rarely done by a computerized spirometer (58).

D. What Is a Significant Change?

The FEV_1 is the most reproducible PF test; however, normal ranges even for the FEV_1 are wide, so measurement of a therapeutic response in an individual patient requires a baseline FEV_1, obtained prior to the drug therapy, for comparison with a follow-up FEV_1. Since a primary characteristic of asthma is intermittent airways obstruction, the short-term, within-subject variability of any PF measure will be higher in patients with asthma, so the range of repeatability seen in healthy persons (a 5–10% change in FEV_1, for instance) cannot be applied to patients with asthma.

A statistically "significant" change in any PF test parameter is defined as one that is unlikely to be due only to measurement variability (noise). The measurement noise is optimally determined for each patient by retesting after a short time interval without any intervention. Determining FEV_1 repeatability for each patient or for a control group may be practical in a research setting or formal clinical trial; however, the time required and the imperative to treat the disease usually make this impractical in clinical practice. For example, confident interpretation of the increase seen in FEV_1 in an individual elderly patient with asthma after a month of inhaled corticosteroid therapy requires knowledge of FEV_1 repeatability from a group of elderly patients with asthma. The short-term within-individual repeatability of a measurement is best summarized as the amount of change that includes 95% of the changes: the 95th percentile confidence interval (CI).

The FEV_1 reproducibility obtained within a spirometry test session may be used as an indicator of the expected between-visits FEV_1 repeatability. The largest difference between the highest and second highest FEV_1 within the two test sessions (baseline and follow-up exam) is a fair estimate of the between-visits measurement noise for that patient. For instance, if the highest and second highest FEV_1s at the baseline exam were 2.2 and 1.8 L and those for the follow-up exam were 2.5 and 2.2 L, the patient's within-test session measurement noise of 0.4 L exceeds the between-visits change in FEV_1 (2.2 to 2.5 L); therefore the 0.3-L visit-to-visit increase should not be considered significant.

Serial assessments of airway responsiveness (methacholine challenge tests) have been used to measure the effectiveness of asthma interventions in drug studies (59,60), but they are rarely used clinically for this purpose.

XIII. Summary

Static lung volumes change with aging in healthy subjects: residual volume increases, causing a decrease in vital capacity, while total lung capacity remains constant. Maximum expiratory flows, especially at low lung volumes, decrease due to a gradual loss of lung elastic recoil. This causes a linear decline in FEV_1 and the FEV_1/FVC ratio with aging. Respiratory muscle strength also decreases with aging, along with general skeletal muscle strength. Diffusing capacity and arterial oxygen tension and saturation decrease with age, but mean Pao_2 becomes stable after age 60 in healthy persons, probably due to a survival effect.

In elderly patients with symptoms suggesting asthma, baseline airways obstruction (a low FEV_1/FVC) along with a large response to inhaled bronchodilator (FEV_1 increases into the normal range) help to confirm the diagnosis of asthma. In patients with asthma symptoms but normal baseline spirometry, a negative methacholine challenge test rules out asthma and a positive methacholine challenge or increased ambulatory PEF lability will help to confirm the diagnosis of asthma, but both of these indices of airways hyperreactivity have increased variability in the elderly and are not specific for asthma. A low diffusing capacity in an elderly former cigarette smoker with airways obstruction suggests that the obstruction is due to emphysema, not asthma. A 20% or larger improvement in the

FEV_1 from visit to visit (assuming good-quality spirometry) is the best objective measure of the efficacy of asthma therapy.

Abbreviations

ATS	American Thoracic Society
BD	bronchodilator
BHR	bronchial hyperreactivity
BMI	body mass index
COPD	chronic obstructive pulmonary disease
DL_{CO}	diffusing capacity of the lungs
ECG	electrocardiogram
ERS	European Respiratory Society
ERV	expiratory reserve volume
F-V curve	flow-volume curve
FRC	functional residual capacity
FVC	forced vital capacity
MCT	methacholine challenge test
MDI	metered-dose inhaler
MIP	maximal inspiratory pressure
PC-20	methacholine challenge test endpoint
PEF	peak expiratory flow
PF	pulmonary function
RV	residual volume
TLC	total lung capacity
VC	vital capacity

References

1. Bates DV, Christie RV. Effects of ageing on respiratory function in man. In: Wolstenholme EV, Cameron MF, eds. Ciba Foundation Colloquia on Ageing: General aspects. Boston: Little Brown, 1955: 58.
2. Quanjer PhH, Tammeling GJ, Cotes JE, et al. Lung volumes and forced ventilatory flows. Eur Respir J 1993; 6(suppl 16):5–40.
3. Enright PL, Kronmal RA, Schenker M, et al. Correlates of respiratory muscle strength, and maximal respiratory pressure reference values in the elderly. Am Rev Respir Dis 1994; 149:430–438.
4. Knudson RJ, Clark DF, Kennedy TC. Effect of aging alone on mechanical properties of the normal adult human lung. J Appl Physiol 1977; 43:1054–1062.
5. Anthonisen NR, Danson J, Robertson PC. Airway closure as a function of age. Respir Physiol 1970; 8:58–65.

6. Knudson RJ. Physiology of the aging lung. In: Crystal RG, West JB, et al. eds. The Lung. New York: Raven Press, 1991:1749–1759.

7. Enright PL, Kronmal RA, Higgins M, et al. Spirometry reference values for women and men 65–85 years of age: Cardiovascular Health Study. Am Rev Respir Dis 1993; 147:125–133.

8. West JB. Respiratory Physiology, 4th ed. Baltimore: Williams & Wilkins, 1990.

9. American Thoracic Society. Lung function testing: Selection of reference values and interpretive strategies. Am Rev Respir Dis 1991; 144:1202–1218.

10. American Thoracic Society. Standardization of spirometry: 1994 update. Am J Respir Crit Care Med 1995; 152:1107–1136.

11. Niewoehner DE, Klienerman J. Morphologic basis of pulmonary resistance in the human lung and effects of aging. J Appl Physiol 1974; 36:412–418.

12. Enright PL, Arnold A, Manolio TA, Kuller LH. Spirometry reference values for healthy elderly blacks. Chest 1996, 110:1416–1424.

13. Tolep K, Kelsen SG. Effect of aging on respiratory skeletal muscles. Clin Chest Med 1993; 3:363–378.

14. Black LF, Hyatt RE. Maximal static respiratory pressures: Normal values and relationship to age and sex. Am Rev Respir Dis 1969; 99:696–702.

15. Sorbini CA, Grassi V, Solinas E, Muiesan G. Arterial oxygen tension in relation to age in healthy subjects. Respiration 1968; 25:3–13.

16. Siggard-Andersen O, Wimberley PD, Fogh-Andersen N, Gothen IH. Arterial oxygen status determined with routine pH and blood gas equipment and multi-wavelength hemoximetry: Reference values, precision, and accuracy. Scand J Clin Lab Invest 1990; 50 (suppl 203):57–66.

17. Shapiro BA, Harrison RA, Cane RD, Templin RK. Clinical Application of Blood Gases, 4th ed. Chicago: Year Book, 1989:82.

18. Blom H, Mulder M, Verweij W. Arterial oxygen tension and saturation in hospital patients: Effect of age and activity. Br Med J 1988; 297:720–721.

19. Cerveri I, Zoia MC, Spagnolatti L, et al. Reference values of arterial oxygen tension in the middle-aged and elderly. Am J Respir Crit Care Med 1995; 152:934–941.

20. American Thoracic Society. Single breath carbon monoxide diffusing capacity (transfer factor): Recommendations for a standard technique. Am Rev Respir Dis 1987; 136:1299.

21. American Thoracic Society. Single-breath carbon monoxide diffusing capacity (transfer factor): Recommendations for a standard technique—1995 update. Am J Respir Crit Care Med 1995; 152:2185–2198.

22. Morrison NJ, Abboud RT, Ramadan F, et al. Comparison of DLCO and pressure-volume curves in detecting emphysema. Am Rev Respir Dis 1989; 139:1179–1187.

23. Gould GA, Redpath AT, Ryan M, et al. Lung CT density correlates with measurements of airflow limitation and diffusing capacity. Eur Respir J 1991; 4:141–146.

24. Crapo RO, Morris AH. Standardized single breath normal values for DLCO. Am Rev Respir Dis 1981; 123:185–189.

25. Paoletti PG, Viegi G, Pistelli G, et al. Reference equations for the single-breath diffusing capacity: A cross-sectional analysis and effect of body size and age. Am Rev Respir Dis 1985; 132:806–813.

26. Miller A, Thornton JC, Warshaw R, et al. Single breath diffusing capacity in a representative sample of the population of Michigan, a large industrial state. Am Rev Respir Dis 1983; 127:270–277.

27. Neas LM, Schwartz. The determinants of pulmonary diffusing capacity in a national sample of U.S. adults. Am J Respir Crit Care Med 1996; 153:656–664.

28. Lipworth BJ, Clark RA, Dhillon DP, McDevitt DG. Comparison of the effects of prolonged treatment with low and high doses of inhaled terbutaline on beta-receptor responsiveness in patients with COPD. Am Rev Respir Dis 1990; 142:338–342.

29. Dales RE, Spitzer WO, Tousignant P, et al. Clinical interpretation of airway response to a bronchodilator: Epidemiologic considerations. Am Rev Respir Dis 1986; 138:317–320.

30. Kradjan WA, Driesner NK, Abuan TH, et al. Effect of age on bronchodilator response. Chest 1992; 101:1545–1551.

31. Casaburi R, Adame D, Hong CK. Comparison of albuterol to isoproterenol as a bronchodilator for use in pulmonary function testing. Chest 1991; 100:1597–1600.

32. Eliasson O, DeGraff AC. The use of criteria for reversibility and obstruction to define patient groups for bronchodilator trials. Am Rev Respir Dis 1985; 132:858–864.

33. Tashkin DP, Altose MD, Connett JE. Airway responsiveness to inhaled methacholine in smokers with early chronic obstructive pulmonary disease. Am Rev Respir Dis 1992; 145:301–310.

34. O'Connor GT, Sparrow D, Segal MR, Weiss ST. Smoking, atopy, and methacholine airway responsiveness among middle-aged and elderly men: The Normative Aging Study. Am Rev Respir Dis 1989; 140:1520–1526.

35. Bakke PS, Baste V, Gulsvik A. Bronchial responsiveness in a Norwegian community. Am Rev Respir Dis 1991; 143:317–322.

36. Peat JK, Salome CM, Woolcock AJ. Factors associated with bronchial hyperresponsiveness in Australian adults and children. Eur Respir J 1992; 5:921–929.

37. Rijcken B, Schouten JP, Mensinga TT, et al. Factors associated with bronchial responsiveness to histamine in a population sample of adults. Am Rev Respir Dis 1993; 147:1447–1453.

38. Paoletti P, Carrozzi L, Viegi G, et al. Distribution of bronchial responsiveness in a general population: Effect of sex, age, smoking, and level of pulmonary function. Am J Respir Crit Care Med 1995; 151:1770–1777.

39. Woolcock AJ, Peat JK, Salome CM, et al. Prevalence of bronchial hyperresponsiveness and asthma in a rural adult population. Thorax 1987; 42:361–368.

40. Brand PLP, Kerstjens HAM, Postma DS, et al. Long-term multicentre trial in chronic nonspecific lung disease: Methodology and baseline assessment in adult patients. Eur Respir J 1992; 5:21–31.

41. American Thoracic Society. Guidelines for the evaluation of impairment/disability in patients with asthma. Am Rev Respir Dis 1993; 147:1056–1061.

42. Eurpoean Respiratory Society. Airway responsiveness: Standardized challenge testing with pharmacological, physical, and sensitizing stimuli in adults. Eur Respir J 1993; 6(suppl 16):53–83.

43. Cherniack RM. Physiologic diagnosis and function in asthma. Clin Chest Med 1995; 16:567–581.

44. Newnham DM, Dhillon DP, Winter JH, et al. Bronchodilator reversibility to low and

high doses of terbutaline and ipratropium bromide in patients with COPD. Thorax 1993; 48:1151–1155.

45. Berger R, Smith D. Acute postbronchodilator changes in pulmonary function parameters in patients with chronic airways obstruction. Chest 1988; 93:541–546.

46. Kesten S, Rebuck AS. Is the acute response of FEV_1 to inhaled bronchodilator sensitive and specific distinguishing feature between asthma and COPD (abstr)? Am Rev Respir Dis 1995; 4(suppl):A500.

47. Gross NJ. COPD: A disease of reversible airflow obstruction. Am Rev Respir Dis 1986; 133:725–726.

48. Guyatt GH, Townsend M, Nogradi S, et al. Acute response to bronchodilator: An imperfect guide for bronchodilator therapy in chronic airflow limitation. Arch Intern Med 1988; 148:1949–1952.

49. Kerstjens HAM, Overbeek SE, Schouten JP, et al. Predicting response in FEV_1 on inhaled corticosteroids in obstructive airways disease: the independent influence of baseline PC-20, reversibility, and smoking status (abstr). Am Rev Respir Dis 1995; 4(suppl):A501.

50. Kawakami Y, Kishi F, Dohsaka K, et al. Reversibility of airway obstruction to prognosis in COPD. Chest 1988; 92:49–53.

51. Anthonisen NR, Wright EC, and the IPPB Trial Group. Bronchodilator response in COPD. Am Rev Respir Dis 1986; 133:814–819.

52. Dompeling E, van Schayck CP, Molema J, et al. A comparison of six different ways of expressing the bronchodilating response in asthma and COPD: Reproducibility and dependence of prebronchodilator FEV_1. Eur Respir J 1992; 5:975–981.

53. Enright PL, Lebowitz MD, Cockroft DW. Asthma Outcome Measures Workshop: Pulmonary function tests. Am Rev Respir Dis 1994; 149(part 2):S9–S18.

54. Traver GA, Cline MG, Burrows B. Asthma in the elderly. J Asthma 1993; 30:81–91.

55. Enright PL, LR Johnson, JE Connett, et al. Spirometry in the Lung Health Study: 1. Methods and Quality Control. Am Rev Respir Dis 1991; 143:1215–1223.

56. Krowka MJ, Enright PL, Rodarte JR, Hyatt RE. Effect of effort on measurement of forced expiratory volume in one second. Am Rev Respir Dis 1987; 136:829–833.

57. Gautrin D, D'Aquino LC, Gagnon G, et al. Comparison between PEF and FEV_1 in the monitoring of asthmatic subjects at an outpatient clinic. Chest 1994; 106:1419–1426.

58. Hansen JE, Casaburi R, Goldberg AS. A statistical approach for assessment of bronchodilator responsiveness in PF testing. Chest 1993; 104:1119–1126.

59. Woolcock AJ, Jenkins CR. Assessment of bronchial responsiveness as a guide to prognosis and therapy in asthma. Med Clin North Am 1990; 74:753–765.

60. Dinh Xuan AT, Lockhart A. Use of nonspecific bronchial challenges in the assessment of antiasthmatic drugs. Eur Respir Rev 1991; 1:19–24.

5

Differential Diagnosis of Asthma in the Elderly

**TAHIR AHMED and
BRUCE P. KRIEGER**

Mount Sinai Medical Center
Miami Beach, Florida

ADAM WANNER

University of Miami School of Medicine
Miami, Florida

I. Introduction

Bronchial asthma is a common disease, with an overall prevalence of 6–8% in the general population (1). Despite this high incidence, asthma is a diagnosis that tends to be overlooked in the elderly (2). Most patients develop asthma at a younger age, which has led to the inaccurate assumption that occurrence of asthma in the elderly is rare. New onset of asthma can develop at any age, even in the eighth and ninth decades of life (3), and may go undetected because elderly patients associate their poor lung function with their advancing age. It is equally important to realize that asthma may also be misdiagnosed. Generally, episodic wheezing with dyspnea is considered synonymous with asthma, but in the elderly the symptoms that commonly occur—such as "cough," "sputum production," and "shortness of breath"—can quite easily be mistaken for chronic bronchitis, occupational lung disease, or decompensated heart failure, conditions that often coexist (4–6). Sir William Osler (7) recognized that dyspnea from heart failure can present with typical symptoms of asthma, including wheezing, chest tightness, and paraoxysmal attacks in the early morning hours; this had been termed "cardiac asthma" (8). Thus, it is important to make an accurate diagnosis of these

"

conditions early on, not only for therapeutic reasons but also for prognostic implications.

On both clinical and physiological grounds, asthma in the elderly can pose a special problem for the general physician. Besides chronic bronchitis, emphysema, and congestive heart failure, symptoms of asthma in the elderly may also be mimicked by other conditions including aspiration pneumonia, vocal cord dysfunction, endobronchial tumors, and drug-induced bronchial hyperreactivity (Table 1). Aging is associated with a decline in lung function, which may lead physicians to minimize the importance of their older patients' symptoms (3,4). Thus, characterizing this group of patients by their symptomatology is inadequate and may contribute to misdiagnosis. As many of the elderly live alone, they may not recognize symptoms or a decline in their condition. Even when cognizant of their symptoms, older patients may ascribe their disability to smoking habits, occupational-environmental exposures, or simply part of old age.

In the elderly, functional status has a great influence on everyday life, particularly in the presence of a chronic disease. In elderly asthmatics, delaying the onset of dependency and disability is essential to improving the quality of life. Dyspnea has been found to be an important aggravating factor of disability in the elderly, the appropriate treatment of which can result in improved quality of life (9,10).

Table 1   Diseases that Mimic the Symptoms of Asthma in the Elderly

Wheeze	Cough
Chronic obstructive pulmonary disease	Chronic obstructive pulmonary disease
Congestive heart failure	Bronchiectasis
Endobronchial or endotracheal obstruction	Recurrent aspiration
	Postnasal drip
Tumors	Tracheomalacia
Foreign bodies	Drugs
Postradiation stenosis	Dyspnea
Tracheal stenosis	Chronic obstructive pulmonary disease
Descending aortic aneurysm	Coronary artery disease
Endobronchial granulomas	Pulmonary emboli
Aspiration with mucosal edema	Aspiration syndromes
Gastroesophageal reflux disease	Upper airways obstruction
Pulmonary emboli	Pulmonary neoplasms
Vocal cord dysfunction	Vocal cord dysfunction
Carcinoid syndrome	Chest bellows disease
Drugs	Gastroesophageal reflux disease
	Primary pulmonary hypertension

II. Definitions

The prevalence of asthma in the elderly has not been reliably determined, largely because of the uncertainties regarding the definition of the disease. The National Asthma Education Expert Panel Report (11) developed a working definition of asthma that included the following characteristics: "(1) airway obstruction that is reversible (but not completely so in some patients) either spontaneously or with treatment; (2) airway inflammation; and (3) increased airway responsiveness to a variety of stimuli." The term *asthma* is not appropriate for the bronchial narrowing that results solely from widespread bronchial infection, e.g., acute or chronic bronchitis, from destructive disease of the lung, e.g., pulmonary emphysema, or from cardiovascular disorders. Asthma may occur in subjects with other bronchopulmonary or cardiovascular diseases, but in these instances the airways obstruction is not causally related to these diseases. Strict adherence to such a definition of asthma in the elderly is especially important because of a high incidence of cardiovascular disease and chronic obstructive pulmonary disease (COPD), which may pose diagnostic problems.

Asthma is difficult to diagnose in the elderly because it is usually intrinsic and lacks the allergic characteristics that often distinguish it in the younger patients. The airways obstruction that characterizes asthma is often referred to as being the physiological opposite of the obstruction associated with chronic bronchitis. When viewed as a clinical spectrum, asthma is synonymous with "reversible" airways obstruction, while chronic bronchitis refers to "irreversible" airways obstruction. However, many patients with COPD have both a reversible and an irreversible component. Therefore, perhaps a more appropriate definition of asthma in the elderly should be based on its pathophysiological hallmark of "reversible airways obstruction" either spontaneously or by therapy. Because some patients with COPD show partial reversibility of airflow obstruction and because some patients with asthma show limited reversibility after treatment, the distinction between these diseases may be difficult. Yet it is very important to make this distinction, because the symptoms of asthma are typically more reversible than those of COPD. In one study, at least 40% of the elderly subjects with obstructive airways disease were found to have reversible component, thus indicating potential benefit from therapy (2). Therefore, in clinical practice it is clearly important to identify a reversible component, not only to prevent a life-threatening situation but also to improve the quality of everyday life with regular inhaled bronchodilator or steroid therapy.

The differential diagnosis of acute, severe dyspnea is of paramount importance when the first attack of "status asthmaticus" occurs in the elderly. Status asthmaticus is the critical clinical expression of bronchial asthma. The therapy is more complex than that required to manage stable asthma or acute episodic attacks. Because the severe gas exchange defects occurring in status asthmaticus result in a life-threatening condition associated with increased mortality, immediate hospitalization of the patient is essential (12). In elderly patients, status asthmaticus with refractoriness to therapy may be difficult to differentiate from an exacerbation of COPD or left ventricular failure. In most cases, however, appropriate clinical history, therapeutic trial, and ultimate reversibility guide the physician to an accurate diagnosis.

III. Pathophysiological Characteristics

Several lines of evidence suggest that the pathophysiology of late-onset asthma differs from that of asthma beginning earlier in life. Asthma developing later in life is less likely to be accompanied by atopy, as assessed by allergy skin testing and serum concentration of total IgE, than is asthma occurring at an earlier age (13). In addition, asthma diagnosed for the first time among older subjects is more likely to be preceded by a diagnosis of chronic bronchitis or emphysema. Elderly asthmatics are likely to have a greater degree of airflow obstruction with limited reversibility after inhaled bronchodilators. This suggests that long-standing asthma may lead to chronic persistent airflow obstruction and thereby may mimic COPD (13).

A. Pulmonary Function

Pulmonary function in elderly asthmatics generally demonstrates evidence of chronic airflow obstruction. There is increasing evidence that the airways function of young and middle-aged asthmatics declines at a greater rate than that of normal subjects (14,15). In an 18-year study, Peat et al. (14) compared a population of nonsmoking adult asthmatics from ages 22–69 years against normal control population. They found that the mean loss of FEV_1 in men with asthma was 50 ml per year, compared with 35 ml per year in normals matched for height. However, the rate of decline of FEV_1 was variable, and not all subjects showed a steeper rate of decline. The precise reasons for this individual variability have not been defined, although there is evidence that atopy and marked bronchial hyperresponsiveness are two risk factors for an accelerated decline in lung function and fixed airways obstruction in later adult life (15). There is also evidence that some nonsmoking patients with chronic asthma may develop severe "fixed" airway obstruction, even after maximum therapeutic intervention with bronchodilators and corticosteroids. It is believed that the persistent airflow obstruction of asthma may be a function of the duration and severity of previous disease (16). In a study of elderly nonsmoking asthmatic patients, those with long-standing asthma and a mean duration of symptoms of 31 years, had a significantly greater degree of airflow obstruction in both pre- and postbronchodilator pulmonary function testing than those with recently acquired disease (13). Following an inhaled bronchodilator, those with long-standing asthma had a mean percent predicted FEV_1 of 58%, compared with 75% in the late-onset asthma group, who had a mean duration of symptoms of only 5 years (13). The cause of chronic persistent airflow obstruction in asthma has not been explained. Sobonya (17) found no structural changes of emphysema in the autopsied lungs of six elderly patients with chronic asthma who died of nonasthmatic causes. Airways smooth muscle hypertrophy, bronchial gland hyperplasia, and mucous plugging, which are common findings in patients dying of status asthmaticus, were not greater in the elderly group than in controls.

Burr et al. (5) also reported airflow obstruction and a significant bronchodilator response in elderly asthmatics. In a group of newly diagnosed elderly asthmatics, airflow obstruction did not respond to bronchodilators alone but did show improvement after addition of corticosteroids, with more than 75% of subjects attaining an FEV_1 within 80% of predicted (4). In the Tucson epidemiological study (18,19), the degree of reduction in FEV_1 was closely related to the severity of the wheezing complaints, especially in the elderly as compared with younger asthmatics (Fig. 1). Although some elderly asthmatics may have relatively fixed airflow obstruction, the course of the disease is dramatically different than that of COPD, where the rate of decline of FEV_1 is very high. Perhaps early identification of these subjects and appropriate therapy will be able to improve baseline pulmonary function and halt further loss of function.

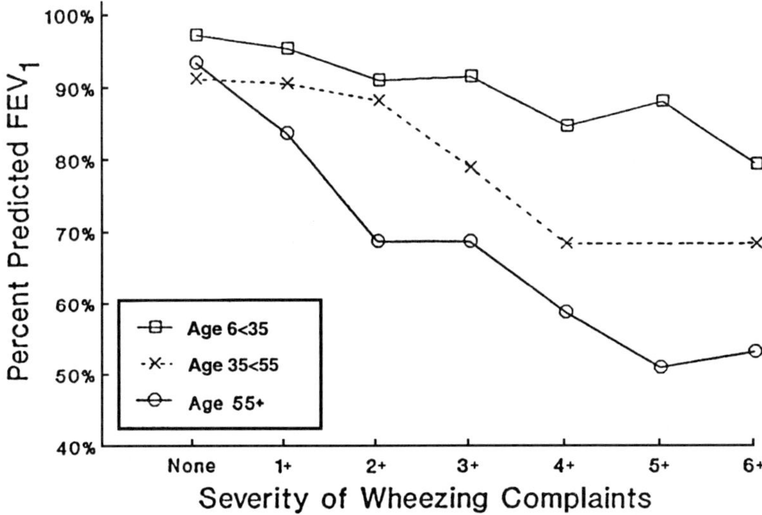

Figure 1 The relationship of wheezing complaints to precent predicted FEV_1 in asthmatics by age group. Those with no wheezing are ex-asthmatics. (From Ref. 19.)

B. Role of Allergy

The relationship of allergy to asthma in the elderly has not been consistent among various studies. Burr et al. (5) reported that approximately 50% of the elderly asthmatics in their study had a family history of allergy, and those with asthma were more likely to have allergic rhinitis. Braman et al. (13) observed that elderly asthmatics who had acquired their asthma prior to age 65 had higher incidence of other allergic diseases. Of those patients who had acquired the disease as young adults, 62% reported a previous history of eczema and allergic rhinitis. None of the patients who had acquired asthma after age 60 had this previous history of atopy. Serum levels of IgE are often but not always elevated in the elderly asthmatics. In an 8-year epidemiological survey in Tucson of new-onset asthma in the elderly, a much higher rate of allergic rhinitis was also reported (20). Increased levels of IgE were found to be closely related to the likelihood of a subsequent diagnosis of asthma (20). A comparison of those elderly patients with newly diagnosed asthma and those with COPD also demonstrates the association between asthma and IgE levels (18,20). There were no new diagnosis of asthma in those subjects with the lowest IgE levels, while in the highest-IgE groups the asthma diagnosis markedly exceeded the diagnosis of COPD. Several studies have reported significant blood eosinophilia in many elderly asthmatics, but the majority of subjects do not demonstrate eosinophilia (4,5,20). Although atopy may be important in the pathogenesis of asthma in some of the elderly subjects, it is uncommon to find clinical provocation by aeroallergens in this age group.

C. Socioeconomic Factors

Asthma does not affect everyone equally. In particular, asthma is especially likely in a setting of poverty (21,22). Many components of poverty may contribute to the increased risk, including poor access to appropriate and high-quality health care, lack of continuity of care, decreased likelihood of treatment with anti-inflammatory drugs, dismal housing with high levels of antigen and pollutant exposure, poor systems of social support, and low levels of education (23,24). The growing morbidity and mortality may also reflect increases in exposure to outdoor pollutants and indoor aeroallergens, including dust mites, cat dander, cockroach antigen, and molds in the poor inner-city households (25,26). It is possible that risk factors of age, race, and ethnic background may be surrogate markers for poverty (27). In a recent study by Lang and Polansky, fatal asthma was found to be significantly more common in census tracts with higher percentages of blacks, Hispanics, women, and people living below the poverty level (24). This report provides further confirmation that in the United States deaths from asthma are disproportionately common among minority groups and in inner cities. These socioeconomic and environmental factors could certainly aggravate the health care of the elderly in general and asthma management in particular.

D. Bronchial Hyperreactivity

There is evidence that some functions of the sympathetic and parasympathetic nervous systems deteriorate with age (28). Although worsening of bronchial reactivity to methacholine remains controversial (29,30), there is increasing evidence that a progressive decline of β-receptor function occurs with aging (15,31). The molecular basis for this is not well understood. The receptor number appears to remain unchanged with advancing age (32), but receptor affinity seems to be decreased (33). Kendall and Woods (34) evaluated both airways and cardiac responses with intravenous terbutaline in younger and older subjects with asthma. Older subjects demonstrated smaller increases in peak flow rates as well as less tachycardia. These findings have been confirmed in in vivo and in vitro studies (35). The diminished β-receptor function in the elderly can result in reduced bronchodilator response and potential worsening of bronchial hyperreactivity. Connolly et al. (36) have demonstrated a reduction of leukocyte β-receptor affinity without loss of receptor density with aging. They have shown that in comparison with young normal subjects, mononuclear leukocytes from elderly asthmatic patients have further reduction in affinity without a reduction in receptor density. The investigators also observed an inverse correlation between non-specific bronchial reactivity to methacholine and receptor affinity (36). These findings suggested that the mechanisms responsible for β-receptor dysfunction in late-onset asthma are similar to those seen during aging and may represent an extreme spectrum of age-associated β-receptor dysfunction. It has also been suggested that an inflammatory mechanism involving basophils may be important in the development of worsening bronchial reactivity during aging (37).

E. Mucociliary Dysfunction

Marked pathophysiological changes in mucociliary transport in bronchial asthma have been observed (38). Mucociliary transport has been found to be depressed in experimental as well as human asthma; during acute antigen-challenge, a further reduction in mucociliary transport is observed. There is evidence to support that leukotrienes might play an important role in the mediation of mucociliary dysfunction in asthma (39). The abnormal mucociliary transport certainly could contribute to the physiological abnormalities in airways function. It has been suggested that cough and residual airways dysfunction found in patients with asthma in remission is partly related to the presence of excessive mucus in the peripheral airway. It is possible that this excess mucus in the elderly may partly contribute to symptoms of cough and to poor reversibility of airway function. The postmortem finding of widespread mucous plugging in the airways of patients who die in status asthmaticus has long been considered to represent the major cause of death. We have aspirated a bronchial mucous plug obstructing the whole left bronchial tree in an elderly patient with severe asthma (Fig. 2). The patient did

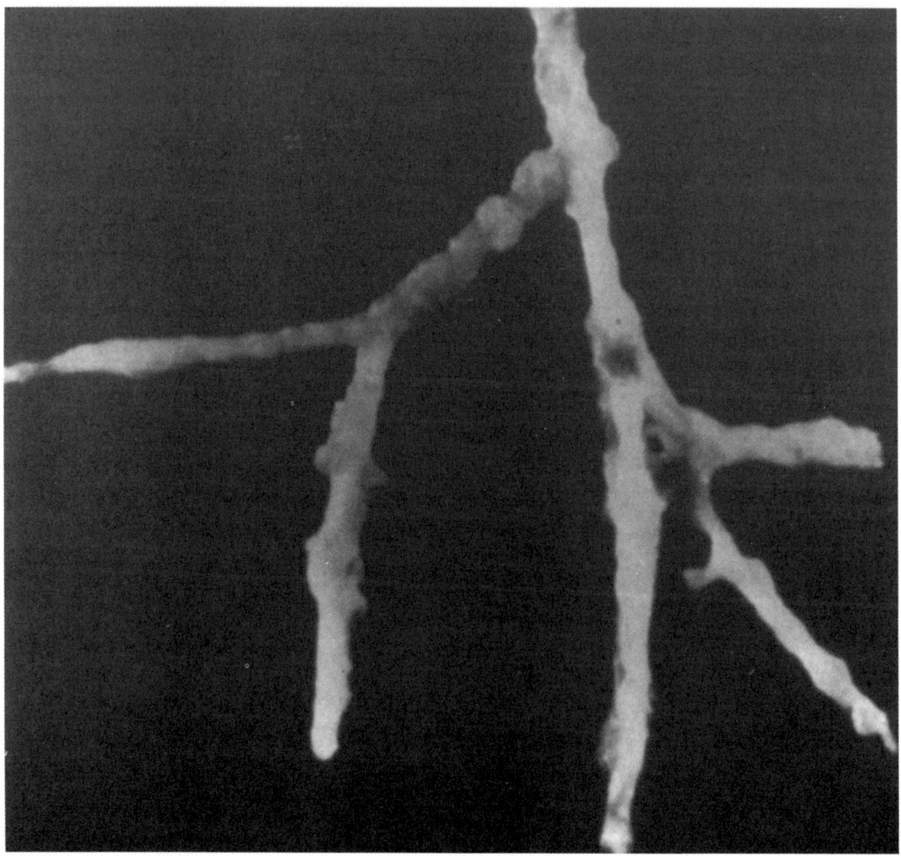

Figure 2   Large mucous plug obstructing the left bronchial tree of an elderly patient in status asthmaticus. The plug was removed by bronchoscopic aspiration.

not respond to medical therapy until the mucous plug was removed with a fiberoptic bronchoscope. Besides contributing to symptoms of cough and airflow obstruction, the mucociliary dysfunction may also predispose elderly asthmatics to respiratory infections, which may contribute to the chronicity of the disease.

F. Cardiovascular Function

Compared with younger patients, elderly asthmatics tend to have a slower heart rate during exacerbations of asthma (40). Petheram et al. (41) showed that during acute exacerbations of asthma, elderly patients have less pronounced pulsus paradoxus and tachycardia than younger patients with similar airways obstruction and hypoxemia. Cardiovascular responses to hypoxemia also diminish with age (42), which may partly explain why heart rate and pulsus paradoxus, which are reliable guides to severity of asthma in younger patients, are less helpful signs in the elderly. This might theoretically result in undertreatment of elderly asthmatics during acute attack and contribute to poor prognosis.

G. Impaired Perception of Dyspnea

Elderly people have impaired perception of externally applied restrictive and elastic respiratory loads (43–45), with reduced sensation of breathlessness, which is consistent with an age-related decline of both sympathetic and parasympathetic functions (28). Others have observed a blunted hypoxic ventilatory drive in older subjects and less hyperventilation in response to the development of bronchial narrowing, which is so characteristic of an acute attack (46–48). Hence, alveolar hypoventilation may develop rapidly in the elderly, even with a moderate degree of airflow obstruction. It has been shown that the perception of dyspnea during resistive loading was significantly decreased in patients with a history of near fatal asthma as compared with normal subjects and patients who had asthma of similar severity but without a previous history of such attacks (46). Kikuchi et al. also found a significant reduction in hypoxic, but not hypercapnic respiratory drive in patients with asthma who had near fatal attacks (46). Such impaired perception and blunted respiratory drive may be pronounced in the elderly. It has also been shown that, compared with younger subjects, elderly asthmatics have impaired perception of methacholine-induced bronchoconstriction, which may delay self-referral at the onset of an acute asthma attack (49). Elderly asthmatic patients tend to deteriorate for longer periods at home before hospital admission (41); when challenged with methacholine, they do not report dyspnea or wheeze to be troublesome despite a significant bronchoconstriction (50). This is especially likely to occur in the elderly with impaired brain function. A recent case report has shown an elderly demented asthmatic patient to be symptomless during a 40% fall in peak expiratory flow (51).

IV. Clinical Presentation of Asthma in the Elderly

Bronchial asthma is frequently underdiagnosed in elderly subjects. Declining mental status and the "acceptance" of chronic symptoms by older patients may contribute to the underreporting of symptoms and therefore underdiagnosis of asthma in the elderly (2). The symptoms of wheeze, cough, and dyspnea were less commonly reported in older asthmatics (age >60 years) compared with younger patients (52). These classical symptoms are frequently noted by nonasthmatic elderly subjects; therefore the diagnosis may be camouflaged (53). A study of 82 randomly selected elderly subjects who demonstrated acute improvement (>15%) in peak expiratory flow rates following inhaled albuterol noted that the incidence of wheeze, cough, and dyspnea was no different than in 113 subjects who showed no significant response to bronchodilators (2). The symptoms of asthma overlap with the symptoms of other commonly diagnosed geriatric diseases (Table 1), such as congestive heart failure (dyspnea, nocturnal awakenings, wheeze), chronic obstructive pulmonary disease (dyspnea, cough, sputum production), and angina pectoris (chest tightness and dyspnea). This overlap may further confuse the diagnosis of asthma and thus contribute to the underdiagnosis of asthma in the elderly. The following section scrutinizes the differential diagnoses of the common asthmatic symptoms (wheeze, cough, and dyspnea).

A. Wheeze

Although wheezing is often equated with bronchospasm, other causes besides bronchospasm can generate enough rapid flow of air through narrowed airways to produce a wheeze (54). Wheezes are usually more audible and musical in quality than crackles and occur more frequently during the expiratory phase of respiration. Wheezes are generated by regular vibration of the airway wall as turbulent airflow increases in velocity through a narrowed aperture (55). Therefore, any process that significantly narrows the endobronchial lumen can provoke wheezing. This was recognized by Cheval Jackson at the beginning of the twentieth century, when he formulated the adage "All that wheezes is not asthma" (55,56). Any process that causes airway limitation can induce wheezing, such as bronchospasm, bronchial edema, excessive airway secretions, laryngospasm, tracheal or endobronchial stenosis, tracheomalacia, endobronchial obstruction due to tumors, granulomas, foreign bodies, or extrinsic compression of the airways (tumors or enlarged lymph nodes).

Wheezing and Asthma

In the Tucson epidemiological study of obstructive lung disease, wheezing was the most common symptom reported by elderly patients who developed asthma (18,20). This symptom is reported as frequently in elderly asthmatics as it is in younger patients with asthma (2,13). As discussed under the pathophysiology of asthma (Sec. III), there are multiple reasons for wheezing to occur in asthmatics. The wheezing that accompanies asthma, as opposed to chronic obstructive lung disease, is episodic and usually completely reversible spontaneously or with appropriate therapy. However, wheezing is not a necessary requirement for the diagnosis of asthma and frequently is not a prominent symptom in elderly asthmatics (57). Contrary to the wheezing that occurs in other disease states, patients with asthma are often able to define precipitating causes that provoke the onset of wheezing, such as inhalational agents (noxious fumes, changes in humidity, nonspecific chemical agents), bronchial infections (viral or bacterial bronchitis), ingested materials (certain drugs such as beta blockers, aspirin, metabisulfite), allergens, or aspirated material (postnasal drip, gastroesophageal reflux, foreign bodies).

Pulmonary function testing is useful in determining whether the presence of wheezing indicates asthma. A reduction in the forced expiratory volume exhaled in one second (FEV_1) in association with an FEV_1/FVC ratio of $< 70–75\%$ is defined as an obstructive airways defect. Good physiological evidence for the diagnosis of asthma (National Institutes of Health criteria) includes an improvement in FEV_1 by $\geq 15\%$ after the inhalation of a beta$_2$-adrenergic bronchodilator and an $FEV_1 \geq 75\%$ of predicted. However, as Braman et al. reported (13), elderly patients with long-standing asthma (31.4 years) did not bronchodilate to a normal FEV_1 (mean, 58.5%). This is in distinction to a group of elderly patients from the same clinic who had newly diagnosed asthma in which the FEV_1 improved to 75.3% of predicted. The former group of earlier-onset elderly asthmatics had physiology that was more consistent with chronic obstructive pulmonary disease, although they all had documented asthma. Pulmonary function testing may be completely within normal limits during stable periods. Laboratory confirmation of asthma then requires bronchoprovocation testing using various agents. Bronchoprovocation with methacholine or water has been shown to be useful and safe in the diagnosis of asthma in the elderly (49–51,58).

Wheezing and Left Ventricular Failure

The association of wheezing with congestive heart failure (CHF) has been recognized for over 150 years (7,8,55,59). Although Snashall and Chung suggest avoiding the term *cardiac asthma*, the two diseases have many similarities, which will perpetuate the use of this terminology (59). Wheezing is a prominent symptom in both conditions. In asthma, this is due mainly to mediator release, whereas in CHF, it appears more likely that this response is hemodynamically mediated (60) (Fig. 3). The classic explanation is that the pulmonary and bronchial venous hypertension that accompanies CHF causes bronchial wall edema, resulting in airway narrowing in bronchi distal to the trachea (61). Recently, Baier et al. used a multiple-gas technique to demonstrate that mucosal edema extended into the trachea as well (62). The narrowing is further worsened by congestion from an increase in airways secretions and foam (59). A recent extensive review of airways obstruction and bronchial hyperresponsiveness in left ventricular failure concluded that airways narrowing in CHF is mainly a consequence of reflex bronchoconstriction, which is mediated by juxtacapillary endings (J fibers) via the vagus nerve (59). Although bronchial mucosal swelling may contribute, decreased

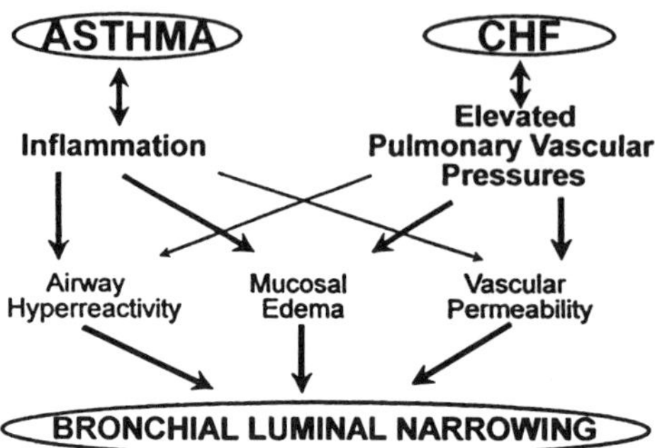

Figure 3 Mechanisms of airway narrowing shared by asthma and congestive heart failure (CHF). Bold arrows indicate major mechanism; thin arrows (crossing in center) represent less important or controversial pathways.

lung volumes due to pulmonary edema may be more important in causing narrowing of the airways (63).

Whereas the response to methacholine bronchoprovocation in patients with asthma is usually positive, the response in CHF is variable. Eichacker et al. (64) noted a positive response to inhalation challenge in only one of nine patients with chronic CHF (New York Heart Association functional class IV), whereas Cabanes et al. showed marked bronchial hyperresponsiveness in 21 of 23 patients, all of whom were class III with a left ventricular ejection fraction < 35% (61). Cabanes et al. further characterized the etiology of the hyperresponsiveness by using pharmacological agents to separate vasomotor from bronchomotor responses (61). Administration of albuterol was partially effective in reversing the methacholine-induced bronchoconstriction, while pretreatment with methoxamine, a potent alpha-adrenergic agonist and vasoconstrictor, completely prevented the decrease in FEV_1 from methacholine. This protective effect was negated when the alpha-adrenergic antagonist phentolamine was also administrated. Cabanes et al. therefore concluded that bronchial vasodilation is a major contributor to the wheezing in patients with pulmonary edema (61).

The airways obstruction associated with CHF is often difficult to distinguish from asthma in the elderly, since both conditions present with similar symptoms of nocturnal awakening, chest pressure, wheezing, dyspnea, and accessory muscle use (55,56,65). Further complicating the distinction between CHF and asthma is the favorable clinical response to inhaled bronchodilators in some patients with "cardiac asthma" (61), even though, theoretically, beta-adrenergic agonists could worsen small airways obstruction in CHF due to their vasodilatory properties. Therefore, the distinction between "cardiac asthma" and asthma in the elderly frequently rests on the appropriate history and associated findings of left ventricular failure (S_3 gallop, jugular venous distension, and cardiomegaly) along with the presence of a pulmonary edema pattern on the chest radiograph (cardiomegaly, redistribution of pulmonary blood flow, Kerley B lines, hilar haziness, and fluffy diffuse pulmonary infiltrates). Intravenous aminophylline was frequently used to treat CHF two decades ago, although its benefit may be a consquence of its inotropic and diuretic properties rather than its weak bronchodilating effects.

Wheezing Due to Endotracheal or Endobronchial Obstruction

Endotracheal or endobronchial obstruction induces wheezing due to the increased airflow velocity promoted through a narrowed orifice. If the site of narrowing is in the trachea but extrathoracic (cephalad to the sternal notch), then inspiratory wheezing (stridor) results. This can be demonstrated in the laboratory by attenuation and flattening of the inspiratory limb of a flow-volume loop (66). Many diseases prevalent in the elderly may result in upper airways obstruction. These include tracheal tumors, of which squamous cell carcinoma and adenoid cystic carcinoma are the most common (67,68); tracheal stenosis following intubation or tracheostomy (69); radiation-induced tracheal stenosis (70); substernal goiter (71); and descending aortic aneuryms.

Lower endotracheal obstruction or endobronchial obstruction is associated with predominantly expiratory wheezing along with an attenuation and flattening of the expiratory limb of the flow-volume loop. However, if an intrathoracic or extrathoracic upper airways obstruction is fixed, both inspiratory and expiratory wheezing along with flattening of the inspiratory and expiratory limbs on flow-volume loop testing are seen (Fig. 4). The causes of intrathoracic upper airways obstruction and endobronchial obstruction in the elderly include pulmonary neoplasms or endobronchial metastases from nonpulmonary malignancies (breast, colon, kidney), lymphoma, aspirated foreign bodies, postradiation stenosis (70), endobronchial tuberculosis, severe mucosal edema from aspiration, herpetic tracheobronchitis (72), or bronchial torsion after pulmonary resection.

The differentiation of upper airways obstruction or endobronchial obstruction from asthma in the elderly is accomplished by a combination of appropriate history taking, radiographs, pulmonary physiological studies, and a physical exam, which often shows a focal increased intensity of wheezing over the involved area. Baughman and Loudon recorded lung sounds over the neck and chest in 30 adult patients with obstructive airways disease and compared these with 5 patients with extrathoracic upper airways obstruction (73). Fast Fourier transformation was used to analyze these sounds. The best discrimination between wheeze and stridor was the timing during the respiratory cycle (expiratory, wheeze; inspiratory, stridor) and location of greatest intensity (chest, wheeze; neck, stridor).

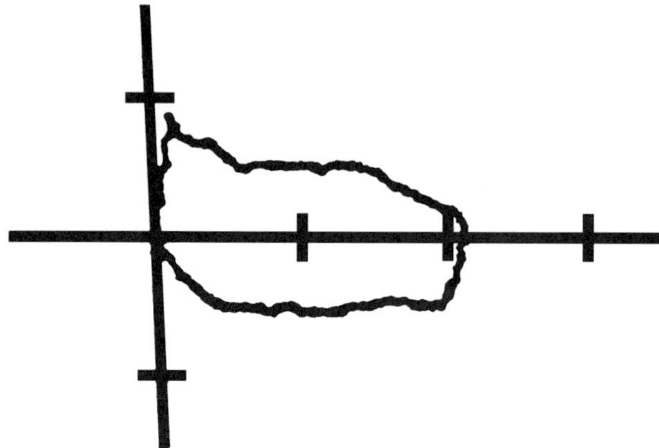

Figure 4 Flow-volume loop demonstrating a fixed upper airway obstruction. This was recorded from a 72-year-old man who was referred for "steroid-dependent asthma." Squamous cell carcinoma arising from the carina with 75% obstruction of both mainstem bronchi was diagnosed during fiberoptic bronchoscopy. Vertical axis, flow; horizontal axis, volume.

Wheezing Associated with Aspiration Syndromes

Aspiration occurs frequently in older individuals (55,74–77). There are various factors contributing to this predisposition, including (1) diminished laryngeal gag reflex; (2) esophageal dysfunction, including gastroesophageal reflux and presby-esophagus; (3) decreased laryngeal gag reflex; and (4) neurological diseases, which may cause abnormal deglutition (e.g., previous strokes, Parkinson's disease, altered levels of consciousness). In a study of normal subjects (age >65 years), 22% had an abnormal cricopharyngeal response to swallowing (55). Depending on the consistency and the amount of material aspirated, wheezing can occur. Particulate matter or foreign bodies can cause wheezing due to endotracheal or endobronchial obstruction, as discussed above. Endobronchial findings after aspiration are notable for diffuse mucusal erythema and edema, which may be localized or diffuse, depending on the extent of the involvement. The associated airways narrowing and increased respiratory and airflow rates promote wheezing after aspiration even in nonasthmatic patients. More common is the association of asthma and gastroesophageal reflux disease (GERD), which does not necessarily require aspiration into the tracheobronchial tree. The mere presence of an acidic pH in the esophagus can cause reflux bronchoconstriction via cholinergic pathways (76,77). Ayres and Miles infused acid into the esophagus of patients with GERD-related cough (76). The cough induced by the acid infusion was almost

Table 2 Drugs Associated with Wheeze or Cough

Cardiovascular agents
  Beta blockers
  Angiotensin-converting enzyme inhibitors
Anti-inflammatory agents
  Aspirin
  Nonsteroidal anti-inflammatory agents
  Hydrocortisone
Miscellaneous
  Contrast media
  Propellants in metered-dose inhalers

---

completely eliminated when the patients were treated with inhaled ipratropium bromide or esophageal-infused lidocaine but not by esophageal-infused ipratropium. These data suggest that GERD-related asthmatic symptoms are mediated via a cholinergic reflex in the lower esophagus.

Drug-Induced Wheezing

Multiple drugs commonly used in the geriatric population have been associated with bronchospasm or cough (Table 2). It has long been recognized that beta blockers (propranolol, etc.) can induce bronchospasm in patients with airways hyperreactivity (78). However, wheezing has also been reported in patients without a history of asthma or COPD (79). When used as ophthalmic solutions for the treatment of glaucoma, beta blockers can induce life-threatening bronchospasm within minutes of administration (80). This does not appear to be a dose-related phenomenon but rather an enhancement of airway cholinergic tone or release of mast cell mediators (78).

Angiotensin-converting enzyme (ACE) inhibitors are associated with cough and airways hyperreactivity, but overt wheezing is rarely encountered (81–83).

Aspirin is also commonly prescribed for elderly patients and is well recognized to provoke wheezing in a minority of asthmatics. Usually, this develops in young adults. There is cross-reactivity with other nonsteroidal anti-inflammatory medications (84).

Miscellaneous Causes of Wheezing

Other diseases commonly seen in the elderly and rarely associated with wheezing include sepsis, lymphangitic carcinomatosis, pulmonary embolism, and factitious wheezing.

Although bronchoconstriction can be demonstrated on pulmonary function testing in patients suffering from acute pulmonary emboli, wheezing is rarely auscultated (85). As to its mechanism, the bronchoconstriction in pulmonary emboli is thought to be due to release of various mediators such as platelet-derived cyclooxygenase products, histamine, and serotonin (86). Supporting the theory that platelet-derived factors are the cause of bronchosconstriction in pulmonary emboli is the observation that heparin can reverse the wheezing by preventing mediator release from platelets. When present, the wheezing is usually a focal and transient finding that helps to differentiate it from asthma in the elderly (85).

Factitious wheezing is due to adduction of the vocal cords and may be difficult to differentiate from asthma on clinical exam. This entity is seen more frequently in younger and psychologically unstable patients (87). The flow-volume loop demonstrates an upper airway obstruction that often is not reliably reproduced. This physiological pattern distinguishes factitious wheezing from asthma (88).

Carcinoid tumors are the most frequent benign tumors of the airways and can cause localized wheezing due to endobronchial obstruction (89). Rarely, these tumors produce high levels of 5-hydroxytryptamine, which cause the "carcinoid syndrome." Manifestations of carcinoid syndrome include episodic flushing and bronchospasm.

B. Cough

Cough is a very frequent complaint in elderly patients. In a questionnatire to more than a thousand elderly subjects without asthma, 15.6% reported the presence of a chronic cough (18). A random sample of over a hundred elderly patients in assisted-living facilities in the United Kingdom reported a 51% incidence of cough (2), which was the most common presenting symptom in elderly asthmatics (57).

Cough and Asthma

Just as cough can be the only manifestation of asthma in younger persons (90), so too can "cough-variant" asthma be the source of chronic cough in elderly persons. We reviewed the records of 38 patients who presented with persistent (mean 13.9 months), unexplained cough. They all had normal spirometry and no explanation for their cough on physical exam or chest radiographs. Of the total, 20 subjects were lifetime nonsmokers and 18 former smokers who had stopped smoking for a minimum of 8 years prior to their evaluation. Following bronchoprovocation testing using ultrasonically nebulized distilled water (91), 22 subjects showed evidence of airways hyperreactivity (responders), while 16 patients showed no evidence of airway hyperreactivity (nonresponders) (Fig. 5). All patients were treated with inhaled beta$_2$-agonists and inhaled or oral corticosteroids. Of the 18

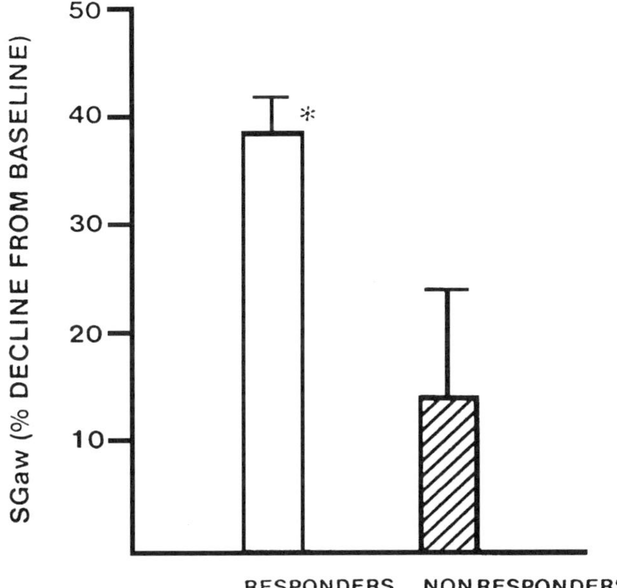

Figure 5 Change in specific airway conductance (SGaw) after bronchoprovocation with ultrasonically nebulized distilled water expressed as percent decrease (mean ± S.D.) from baseline SGaw prior to bronchoprovocation. *p < 0.001. Reactors, who demonstrate a greater than 35% decrease in SGaw, have a greater chance of showing improvement in symptoms of cough with inhaled or oral corticosteroids.

responders, 17 reported improvement of their cough within 1 month of instituting inhaled therapy, while only 1 of the 12 nonresponders noted subjective improvement in the frequency or intensity of their cough. Thus prolonged unexplained cough in the elderly associated with airway hyperreactivity may respond well to asthma therapy.

Bucca et al. questioned whether "asthma-like symptoms" such as cough were due to bronchial or extrathoracic airways dysfunction (92). Histamine bronchoprovocation was performed on 441 patients who presented with at least one of three symptoms (cough, wheeze, dyspnea). A 20% or greater fall in FEV_1 with ≤ 8 mg/ml was defined as bronchial hyperresponsiveness while a ≥ 25% fall in maximal midinspiratory flow was used to define extrathoracic airways hyperresponsiveness (Fig. 6). In 34% of the patients who presented solely with cough, a significantly greater incidence of extrathoracic upper airway hyperresponsiveness was observed, whereas the combination of cough plus wheeze and/or dyspnea was associated with both extrathoracic upper airways and bronchial hyperresponsive-

Ahmed et al.

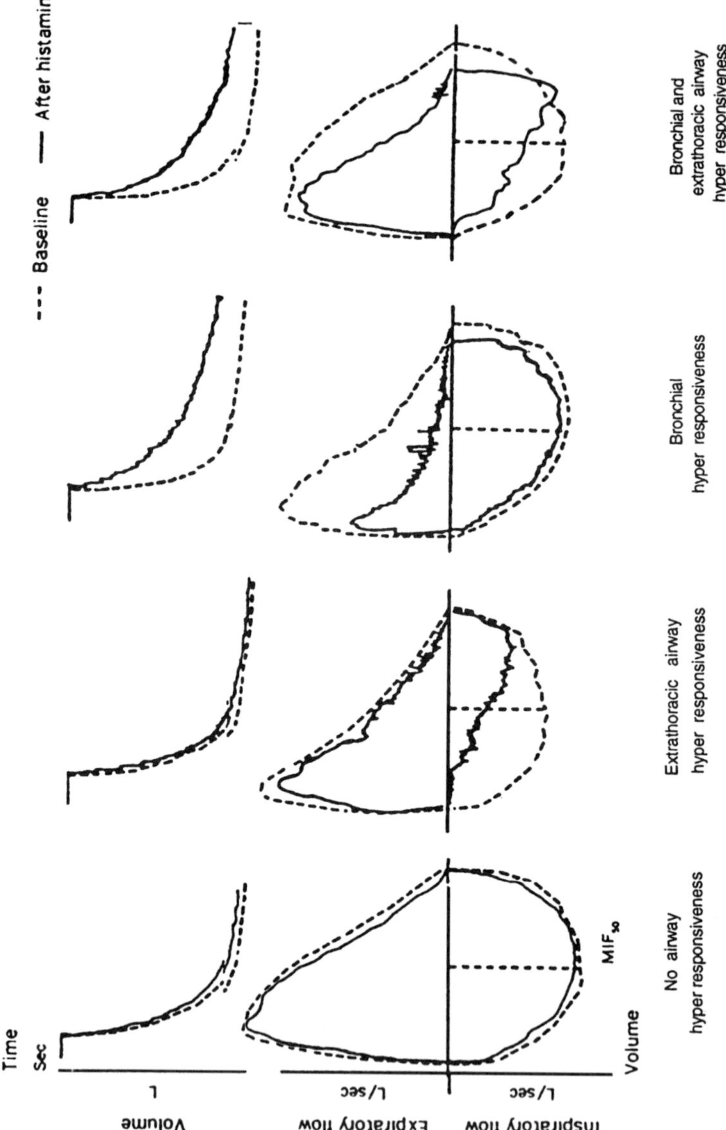

Figure 6 Changes in FEV_1 ($\geq$ 20% decline) and maximal midinspiratory flow (MIF_{50} decrease $\geq$ 25%) after exposure to histamine challenge ($\leq$ 8 mg/ml) were defined as bronchial and extrathoracic upper airways hyperresponsiveness, respectively. (From Ref. 92.)

ness. The authors concluded that extrathoracic dysfunction may account for cough-variant asthma in patients who have no other respiratory symptoms.

Cough and Chronic Obstructive Lung Disease

Chronic cough is frequently diagnosed inappropriately as chronic bronchitis in elderly patients with reversible obstructive airways disease. Six of 15 patients who developed asthma at the age of 60 were misdiagnosed as chronic bronchitis for up to 22 years (4). The authors of the Tuscon epidemiological study questioned whether the patients with chronic cough who were diagnosed as having asthma did not also have chronic bronchitis (18). Of the elderly asthmatics in their study, 46% had a diagnosis by their physicians of chronic bronchitis as well. This highlights that the differentiation between asthma and COPD is not always clear-cut, especially when cough is a prominent symptom and patients have a past history of smoking. The difficulty in distinguishing between these diseases has led to the clinical use of the term *asthmatic bronchitis.* Pulmonary function testing with assessment of the response to bronchodilator or bronchoprovoking agents is often necessary to distinguish between COPD and asthma when cough is a prominent symptom.

Bronchiectasis can also mimic asthma because of the symptoms of a productive cough and dyspnea (93). High-resolution computed tomography often establishes this diagnosis (94).

Drug-Induced Cough

Angiotensin-converting enzyme (ACE) inhibitors are commonly prescribed in the geriatric population. Cough is a frequent side effect, with a reported incidence of approximately 15% (81). However, asthma exacerbation has not been reported, which prompted questions as to the role of bronchial hyperreactivity in ACE-related cough (82). Kaufman et al. reported a positive response to methacholine in 8 of 9 patients who had cough while taking ACE inhibitors, whereas none of 8 noncoughing patients had a positive methacholine test (83). After stopping the medication for at least 8 weeks, 6 of 8 patients still had airways hyperreactivity. This suggests that the patients who developed ACE-related cough either had underlying airway hyperreactivity or developed hyperreactivity in association with the use of ACE inhibitors.

Similarly, beta blockers can induce cough in asthmatic patients by triggering bronchospasm. Most studies have emphasized the symptoms of wheeze and dyspnea and not just cough (78,79).

Cough Associated with Gastroesophageal Reflux Disease

Cough may be the presenting symptom of gastroesophageal reflux disease (GERD) (76,95). The prevalence of GERD is higher in asthmatics than in the normal population (96). The elderly have a high incidence of hiatal hernia, thus predisposing them to reflux when the hernia is of the sliding variety (55). The association of asthma and GERD was described a century ago by Sir William Osler (97). Typical symptoms of asthma and GERD may be absent in the elderly patient. However, unexplained cough, especially when nocturnal or associated with the supine position, may suggest the diagnosis (55).

The finding of reflux in a patient with cough does not necessarily establish a diagnosis of asthma. Indeed, acid infusion into the esophagus of nonasthmatics caused a decrease in peak expiratory flow rates (PEFR), which normalized after subsequent saline infusion (98). This normalization of PEFR distinguished the group of asthmatics who also had GERD, since neither their PEFR nor airways resistance measurement statistically improved following subsequent saline infusion (77,98).

Neoplasm and Miscellaneous Causes of Cough

Other diseases that present with cough and affect the elderly include interstitial pneumonitides, pneumonia, recurrent aspiration, postnasal drip, tracheomalacia, and neoplasm. If cough is caused by a pulmonary neoplasm, usually there are associated radiographic abnormalities (67). However, an endobronchial or endotracheal lesion may be radiographically occult or require sophisticated techniques to image and present solely as a cough syndrome.

C.   Dyspnea and Chest Discomfort

There are multiple causes, with or without chest discomfort, that can produce symptoms of dyspnea in elderly patients. They include COPD, CHF, angina pectoris, upper airways obstruction, pulmonary thromboembolic disease, aspiration syndrome, bronchogenic neoplasms, benign pulmonary neoplasms, vocal cord dysfunction, chest bellows disease (neuromuscular disease or chest wall deformities), interstitial pneumonitides, primary pulmonary hypertension, and gastroesophageal reflux disease. Although the combination of wheezing, dyspnea, and chest tightness is a classical presentation of asthma, dyspnea can also be the sole manifestation of asthma in the elderly (56). Frequently patients will undergo a cardiac evaluation to determine the source of dyspnea before asthma is considered as a possibility. Symptoms that suggest the possibility of asthma include a familial atopic or asthmatic history, a history of any type of "respiratory trouble" before the age of 16, identifiable triggers for the dyspnea, an atopic history, or an elevated IgE level (18). Although nocturnal awakenings may point toward the diagnosis of asthma, this is also a manifestation of angina pectoris and aspiration syndromes. If the elderly patient maintains a sedentary lifestyle, dyspnea may not be evident and may be underreported. Primary pulmonary hypertension has been reported in elderly patients and can be confused with asthma because of the symptom of dyspnea (99).

V. Near Fatal Asthma

Some patients with asthma are at a particularly high risk of dying of this disease. Patients who develop asthma in adult life have predominantly intrinsic-type disease, which tends to be resistant to the usual form of therapy. Status asthmaticus is more common in this group than in patients with extrinsic asthma, and it has been shown that elderly asthmatics, like the younger patients, can suffer severe exacerbations of their disease, leading to near fatal or fatal episodes (41,100). Patients at high risk for near fatal attacks of asthma include (1) those with unexpected episodes of severe, overwhelming asthma; (2) those with chronic, progressive worsening of asthma symptoms requiring long-term oral steroid use; and (3) those who fit neither of these categories but who had extremely poor control of their asthma in the months before a near fatal or fatal asthma attack (26,101–103). About 80% of patients who die with status asthmaticus have had asthma for more than 5 years, and about one-half have had asthma for less than 10 years. Most patients who die with status asthmaticus have asthma that started after age 40. Thus, the prognosis of patients whose asthma starts at age 40 or beyond is worse than that of those whose asthma begins before age 40, as they are most likely to terminate in status asthmaticus.

The mechanism by which fatal and near fatal attacks develop are not yet known, but it is likely that the essential ingredients consist of the degree of airways lability, the severity of preexisting airways obstruction, the magnitude of the stimulus applied, and the patient's ability to respond to extreme airways narrowing. The only accepted criterion in predicting which patient is likely to develop a life-threatening episode of status asthmaticus is a previous history of an episode of status asthmaticus. Approximately 50% of the patients who have been in status asthmaticus suffer another episode within a 2-year period (12). As with other aspects of severe asthma, there are surprisingly few data indicating the precipitating factors and pathogenesis of a life-threatening attack. The stimuli most often associated with fatal or near fatal airway narrowing are profound emotional upset, environmental allergens, air pollutants, the use of beta blockers, and the ingestion of aspirin or other nonsteroidal anti-inflammatory agents in sensitive patients (103,104).

The identification of patients at high risk for a fatal attack of asthma continues to be a difficult problem and a challenge for the physicians. If high-risk patients are identifiable, then appropriate and timely intervention can reduce their risk of hospitalization and sudden death. Retrospective analyses have highlighted several clinical characteristics of patients who die from asthma (105). These include (1) severe asthma, (2) poor compliance with therapy and problems with self-management, (3) denial of disease, (4) delay in seeking or delivering medical help, (5) poor family support system, (6) instability of airways function, (7) psychological factors, (8) recurrent emergency room visits and/or hospitalization, (9) previous occurrences of life-threatening attacks, and (10) poor medical care (102,106).

Elderly patients may be especially prone to near fatal asthma because of a blunted perception of dyspnea. In the elderly, an acute attack of asthma may be very rapidly fatal (100) and carries a worse prognosis than in the young (107). Thus, when they report breathlessness and wheezing, they may be close to death. Of the many potential reasons for the higher mortality from asthma in old age, the possibility of impaired awareness of the severity of an acute asthmatic attack by the elderly patient, the physician, or both may be possible. In addition, the diminished pulmonary and cardiovascular reserves in the elderly predispose them to more severe disease. These observations have important implications for the prevention of morbidity and mortality from asthma. Elderly asthmatics may be at a higher mortality risk because of their blunted perception of dyspnea and should be monitored closely. A history of a prior acute, severe asthma attack should be taken as a warning that a life-threatening attack may occur. It is important to remember that delayed access to medical care and undertreatment rather than overtreatment are the most important factors for an asthmatic to be at risk for death, which is more likely to happen in the elderly. The vast majority of deaths from asthma are preventable and result from a failure of the physician, the patient, or both to recognize the seriousness of the episode.

VI. Economic Impact

The potential for benign neglect is an unintentional reality for the elderly in our health-care system. In our currently evolving system of managed care, widespread interest in cost containment among the health-care providers (a misnomer for physicians) and the health-care industry is likely to aggravate this age-based bias.

Asthma, being a common illness, is estimated to result in 2–3 million emergency room visits and 0.5–1 million hospitalizations annually in the United States (108,109). One important component of morbidity caused by asthma in the United States is its economic impact. In 1990, the cost of illness related to asthma was estimated to be $6.2 billion (the 1995 estimate is $10 billion). Because of inefficient preventive care, 43% of the economic impact was asociated with emergency room use and hospitalization costs, which can be greatly reduced (110). The potential savings from the shift from more expensive hospital/ emergency room care to less expensive preventive ambulatory care is readily apparent. Therefore, if the costs of asthma are to be reduced, any future efforts to direct health policy toward improvement in asthma care must emphasize improving the effectiveness of primary preventive care of asthma in the ambulatory setting (111,112). By using a vigorous medical regimen and an intensive educational program, reduced hospital use among adult asthmatics—who had previously required repeated readmissions for severe asthma exacerbation—has been clearly demonstrated (113).

Cost-effective preventive care is especially important for high-risk elderly patients with asthma who required intubation and mechanical ventilation. An asthma management program after discharge from the hospital could effectively reduce the total cost from over \$40,000 to \$5000 and inpatient costs from approximately \$40,000 to \$2000. This suggests that "active intervention"— including patient education, specialist care, regular outpatient visits, and an access to emergency call service—can significantly reduce the cost of asthma care and morbidity in the high-risk patient. It is reasonable to assume that careful and regular preventive management of elderly asthmatics should result in much better quality of life and patient well-being; the likely decrease in emergency room visits or hospitalization could result in a substantial decrease in health-care costs associated with long-term care.

References

1. Speizer FE. Epidemiology and mortality patterns in asthma. In: Weiss EB, ed. Status asthmaticus. Baltimore: University Park Press, 1978:13–18.
2. Banerjee DK, Lee GS, Malik SK, Daly S. Under-diagnosis of asthma in the elderly. Br J Dis Chest 1987; 81:23–29.
3. Braman SS. Asthma in the ederly patient. Clin Chest Med 1993; 14:413–422.
4. Lee HY, Stretton TB. Asthma in the elderly. Br Med J 1972; 4:93–95.
5. Burr ML, Charles TJ, Roy K, Seaton A. Asthma in the elderly: An epidemiological survey. Br Med J 1979; 1:1041–1044.
6. Lal S, Mandaleson K, Norman A. Asthma in the elderly. Res Clin Forms 1984; 6: 17–22.
7. Osler W. Lectures on Angina Pectoris and Allied States. New York: Appleton, 1897:81.
8. Hope JA. Treatise on Diseases of the Heart and Great Vessels. Vol. 1. London: William Kidd, 1833.
9. Nejjari C, Tessier JF, Bargerger-Gateau P, et al. Functional status of elderly people treated for asthma-related symptoms: A population based case-control study. Eur Respir J 1994; 7:1077–1083.
10. Chang JT, Moran MB, Cugell DW, Webster JR. COPD in the elderly: A reversible cause of functional impairment. Chest 1995; 108:736–740.
11. National Asthma Educational Program Expert Panel Report. Guidelines for the Diagnosis and Management of Asthma. Bethesda, MD: U.S. Department of Health and Human Services Publication No. 91-3042, 1991.
12. Ahmed T, Chediak AD. Status asthmaticus. In: Dantzker DR, Scharf SM, eds. Cardiopulmonary Critical Care. New York: Saunders. In press 1997.
13. Braman SS, Kaemmerlen JT, Davis SM. Asthma in the elderly: A comparison between patients with recently acquired and long standing disease. Am Rev Respir Dis 1991; 143:336–340.
14. Peat JK, Woodcock AJ, Cullen K. Rate of decline of lung function in subjects with asthma. Eur J Respir Dis 1987; 70:171–179.

15. Van Schayck CP, Dompeling E, Van Herwaarden CLA, et al. Interacting effects of atopy and bronchial hyperresponsiveness on the annual decline in lung function and the exacerbation rate in asthma. Am Rev Respir Dis 1991; 144:1297–1301.

16. Brown PJ, Greville HW, Finucane KE. Asthma and irreversible airflow obstruction. Thorax 1984; 39:131–136.

17. Sobonya RE. Quantitative structural alterations in longstanding allergic asthma. Am Rev Respir Dis 1984; 130:289–292.

18. Burrows B, Barbee RA, Cline MG, et al. Characteristics of asthma among elderly adults in a sample of the general population. Chest 1991; 100:935–942.

19. Traver GA, Cline MG, Burrows B. Asthma in the elderly. J Asthma 1993; 30:81–91.

20. Burrows B, Lebowitz MD, Barbee RA, Cline MG. Findings before diagnoses of asthma among the elderly in a longitudinal study of a general population sample. J Allergy Clin Immunol 1991; 88:870–877.

21. Coultas DB, Gong H Jr, Grad R, et al. Respiratory disease in minorities of the United States. Am J Respir Crit Care Med 1994; 149:S93–S131.

22. Weiss KB, Gergen PJ, Crain EF. Inner city asthma: The epidemiology of an emerging U.S. Public health concern. Chest 1992; 101:362S–367S.

23. Buist AS, Vollmer WM. Preventing deaths from asthma (editorial). N Engl J Med 1994; 331:1584–1585.

24. Lang DM, Polansky M. Patterns of asthma mortality in Philadelphia from 1969 to 1991. N Engl J Med 1994; 331:1542–1546.

25. Schwartz J, Slater D, Larson TV, et al. Particulate air pollution and hospital emergency room visits for asthma in Seattle. Am Rev Respir Dis 1993; 147:826–831.

26. O'Hallaren MT, Yunginger JW, Offord KP, et al. Exposure to an aeroallergen as a possible precipitating factor in respiratory tract in young patients with asthma. N Engl J Med 1991; 324:359–363.

27. Marder D, Targonski P, Orris P, et al. Effect of racial and socioeconomic factors on asthma mortality in Chicago. Chest 1992; 101:426S–429S.

28. Pfeifer MA, Weinberg CR, Cook D. Differential changes of autonomic nervous system functions with age in man. Am J Med 1983; 75:249–254.

29. Davis PB, Byard PJ. Relationship among airway reactivity, pupillary α-adrenergic and cholinergic responsiveness, and age. J Appl Physiol 1988; 65:200–204.

30. Hopp RJ, Bewtra A, Nair NM, Townley RG. The effect of age on methacholine response. J Allergy Clin Immunol 1985; 76:609–613.

31. Ullah MI, Newman GB, Saunders KB. Influence of age on response to ipratropium and salbutamol in asthma. Thorax 1981; 36:523–529.

32. Abrass IB, Scarpace PJ. Human lymphocyte β-adrenergic recptors are unaltered with age. J Gerontol 1981; 36:298–301.

33. Feldman RD, Limbird LE, Nadeau J, et al. Alterations in leukocytes β-receptor affinity with aging: A potential explanation for altered β-adrenergic sensitivity in the elderly. N Engl J Med 1984; 310:815–819.

34. Kendall MJ, Woods KL. Responsiveness to β-adrenergic receptor stimulation: The effects of age are cardioselective. J Clin Pharmacol 1982; 14:821–827.

35. Hamelin BA, Blouin RA, Wolf KM, et al. In vivo and in vitro β_2-adrenergic receptor responsiveness in young and elderly asthmatics. Pharmacotherapy 1992; 12: 376–382.

36. Connolly MJ, Crowley JJ, Nielson CP, et al. Peripheral mononuclear leucocyte β-adrenoceptors and nonspecific bronchial responsiveness to methacholine in young and elderly normal subjects and asthmatic patients. Thorax 1994; 49:26–32.

37. Sparrow D, O'Connor GT, Rosner B, Weiss ST. Predictors of longitudinal change in methacholine airway responsiveness among middle-aged and older men. Am J Respir Crit Care Med 1994; 149:376–381.

38. Wanner A. Allergic mucociliary dysfunction. J Allergy Clin Immunol 1983; 72: 347–350.

39. Ahmed T, Greenblatt DW, Birch S, et al. Abnormal mucociliary transport in allergic patients with antigen-induced bronchospasm: Role of slow reacting substance of anaphylaxis. Am Rev Respir Dis 1981; 124:110–114.

40. Cooke NJ, Crompton GK, Grant IWB. Observation on the management of acute bronchial asthma. Br J Dis Chest 1979; 73:157–163.

41. Petheram IS, Jones DA, Collin JV. Assessment and management of acute asthma in the elderly: A comparison with younger asthmatics. Postgrad Med J 1982; 58: 149–151.

42. Kronenberg RS, Drage CW. Attenuation of the ventilatory and heart rate responses to hypoxia and hypercapnia with aging in normal men. J Clin Invest 1973; 52:1812–1819.

43. Tack CM, Altose MD, Cherniack NS. Effect of aging on the perception of resistive ventilatory loads. Am Rev Respir Dis 1982; 126:463–467.

44. Tack CM, Altose MD, Cherniack NS. Effect of aging on respiratory sensations produced by elastic loads. J Appl Physiol 1981; 50:844–850.

45. Altose MD, Leitner J, Cherniak NS. Effects of age and respiratory efforts in the perception of resistive ventilatory loads. J Gerontol 1985; 40:147–150.

46. Kikuchi Y, Okabe S, Tamua G, et al. Chemosensitivity and perception of dyspnea in patients with a history of near fatal asthma. N Engl J Med 1994; 330:1329–1334.

47. Gibson GJ. Perception, personality and respiratory control in life-threatening asthma. Thorax 1995; 50:S2–S4.

48. Barnes PJ. Blunted perception and death from asthma (editorial). N Engl J Med 1994; 330:1383–1384.

49. Connolly MJ, Crowley JJ, Charan NB, et al. Reduced subjective awareness of bronchoconstriction provoked by methacholine in elderly asthmatic and normal subjects as measured on a simple awareness scale. Thorax 1992; 47:410–413.

50. Connolly MJ, Kelly C, Walters EH, Hendrick DJ. An assessment of methacholine inhalation test in elderly asthmatics. Age Aging 1988; 17:123–128

51. Connolly MJ, Jarvis EH, Hendrick DJ. Late onset asthma in a demented elderly patient: The value of methacholine challenge in diagnosis. J Am Geriatr Soc 1990; 38:539–541.

52. Bailey WC, Richards JM Jr, Brooks CM, et al. Features of asthma in older adults. J Asthma 1992; 29:21–28.

53. McKinney B. Under new management: Asthma and the elderly. J Gerontol Nurs 1995; 21:39–45.

54. Pierson DJ. Asthma in the elderly: Special challenge. Geriatrics 1982; 37:87–100.

55. Braman SS, Davis SM. Wheezing in the elderly: Asthma and other causes. Geriatr Clin North Am 1986; 2:269–283.

56. Parson GH. Asthma in the elderly: Diagnostic and treatment concerns. Geriatrics 1985; 40:89–96.
57. Bardana EJ Jr. Is asthma really different in the elderly patient? J Asthma 1993; 30:77–79.
58. Barrio JL, Krieger BP. Hyperreactive airways disease in elderly patients with normal spirometry (abstr). Chest 1986; 448S.
59. Snashall PD, Chung KF. Airway obstruction and bronchial hyperresponsiveness in left ventricular failure and mitral stenosis. Am Rev Respir Dis 1991; 144: 945–956.
60. Fishman AP. Cardiac asthma—A fresh look at an old wheeze. N Engl J Med 1989; 320:1346–1348.
61. Cabanes LR, Weber SN, Matran R, et al. Bronchial hyperresponsiveness to methacholine in patients with impaired left ventricular function. N Engl J Med 1989; 320:1317–1322.
62. Baier H, Onorato D, Barker J, Wanner A. Tracheal mucosal edema in hydrostatic pulmonary edema. J Appl Physiol 1994; 77:352–356.
63. Noble WH, Kay JC, Obdrzalek J. Lung mechanics in hypervolemic pulmonary edema. J Appl Physiol 1975; 38:681–687.
64. Eichacker PQ, Seidelman MJ, Rothstein MS, Lejemtel T. Methacholine bronchial reactivity testing in patients with chronic congestive heart failure. Chest 1988; 93: 336–338.
65. Fanta CH. Asthma in the elderly. J Asthma 1989; 26:87–97.
66. Kryger M, Bode F, Antic R, Anthonisen N. Diagnosis of obstruction of the upper and central airways. Am J Med 1976; 61:85–93.
67. Weber AL, Grillo HC. Tracheal tremors: A radiological, clinical, and pathological evaluation of 84 cases. Radiol Clin North Am 1978; 16:227–246.
68. Allen MS. Malignant tracheal tremors. Mayo Clin Proc 1993; 68:680–684.
69. Stauffer JL, Olson DE, Petty TL. Complications and consequences of endotracheal intubation and tracheostomy: A prospective study of 150 critically ill adult patients. Am J Med 1981; 70:65–76.
70. Speiser BL, Spratling L. Radiation bronchitis and stenosis secondary to high dose rate endobronchial irradiation. J Radiation Oncol Biol Phys 1993; 25:589–597.
71. Jauregui R, Lilker ES, Bayley A. Upper airway obstruction in euthyroid goiter. JAMA 1977; 238:2163–2166.
72. Sherry MK, Klainer AS, Wolff M, Gerhard H. Herpetic tracheobronchitis. Ann Intern Med 1988; 109:229–233.
73. Baughman RP, Loudon RG. Stridor: Differentiation from asthma or upper noise. Am Rev Respir Dis 1989; 139:1407–1409.
74. Krieger BP. Respiratory tract infections in the elderly. J Geriatr Drug Ther 1995; 10:29–50.
75. Pontoppidan H, Beecher HK. Progressive loss of protective reflexes in the airway with the advances of age. JAMA 1960; 174:2209–2213.
76. Ayres JG, Miles JF. Oesophageal reflux and asthma. Eur Respir J 1996; 9:1073–1078.
77. Harding SM, Schan CA, Guzzo MR, et al. Gastroesophageal reflux-induced bronchoconstriction: Is microaspiration a factor? Chest 1995; 108:1220–1227.

78. Meeker DP, Wiedemann HP. Drug-induced bronchospasm. Clin Chest Med 1990; 11:163–175.

79. Fraley DS, Bruns FJ, Segel DP, Adler S. Propanolol-related bronchospasms in patients without history of asthma. South Med J 1980; 73:238–240.

80. Prince DS, Carliner NH. Respiratory arrest following first dose of timolol ophthalmic solution. Chest 1983; 84:640–641.

81. Sebastian JL, McKinney WP, Kaufman J, Young MJ. Angiotensin-converting enzyme inhibitors and cough: Prevalence in an outpatient medical clinic population. Chest 1991; 99:36–39.

82. Rosenow EC III, Myers JL, Swenson SJ, Pisani RJ. Drug-induced pulmonary disease: An update. Chest 1992; 102:239–250.

83. Kaufman J, Casanova JE, Riendl P, Schlueter DP. Bronchial hyperreactivity and cough due to angiotensin-converting enzyme inhibitors. Chest 1989; 95:544–548.

84. Mathison DA, Stevenson DD, Simon RA. Precipitating factors in asthma: Aspirin, sulfites, and other drugs and chemicals. Chest 1985; 87:50S–54S.

85. Moser KM. Venous thromboembolism. Am Rev Respir Dis 1990; 141:235–249.

86. Moser KM, Fedullo PF. Venous thromboembolism: Three simple decisions. Part I. Chest 1983; 83:117–121.

87. Christopher KL, Wood RP II, Eckert RC, et al. Vocal-cord dysfunction presenting as asthma. N Engl J Med 1983; 308:1566–1570.

88. Newman KB, Mason UG III, Schmaling KB. Clinical features of vocal cord dysfunction. Am J Respir Crit Care Med 1995; 152:1382–1386.

89. Davila DG, Dunn WF, Tazelaar HD, Pairolero PC. Bronchial carcinoid tumors. Mayo Clin Proc 1993; 68:795–803.

90. Corrao WM, Braman SS, Irwin RS. Chronic cough as the sole presenting manifestation of bronchial asthma. N Engl J Med 1979; 300:633–637.

91. Chadha TS, Birch S, Allegra L, Sackner MA. Effects of ultrasonically nebulized distilled water on respiratory resistance and breathing pattern in normal asthmatics. Bull Eur Physiopathol Respir 1984; 20:257–262.

92. Bucca C, Rolla G. Brussino L, et al. Are asthma-like symptoms due to bronchial or extrathoracic airway dysfunction? Lancet 1995; 346:791–795.

93. Barker AF, Bardana EJ Jr. Bronchiectasis: Update of an orphan disease. Am Rev Respir Dis 1988; 137:969–978.

94. Mootoosamy IM, Rezneck RH, Osman J, et al. Assessment of bronchiectasis by computed tomography. Thorax 1985; 40:920–924.

95. Irwin RS, Zawacki JK, Curley FJ, et al. Chronic cough as the sole presenting manifestation of gastroesophageal reflux. Am Rev Respir Dis 1989; 140:1294–1300.

96. Simpson WG. Gastroesophageal reflux disease and asthma: Diagnosis and management. Arch Intern Med 1995; 155:798–803.

97. Harding SM, Richter JE, Guzzo MR, et al. Asthma and gastroesophageal reflux: Acid suppressive therapy improves asthma outcome. Am J Med 1996; 100:395–405.

98. Schan CA, Harding SM, Haile JM, et al. Gastroesophageal reflux–induced bronchoconstriction: An Intraesophageal acid infusion study using state of the art technology. Chest 1994; 106:731–737.

99. Phipps B, Wong B, Chang CH, Dunn M. Unexplained severe pulmonary hypertension in the older age group. Chest 1983; 84:399–402.

100. Macdonald JB, Seaton A, Williams DA. Asthma deaths in Cardiff 1963–1974; 90 deaths outside hospital. Br Med J 1976; 1:1493–1495.
101. Molfino NA, Nannin LJ, Martelli AN, Slutsky AS. Respiratory arrest in near fatal asthma. N Engl J Med 1991; 324:285–288.
102. Molfino NA, Slutsky AS. Near fatal asthma. Eur Respir J 1994; 7:981–990.
103. McFadden ER Jr. Fatal and near fatal asthma (editorial). N Engl J Med 1991; 324:409–411.
104. Benater SR. Fatal asthma. N Engl J Med 1986; 314:423–429.
105. Strunk RC. Identification of the fatality-prone subject with asthma. J Allergy Clin Immunol 1989; 83:477–485.
106. Boulet LP, Deschesnes F, Turcotte H,Gignac F. Near-fatal asthma: Clinical and physiologic features, perception of bronchoconstriction, and psychologic profile. J Allergy Clin Immunol 1991; 88:838–846.
107. Unger L. Chronic bronchial asthma in the older age group. Med Clin North Am 1956; 40:115–134.
108. National Center for Health Statistics, 1984: DHHS Publication No. (PHS) 85-1232. Washington, DC: United States Government Printing Office, December 1984 (emergency room visits).
109. Graves EJ. Detailed diagnosis and procedures, National Hospital Discharge Survey, 1990. Vital Health Stat 1992; 13:16 (hospitalization).
110. Weiss KB, Gergen PJ, Hodgson TA. An economic evaluation of asthma in the United States. N Engl J. Med 1992; 326:862–866.
111. Weiss KB. The health economics of treating mild asthma. Eur Respir Rev 1996; 6: 33, 45–49.
112. Barnes PJ, Jonsson B, Kim JB. The costs of asthma. Eur Respir J 1996; 9:636–642.
113. Mayo PH, Richman J, Harris HW. Results of a program to reduce admissions for adult asthma. Ann Intern Med 1990; 112:864–871.

6

Management Overview
Special Considerations for the Elderly

CONNIE L. KOHLER, E. A. GALLAGHER, RICK PLAYER, and WILLIAM C. BAILEY

University of Alabama at Birmingham
Birmingham, Alabama

I. Introduction

This chapter describes the needs and characteristics of older adults that should be considered in the optimal diagnosis and management of asthma in this population. The National Asthma Education and Prevention Program (NAEPP) of the National Heart, Lung and Blood Institute (NHLBI) published detailed recommendations for asthma management in 1991 (1). More recently, the NHLBI convened a group of experts to address issues specific to elderly patients and their families (2), which resulted in a report intended to supplement the original guidelines. As pointed out in the original guideline publication, specific therapeutic regimens, while based on expert recommendations, must be tailored to individual needs and circumstances of the older patient (3,4).

The purpose of this chapter is to provide a general overview of the *nonpharmacological* management of asthma in older adults and to identify the factors characteristic of this population that influence successful management. The first section of the chapter is a review of the characteristics of older adults and other related factors that contribute to the successful management of asthma. The second section is an outline of the management considerations that result from the characteristics and factors described. The chapter ends with a description of a stepwise approach to therapy for older patients that has been recommended by the Working Group on Asthma in the Elderly.

II. Characteristics of Older Adults and Other Factors that Can Influence Successful Management

Certain personal characteristics, along with social and environmental factors, are altered as patients age. This section details those factors that may influence management choices or outcomes. The reader should bear in mind that the factors described are generalizations and may not apply to even a majority of older adults. However, they do occur to a greater degree in the elderly population than in younger adults and therefore should be considered in an assessment of the older patient's needs.

A. Social and Environmental Factors

The typical day of an older person is characterized by an array of social and environmental circumstances different from those faced by younger adults A majority of older adults are retired or out of the work force for other reasons. Some are disabled and spend their days in social and physical environments atypical of the general population. Social factors that may relate to management and outcomes for asthma patients include the family, social support networks, and institutions available to the patient. Older adults may not live geographically close to family members and, therefore, may experience less frequent family contact. This is especially problematic if a spouse is no longer present (5). In the absence of spouse or families, it is hoped that other social support networks are relied upon— namely, networks such as neighbors, churches, and elder-care programs.

A special case of a social network is the health care staff. The patient's relationship to the providers affects asthma care. Recommendations that both patient and family be a part of the management "team" are of long standing. When family members are also caretakers, they play a very important role, especially if the older patient has communication or cognitive difficulties (6). However, social networks mentioned above may become the intermediary if family members are distant. Also, in the patient-provider relationship, some older adults tend to be less assertive and may not feel comfortable in a role more autonomous than that of the traditional patient (7). Family members or support networks may have to assume this advocacy role in the elder's behalf (8,9).

Older adults are more likely to have fixed or limited financial resources, and this may affect their health insurance options. They may be less likely to fill expensive prescriptions or may try to conserve medications. They may put off doctors' appointments if they consider them to be too costly. They may also have limited access to transportation, which further decreases their level of health care utilization (3). For example, in a university clinical population of adults with asthma, elderly patients were seen to utilize health resources less frequently than younger patients (10).

Environmental factors that influence asthma are largely triggers to attacks (11). A major source of such exposures for the general population is the workplace. Older adults are less likely than their younger counterparts to experience occupational exposures, but they may live in older housing or in assisted living situations that tend to expose them to more irritants such as dust, mildew, and especially institutional cleaning agents (4). Many elderly who remain in their homes are living in older neighborhoods that tend to be closer in to the central city, where higher levels of air pollution may be found (12); but even those in rural areas are at risk of environmental triggers, particularly if they live in older homes.

While many older adults remain independent and active, others, due to illness and living arrangements, may find themselves with less control over their social and physical environment than they once had. They may be under the care of a relative, or living in a relative's home, or under professional nursing care in an institutional setting. They may spend a greater amount of time in environments that allow them to be more sedentary and—because of waning physical strength, chronic illness, and fewer resources—their daily activities may be much more limited (13). All of these factors may constrain the level of autonomy and personal control that an older adult feels.

B. Personal Characteristics

Two types of characteristics that may influence asthma management are reviewed: physical changes and psychological changes. Physical changes are related to both the normal aging process and to chronic diseases that become more evident in older adults. Loss of muscle tone, poor coordination, decreased motor speed, and a diminished gag reflex are characteristics that can affect the use of inhalation devices (14,15). Several of these factors, in combination with increased rigidity of the chest wall, will affect the measurement of peak expiratory flow rates (16). Vision and hearing losses have implications for attending to and following the clinician's recommendations.

Older adults more often suffer from chronic diseases. Elderly asthma patients report more chronic obstructive pulmonary disease (COPD), arthritis, diabetes, and hypertension than younger asthmatics (10). Asthma in the elderly may be associated with severe and persistent ventilatory impairment (17). On the one hand, as asthma patients age, they tend to become less sensitive to inhaled allergens; on the other hand, the older asthma patient may develop incomplete reversibility of airflow obstruction. Additionally, coexisting diseases, such as arthritis, can further affect the patient's ability to use inhalation devices (10), and diabetes and cardiovascular diseases may increase the number of daily medications with which the patient must contend (18). Interestingly, in studies of both asthma and COPD compliance, older adults have demonstrated a better rate of compliance than those under 60 years of age, especially with oral medications (10,19). In another study, older adults admitted to the hospital for an asthma exacerbation were more likely than younger patients to have overutilized bronchodilator inhalers in the preceding 24 hr.

Psychological changes that occur with aging relate to cognitive abilities and affective state. Cognitive functioning may become impaired by a number of factors such as sleep disturbance, stroke, anemia, dementia, electrolyte imbalance, thyroid dysfunction, and medication side effects. Both perceptual and memory difficulties may be present in older adults. Decreased perception of breathlessness among older asthma patients—especially more sedentary patients—may result in failure to recognize and act on dyspnea. Memory loss is most pronounced for short-term memory (20), which can affect the patient's ability to remember and adhere to the clinician's instructions. Older asthmatics are less likely to be high school graduates (10), and, as a group, the elderly are twice as likely to have a lower literacy rate than the general population (21). Other cognitive changes that may occur with aging include confusion; less ability to handle multiple, complex stimuli; slower reaction time; and diminished ability to learn new information as well as to adapt to environmental changes.

The most common change in affective state seen with aging is depression. Depression is a risk factor for fatality-prone asthma (1). Depression in aging may result from a number of factors such as family loss or family disruption when a spouse dies or adult children move away, difficult adjustment to retirement, chronic disease, or medication effects (5,22). Depression can affect both motivation and memory, and it has the potential to affect compliance negatively. Decreased energy levels may result in less aggressive efforts at identifying triggers, monitoring peak flow rates, or using a compliance monitoring system.

Being less assertive is characteristic of both depression and older age, and low assertiveness may have trigger-control implications. In living situations where the perceived level of control is low, as in institutional settings where older adults often depend on attendants, a passive or nonassertive person may be exposed to triggers such as cleaning agents, personal grooming products, dust, and dust mites more often than a person who speaks up about his or her needs (23).

Finally, the physical and cognitive changes described above may result in general functional impairment, such as decreased mobility and fewer normal activities of daily living. These functional impairments also have implications for asthma management (13). For example, decreased mobility may be one explanation for a decrease in health care utilization (10). The next section details asthma management strategies that take these implications into consideration.

III. Management Considerations for Older Patients

The NAEPP goals for management include maintenance of patients' normal activity and of near normal pulmonary function, prevention of symptoms and recurrent exacerbations of asthma, and avoidance of adverse effects from medications (1). In older adults, these goals should be pursued on a more modest level, tempered by consideration for the patient's quality of life (2). For example, a balance must be sought between the quest for normal pulmonary function and the need to keep medication regimens simple. Table 1 lists the general goals of asthma therapy for elderly patients identified by the NAEPP working group on asthma in the elderly (2). The age-associated changes that were outlined in the previous section suggest some ways in which asthma management strategies should be altered for older patients. Of course, the presence of any of the above factors should be confirmed in a patient assessment before altering the therapeutic regimen (24), and such an assessment is the first strategy listed below.

The NAEPP recommends four components of asthma therapy: patient education, environmental control, pharmacological therapy, and objective monitoring of the disease (1). Co-morbidities in older asthma patients and implications for pharmacological management are addressed in other chapters of this volume. This chapter has as its focus the nonpharmacological management strategies related to patient education, environmental control, and disease monitoring. An important goal of nonpharmacological management is to enable patients to "self-manage" their asthma as much as possible (24). Many of the factors identified earlier in this chapter have implications for asthma self-management.

A. General Asthma Management Strategies

Assess the clinical differences that characterize asthma in older adults and adjust treatment as necessary. Clinical differences that affect management—such as incomplete irreversibility of airflow obstruction, poor performance on spirometry

Table 1 General Goals of Asthma Therapy for Elderly Patients

Permit desired level of activity and maintain quality of life
Optimize pulmonary function
Control cough and nocturnal symptoms
Prevent exacerbations
Promote prompt recognition and treatment of exacerbations to avoid hospitalizations or emergency department visits
Avoid aggravating other medical conditions
Minimize adverse effects from medications

Source: Ref. 2.

(25), decreased sensitivity to allergens, and depression—should be assessed rather than assumed. For example, it has been recommended that spirometric assessment takes into account the performance problems the elderly may have, including poor technique, severe obstruction, and bronchoconstriction. In addition, assessment of immunological status should not be routine in elderly patients because it is felt that they are less likely to have allergic reactions (26). On the other hand, in the absence of clinical measures, obtaining an allergy history is important, and for those with allergies, environmental control tends to be more effective than immunotherapy (27). Assessment of cognitive changes, including depression, can be done using simple screening tools such as the Hospital Anxiety and Depression (HAD) scale (28). Similarly, assessments of functional impairment for asthmatics are available (29).

Include key support persons on the asthma team. It is very important to include key members of the patient's social support network in the development and carrying out of asthma management plans. Spouses, adult children who have assumed a caregiving role, and professional caregivers will be able to contribute to the assessment of the patient's special needs and to provide the material support necessary to carry out many of the management activities. Activities in which the support person may play a key role include listening to, interpreting, and remembering clinician instructions; prompting and reminding the patient to take medications; providing transportation to clinic appointments; providing assistance in environmental control measures such as housekeeping; helping the patient recognize signs of an exacerbation and to remain calm; helping the patient plan and manage resources to afford medications or other aspects of asthma care.

Identify social networks that need to be informed about the patient's disease. Older patients may spend significant parts of the day among different social networks, such as church groups, elder-care settings, or neighborhoods. Just as schools and teachers are informed of students' asthma needs, it may be helpful if members of these groups are aware of the patient's disease and the appropriate responses to potential problems such as an asthma attack.

Work at the patient's desired level of autonomy and control. While the goals of asthma therapy are to increase independence and foster self-management of the disease, patients with coexisting conditions, including depression, may desire or require more structure and leadership from the health care provider (30). While the ideal continues to be to encourage patient involvement in care, asthma treatment should not overwhelm the patient who may have limited ability to deal with the demands of self-management.

B. Strategies to Enhance Medication Adherence

Tailor the medication regimen to the patient's typical day. Older patients may take daily medications for more than one health problem and may have less ability to remember what to take when (31). Strategies to overcome these difficulties are to keep dosing times to a minimum and/or to match the dosing schedule for asthma medications to dosing schedules for other medications if possible. Medication schedules should be provided to the patient and support person in writing, and it may be helpful to suggest the use of pill dispensers or other reminder systems (8). However, using pill dispensers can be problematic, because once a pill is removed from its original container, it will be difficult to identify. One solution to this problem is to have separate dispensers for each medicine and to label the dispenser accordingly.

Have patients bring all medications to every visit. Patients may not remember the names or dosing schedules of their medications and may not report changes since their last visit. It is important to ask about all medicines the patient takes, including over-the-counter medicines. For each medicine, ask the patient how many are taken in a day and when. Ask how many have been taken so far that day. This will provide valuable information about the patient's understanding of the dosing schedule. In addition, it will provide evidence if the prescription is being refilled as expected.

Provide the patient with clear verbal and written information on the actions and effects of bronchodilator versus anti-inflammatory agents. Patients' expectations of what a medicine should do has a strong influence on their adherence (31). When patients understand that their inhaled anti-inflammatory medications are not meant to give immediate symptom relief, they are more likely to use their medications correctly. The distinction between "fast acting" or "rescue" medications and "maintenance" medications is a very useful one for patients.

Alter metered-dose inhaler (MDI) use as necessary. Incorrect MDI technique is a major problem in older patients (27). Carefully assess the patient's ability to use an MDI (32). If weakness or other disabilities are noted that cause suboptimal medication delivery, there are several alternatives to consider, such as devices to make activation easier for patients with decreased strength (20), alternative inhalation devices such as breath-actuated inhalers, and spacers or reservoirs. Spacers are also helpful to patients who have trouble holding their breath (32). These patients can take multiple breaths to empty the spacer. Dry powder inhalation devices seem to be as effective as aerosols when used appropriately (33). Teach patients to use the closed-mouth technique with inhalers, especially for using ipratropium, to avoid unintentional spraying in eyes. If patients are using multiple inhalers, they should be easily distinguished—for example, by color-coding canisters with colored stickers. Small-volume nebulizers are another alternative, but they should be used only with unit-dose preparations to avoid mistakes in mixing and filling the nebulizer (7,34). In addition, it is important to take into consideration that repeated nebulized β_2-agonist doses during an asthma exacerbation increases the risk of cardiac arrhythmias (27).

C. Use of a Written Management Plan

Make written materials and instructions "user friendly." To compensate for vision, hearing, and memory difficulties, all patient instructions should be provided in writing. Because of vision difficulty and the greater likelihood of poor literacy, materials should be kept simple, using relatively large print and simple illustrations. Handwritten instructions should be large and legible. The format should be convenient to the patient—single sheet "handouts" can be folded and carried around or posted in the home. With regard to written materials,

1. Provide copies of all such materials to caregivers or support persons.
2. Attach copies of medication instructions to the patient's prescription, with a note asking the pharmacist to review the instructions with the patient when dispensing medications.
3. Include all important information in the written management plan.

Use an asthma management zone system based on the frequency and severity of symptoms and peak expiratory flow rates. This system indicates the appropriate actions for each zone, such as which bronchodilator to take and how to seek medical attention. Include the specific dose of long-term maintenance medication, specific triggers to avoid, and other specific environmental control measures. If diaries are given, make sure patients understand them and can fill them out.

D. Trigger Control Strategies

Tailor environmental control measures so that they are feasible for and acceptable to the patient and that they will not adversely affect his or her quality of life. Older adults will have varying amount of control over their environment depending on their living situations. Older adults who keep house for themselves have the freedom to control triggers, but they may not be aware of or able to control dust and irritants. They may be reluctant to change their lifestyles. For example, they may feel that it is important to use certain types of cleaners that contain irritants, or they may not want to give up a special pet. If trigger control becomes a serious issue for the patients' health, it may be necessary to conduct an inspection or ask for a home health visit to evaluate the home setting and institute appropriate measures. For patients who are not living independently, written guidelines for environmental control should be given to the people responsible for the patient's environment.

To avoid infections, give prophylactic vaccinations. Pneumococcal vaccinations are recommended every 6–10 years and influenza vaccinations yearly (2).

E. Self-Monitoring Strategies

Teach patients to monitor peak expiratory flow rate and/or symptoms. Because of a more sedentary lifestyle, elderly patients may underestimate the severity of their disease, which makes peak expiratory flow rate (PEFR) monitoring more important (9). Alternatively, depending on the patient's abilities and disease, symptom monitoring may be preferable to PEFR monitoring. Patients most likely to benefit from PEFR monitoring are those who experience episodic worsening of symptoms, require emergency department care for exacerbations, or have coexisting heart and lung disease that PEFR may help distinguish (2). Some patients may not have the ability to make sufficient expiratory effort for the peak flowmeter; for them, it would be better to monitor symptoms. In addition, the decreasing level of variability in lung function and degree of irreversible obstruction may make PEFR monitoring less useful. Therefore, in monitoring PEFR, elderly patients should use personal best measures rather than predicted PEFR (35). Patients' ability to perceive their symptoms and judge symptom severity also varies, which can make symptom monitoring a problem. The most common symptoms to monitor include chest tightness; cough; wheeze; dyspnea (2); nocturnal or early morning awakenings with wheeze or cough; increase in use of or diminished response to inhaled β_2-agonist; decrease in tolerance of exercise, including normal daily activities; changes in phlegm; and acute episodes of shortness of breath or wheezing (2). The optimal approach is to have the patient monitor both symptoms and peak flow rate and to assist the patient to correlate symptoms with PEFR (36).

Review and correct peak flow meter technique at each visit. As with inhaler use, peak flow measurement technique may not be correct. Even patients who have been instructed in the proper technique may not consistently use it and may develop incorrect behaviors (37). Observing the technique at each visit can provide a valuable opportunity to correct problems (2).

IV. Summary: Asthma Management via Stepped Care

Given the above considerations and strategies, it has been noted that the overall therapeutic approach to asthma in older patients is not significantly different from that regularly recommended for the general population of asthmatics: determine the patient's level of asthma severity and step treatment up or down accordingly (2).

Mild asthma should be treated with inhaled bronchodilators on an as-needed basis. Preexposure to known triggers should be avoided and advance medication may be indicated for some patients prior to trigger exposure. Influenza and pneumococcus vaccines are recommended. It may be helpful to remind patients that although they may be symptomless for an extended time, the disease is still present, and they must be prepared in case symptoms recur (27).

Table 2 Recommendations for Stepped Care in Patients with Good Reversibility

Administration as needed of short-acting β_2-agonist therapy. Consistent use over three times a day indicates the need for treatment reevaluation.

Administration of inhaled anti-inflammatory therapy if the β_2-agonist is needed daily to control symptoms, if there are acute exacerbations more than twice a week, or if there are nighttime awakenings more than twice a month.

Long-acting bronchodilators to control nighttime symptoms may also be considered. Theophylline should be used with caution, keeping the serum concentration between 8 and 12 μg/ml.

If asthma worsens or does not respond to the anti-inflammatory plus the long-acting bronchodilator therapy, the inhaled corticosteroid dose can be increased up to 1–2 mg daily. Inform patients that the effects of this change may take 4–8 weeks, that inhaled corticosteroids are safer than oral corticosteroids, and that oral side effects can be avoided by using a spacer and rinsing the mouth after dosing.

If necessary administer 7–14 day short courses of systemic corticosteroid therapy. Consider bone densitometry studies and calcium supplementation.

Source: Ref. 2.

Chronic moderate to severe asthma therapy is based on whether or not there is a component of irreversible airway obstruction present, and if so, at what level (2,27). Therapy for older patients with good reversibility does not differ significantly from that recommended for all patients at the same severity level (2). The NAEPP Working Group on asthma in the elderly has recommended the therapeutic elements seen in Tables 2 and 3.

As pharmacotherapy is stepped up, the considerations regarding patient self-management become more critical. As the medication regimen becomes more complex, it is more important to make sure the schedule is given to the patient in writing and that the patient and caregiver both understand the written schedule (8,31). It may be helpful to put into writing a plan that specifies the time and particular activity during which medications will be taken and PEFR measured (19).

Written materials regarding exacerbations should be very specific and reflect any differences in the patient's instructions for responding to exacerbations that may become necessary as care is stepped up (2). These materials should be easy to read and understand. In certain circumstances, tape-recorded instructions may be advisable (37).

Patients whose care has been stepped up significantly or who have an irreversible component may be sicker than other patients. Therefore, the management team should include all caregivers, such as family members, nurses or providers of elder care, primary care physicians, and asthma specialists. The team may also need to include a professional to address issues of depression in the patient. Further, it is very important to determine the patient's level of external control of social and environmental factors. In some settings, such as long-term-

Table 3 Recommendations for Stepped Care in Patients with Irreversibility

Modify treatment goals to reflect decreased response to bronchodilator medication and possibly to corticosteroids.
Administer ipratropium bromide at an earlier point in treatment.
Modify therapeutic endpoints to reflect the decreased reliability of spirometry and peak flow measures and the need to consider qualify-of-life issues.

Source: Ref. 2.

care facilities, the patient may have little control over his or her schedule or social and physical environmental factors. In other settings, as when the patient lives with a caretaker/family member, control and autonomy may be present in the patient's social environment but not in the physical environment. Expectations for effective self-management in these situations may have to give way to a concerted effort to work with the key individuals who can affect the patient's abilities to self-administer medicines, control triggers, and monitor symptoms.

Aging comes with many physical and cognitive changes that affect asthma management and outcomes. In today's society, there is a significant difference in the types of social and physical environments in which older adults operate, and these changes have implications for the degree of control and autonomy of the elderly. While independent living remains a goal of asthma therapy, the potential for independence may be reduced, and the patient's quality of life must always be the primary consideration when one is making management decisions (2).

Treatment for older adults may be the same as for any person with asthma, particularly if they are fortunate enough not to have any of the special circumstances described above. However, at any point in time, an older adult may find a number of these circumstances operating in his or her life. The priority for care of older adults with asthma should be an awareness of and responsiveness to changes in their life circumstances that can affect their care. Thus, every patient visit should include an evaluation of these factors, whether or not they were present in previous visits. Only with such proactive steps can providers truly be responsive to the needs of this population.

References

1. National Heart, Lung and Blood Institute. National Asthma Education and Prevention Program. Guidelines for the Diagnosis and Management of Asthma. Bethesda, MD: NIH Pub. 91–3042, 1991.
2. National Heart, Lung and Blood Institute. National Asthma Education and Prevention Program. Working Group Report: Considerations for Diagnosing and Managing Asthma in the Elderly. Bethesda, MD: NIH Pub. 96-3662, 1996.

3. FitzGerald JM. Psychosocial barriers to asthma education. Chest 1994; 106:260S–263S.

4. Peat JK. The epidemiology of asthma. Curr Opin Pulm Med 1996; 2:7–15.

5. Horne A, Blazer DG. The prevention of major depression in the elderly. Clin Geriatr Med 1992; 8:159–172.

6. Kennedy GJ, Kelman HR, Thomas C, et al. Hierarchy of characteristics associated with depressive symptoms in an urban elderly sample. Am J Psychiatry 1989; 146:220–225.

7. Almy TP. Comprehensive functional assessment for elderly patients. Ann Intern Med 1988; July: 70–72.

8. Clark NM, Gotsch A, Rosenstock IR. Patient, professional, and public education on behavioral aspects of asthma: A review of strategies for change and needed research. J Asthma 1993; 30:241–255.

9. Clark NM, Starr-Schneidkraut NJ. Management of asthma by patients and families. Am J Respir Crit Care Med 1994; 149:S54–S66.

10. Bailey WC, Richards JM Jr, Brooks CM, et al. Features of asthma in older adults. J Asthma 1992; 29:21–28.

11. Hayes JP, Fitzgerald MX. Modern management of asthma in adults. Q J Med 1993; 86:693–696.

12. Weiss KB, Gergen PJ, Crain EF. Inner-city asthma: The epidemiology of an emerging U.S. public health concern. Chest 1992; 101:362S–367S.

13. Nejjari C, Tessier JF, Barberger-Gateau P, et al. Functional status of elderly people treated for asthma-related symptoms: A population based case-control study. Eur Respir J 1994; 7:1077–1083.

14. Altose MD, Leitner J, Cherniack NS. Effect of age and respiratory efforts on the perception of resistive ventilatory loads. J Gerontol 1985; 40:147.

15. Peat JK, Woolcock AJ, Cullen K. Rate of decline of lung function in subjects with asthma. Eur J Respir Dis 1987; 70:171–179.

16. Enright PL, Kronmal RA, Higgins M, et al. Spirometry reference values for women and men 65 to 85 years of age. Am Rev Respir Dis 1993; 147:125–133.

17. Burrows B, Barbee RA, Cline MG, et al. Characteristics of asthma among elderly adults in a sample of the general population. Chest 1991; 100:935–942.

18. Bailey WC, Soong S, Brooks CM, et al. Demographics, comorbidity, and medication in an asthma population. Chest 1987; 92(2):12.

19. Rand CS, Wise RA. Measuring adherence to asthma medication regimens. Am J Respir Crit Care Med 1994; 149:S69–S76.

20. Park DC, Morrell RW, Frieske D, Kincaid D. Medication adherence behaviors in older adults: Effects of external cognitive supports. Psychology Aging 1992;7: 252–256.

21. Kirsch I, Jungeblut A, Jenkins L, Kolstad A. Adult Literacy in America: A First Look at the Results of the National Adult Literacy Survey. Washington, DC: National Center for Educational Statistics, US Department of Education, 1993.

22. Leher PM, Isenberg S, Hochron SM. Asthma and emotion: A review. J Asthma 1993; 30:5–21.

23. Alt HL. Psychiatric aspects of asthma. Chest 1992; 101:415S–417S.

24. Bailey WC, Richards JM, Manzella BA, et al. Promoting self-management in adults with asthma: An overview of the UAB program. Health Ed Q 1987; 14:345–355.
25. Enright PL, Lebowitz MD, Cockroft DW. Physiologic measures: Pulmonary function test, asthma outcome. Am J Respir Crit Care Med 1994; 149:S9–S18.
26. Braman SS. Asthma in the elderly patient. Clin Chest Med 1993; 14:413–422.
27. Barbee RA. Balancing the therapeutic needs of elderly asthmatics. J Respir Dis 1995; 16:114–122.
28. Janson C, Bjornsson E, Hetta J, Boman G. Anxiety and depression in relation to respiratory symptoms and asthma. Am J Respir Crit Care Med 1994; 149:930–934.
29. Richards JM, Hemstreet MP. Measures of life quality, role performance and functional status in asthma research. Am J Respir Crit Care Med 1994; 149:S31–S39.
30. Snadden D, Brown JB. The experience of asthma. Soc Sci Med 1992; 34:1351–1361.
31. Opdycke RA, Ascione FJ, Shimp LA, Rosen RI. A systematic approach to educating elderly patients about their medications. Patient Ed Couns 1992; 19:43–60.
32. Daniels KS, Meuleman J. Importance of assessment of metered-dose inhaler technique in the elderly. J Am Geriatr Soc 1994; 42:82–84.
33. Kesten S, Elias M, Cartier A, Chapman KR. Patient handling of a multidose dry powder inhalation device for albuterol. Chest 1994; 105:1077–1081.
34. Traver GA, Cline MG, Burrows B. Asthma in the elderly. J Asthma 1993; 30:81–91.
35. Burrows B, Lebowitz M, Barbee RA, Cline MG. Findings before diagnoses of asthma among elderly in a longitudinal study of a general population sample. J Allergy Clin Immunol 1991; 88:870.
36. Malo JL. Assessment of peak expiratory flow in asthma. Curr Opin Pulm Med 1996; 2:75–80.
37. Kohler CL, Davies SL, Bailey WC. Self-management and other behavioral aspects of asthma. Curr Opin Pulm Med 1996; 2:16–22.

7

Pharmacological Management of Asthma in the Elderly

JOHN W. BLOOM

University of Arizona College of Medicine
Tucson, Arizona

I. Introduction

The objectives of this chapter are to review the commonly used agents for asthma, examine possible adverse effects associated with their use in the elderly patient, and summarize the pharmacological guidelines for management. The goals for treatment have been outlined in a recent National Heart, Lung and Blood Institute (NHLBI) report for the diagnosis and management of asthma in the elderly patient (1). The overall goal is to maintain quality of life. In order to achieve this objective, specific goals for management were suggested (Table 1). These goals may be particularly difficult to reach in the elderly. Concerns regarding the adverse effects of medications and the possibility of aggravating other medical conditions are particularly relevant in therapy of the elderly patient. In the older asthmatic patient, it is also important to consider that complete reversal of airway obstruction and attainment of normal lung function may not be possible even with maximal pharmacological therapy.

Table 1 Goals of Asthma Therapy in the Elderly Patient

Permit the desired level of activity
Optimize pulmonary function
Control chronic symptoms
Prevent exacerbations
Promote prompt recognition and treatment of exacerbations
Eliminate the need for hospitalizations or emergency department visits
Avoid aggravating other medical conditions
Minimize adverse effects from medications

II. Bronchodilators

Drugs for airways obstructive disease can be divided into broad categories of bronchodilators and anti-inflammatory agents. Bronchodilators, which include β-adrenergic agonists, theophylline, and anticholinergic agents, act primarily to relax airways smooth muscle. However, theophylline may have some anti-inflammatory effects in the airways, and β_2-adrenergic agonists have effects on cells other than airways smooth muscle.

A. β-Adrenergic Agonists

Intracellular Mechanisms of Action

β-adrenergic agonists are the most effective bronchodilators in patients with asthma and are the preferred therapy for the relief of acute symptoms. These agents act by activating β_2-adrenergic receptors in airway smooth muscle and producing functional antagonism of bronchoconstriction in airways of all sizes (2,3). β-adrenergic receptor stimulation activates adenylyl cyclase, resulting in an increase in cyclic AMP, activation of protein kinase A, and relaxation of airways smooth muscle through the cyclic AMP/protein kinase A phosphorylation cascade (4). Recent evidence suggests that additional molecular mechanisms may be involved (5). There are now data from some systems demonstrating that an elevation in cyclic AMP can activate protein kinase G as well as protein kinase A (6). Thus, the bronchodilator effects of β-adrenergic agonists may be partially mediated by cyclic AMP activation of protein kinase G rather than protein kinase A. In addition, other data demonstrate that β-adrenergic agonists at low concentrations can open large-conductance calcium-activated potassium (or maxi-K) channels in airways smooth muscle, suggesting that this may be an important mechanism of bronchodilation (7). Furthermore, maxi-K channels may be opened directly by the alpha subunit of the Gs GTP-binding protein (8–10). This finding suggests the possibility that β-adrenergic agonists can produce relaxation of airways smooth muscle by a cyclic AMP–independent mechanism involving direct coupling of the β-adrenergic receptor to the maxi-K channel. Thus, it now appears that multiple cyclic AMP–dependent and cyclic AMP–independent pathways may be involved in β-agonist–induced bronchodilation, although the relative contributions of the various mechanisms are uncertain (5).

Cellular Localization and Function

β_2-adrenergic receptors have been identified on other cell types in addition to airways smooth muscle, including lung epithelium, nerves, vessels, submucosal glands, and inflammatory cells (11). Action of β-adrenergic agonists on these cells may have additional effects that contribute to their effectiveness. For example, β-adrenergic agonists may inhibit release of bronchoconstrictor mediators from mast cells in the airways by activating β_2 receptors on these cells (12,13). In addition, nonbronchodilator effects of β-adrenergic receptor agonists include inhibition of cholinergic neurotransmission (14), increased ciliary beating and mucociliary clearance (15,16), and enhancement of vascular integrity and inhibition of plasma exudation in the airways (17,18). These actions of β-adrenergic receptor agonists may have acute anti-inflammatory effects, but this is controversial. Certainly, there is good evidence that β-agonists have no significant effect on chronic inflammation and bronchial hyperresponsiveness in asthma (19).

Receptor Function and Aging

There is evidence, particularly in the cardiovascular system, that aging is associated with reduced β-adrenergic receptor responsiveness (20). Functional studies in normal humans, performed mainly using peripheral blood mononuclear cells, demonstrate that β-adrenergic receptor number does not change with age, but receptor affinity declines (21,22). In addition, functional studies show decreases in membrane adenylyl cyclase activity and cellular production of cyclic-AMP in response to β-agonist (23,24). There is also evidence for a decrease in the Gs subunit of the GTP-binding protein with age (25). Taken together, these data are consistent with a decrease in β-adrenergic receptor coupling with aging.

Several investigators have addressed the question of whether the reduction in β-adrenergic receptor responsiveness is also found in the lungs of either healthy elderly individuals or older asthmatics. Connolly and coworkers studied the bronchodilator response in healthy nonasthmatic elderly subjects (26). They found that the bronchodilatory effect of inhaled albuterol after methacholine-induced bronchoconstriction was reduced in elderly subjects compared with healthy young controls. Their conclusion was that airway β_2-adrenergic receptor responsiveness diminished with age in healthy subjects. In several studies involving asthmatic subjects, investigators have reported the effect of age on bronchodilator response. Ullah and coworkers found that the response to albuterol declined significantly with age, whereas the response to the anticholinergic bronchodilator ipratropium bromide did not (27). In contrast, Kradjan and coworkers found no effect of age on the bronchodilator response to β-agonist in asthmatic subjects (28), whereas other investigators have reported small trends toward decreased airway β₂-adrenergic responsiveness that did not reach significance (29,30). These conflicting data suggest that the decline in airway β-receptor responsiveness with aging is small and probably of little clinical importance.

β₂-Adrenergic Agonists

The prototype catecholamine bronchodilator was epinephrine, which activated not only β₂-adrenergic receptors in the airways but also β₁-receptors in the heart and alpha receptors in the vasculature. Although inhalers containing epinephrine are still available as nonprescription medication, the elderly patient theoretically would be at an increased risk of adverse effects from inhaled epinephrine. Structural alterations that produced isoproteronol (Fig. 1) resulted in an agent with β-receptor selectivity but a brief duration of action similar to epinephrine because of susceptibility to the enzyme catechol-O-methyltransferase (COMT) (31). Further structural alterations resulted in longer-acting agents, which are resistant to COMT. These agents, which have a duration of action in the range of 3–6 hr, are also relatively more selective for β₂-adrenergic receptors and include drugs such as albuterol, terbutaline, pirbuterol, and bitolterol. The relatively rapid onset of action makes them the choice for therapy of acute episodes of wheezing and dyspnea. β₂-adrenergic agonists are also useful in prevention of bronchoconstriction resulting from exercise and other stimuli (4).

The long acting β₂-agonists salmeterol and formoterol have recently become available for asthma therapy. Both drugs produce prolonged (> 12 hr)

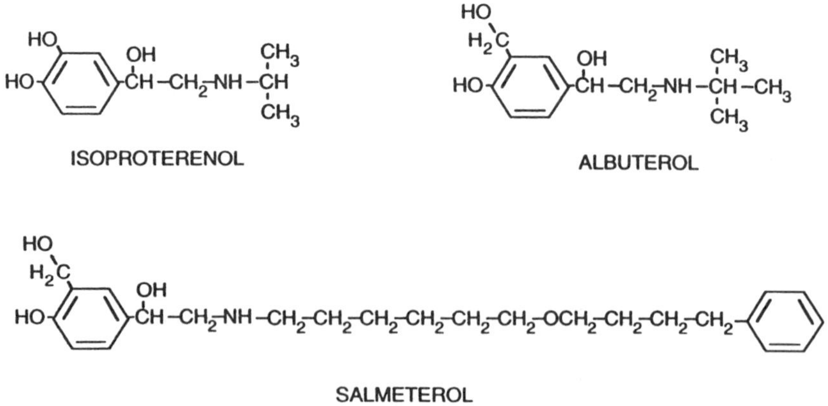

Figure 1 Structures of β-adrenergic agonist bronchodilators.

bronchodilation and protection against bronchoconstrictor challenges, but the onset of action is slower than that of the shorter-acting agents such as albuterol (32,33). Thus, the long-acting agents should not be used for acute bronchospasm. Both salmeterol (Fig. 1) and formoterol have long lipophilic side chains, which stabilize the molecule at the β_2-adrenergic receptor and produce prolonged receptor activation (34).

Tolerance

A theoretical problem of regular use of β_2-adrenergic agonists, particularly the long-acting agents, is the development of tolerance to the bronchodilator effects. Tolerance to the acute bronchodilating effect has been demonstrated in studies with the short-acting agents albuterol and terbutaline (35–37). The effect was apparent after 2–4 weeks of regular use and, at least in one study, affected the duration of bronchodilator response to a much greater degree than the peak of the response (35). In contrast, tolerance has not been demonstrated in other studies with chronic administration of β_2-agonists (38–40). Even in the studies in which tolerance was demonstrated, the effect was small and probably of little clinical significance. There is clearer evidence that tolerance of β_2-agonists does develop to the antibronchoconstrictor effects—that is, the protective effects against induced bronchoconstriction by agents such as allergens, adenosine, cholinergic agonists, exercise, and cold air (41–43).

Because the long-acting β_2-adrenergic agonists salmeterol and formoterol have a sustained contact with the receptor, tolerance could be a significant problem with these agents. In clinical trials of the chronic administration of salmeterol, no significant bronchodilator tolerance has developed (33,44), although some tolerance developed to the antibronchoconstrictor effects (43,45). For formoterol, there is evidence for tolerance to both bronchodilator and antibronchoconstrictor effects (46–48). Despite the demonstration of tolerance for the long-acting β_2-agonists, these agents provided improved symptom control. Thus, as with the short-acting β_2-agonists, the clinical importance of tolerance with the use of long-acting agents is unclear (49).

Glucocorticoids increase β_2-adrenergic receptor density in airway smooth muscle and prevent the development of tolerance in vitro (50–52). Systemic glucocorticoid therapy has been shown to prevent or reverse tolerance (36,53), and inhaled glucocorticoids may also be effective in this regard (54). However, there are some data demonstrating that inhaled glucocorticoids do not prevent tolerance induced by long-acting β_2-agonists (46,47). As noted above, there is evidence for decreased β_2-adrenergic receptor coupling in the elderly. This finding suggests that the development of tolerance may be different in the elderly patient as compared with the younger adult with asthma, but this question has not been investigated.

Clinical Problems

The safety of β-agonists was first questioned in the 1960s, when an increase in asthma mortality was temporally associated with the introduction of a metered-dose inhaler (MDI) delivering a high dose of isoproteronol (55). In the 1970s, epidemiological data provided evidence for an association between the use of the β_2-agonist fenoterol and an epidemic of asthma deaths in New Zealand (56,57). Whether the use of fenoterol was directly related to the increase in mortality is controversial. There are data to support the possibility that undertreatment of asthma was responsible for the excess deaths. Nonetheless, in a subsequent study of asthma morbidity and mortality in Canada, there was a strong association between deaths or near deaths from asthma and the increasing use of inhaled β-agonists (58). The data do not demonstrate a definite causal link between asthma mortality and β-agonist use because patients with more severe and poorly controlled asthma, who are at higher risk of dying from their disease, are more likely to use higher doses of β-agonists (59). Although this controversy has not been resolved, it is clear that patients using large doses of β-agonists should receive anti-inflammatory therapy in an attempt to reduce β-agonist dosage (1,60).

A related but equally controversial issue is whether β-agonists should be administered on a regularly scheduled basis (61–64). There is evidence that scheduled use four times a day of inhaled β-agonists compared to "on demand" or "as needed" use for symptom control may increase asthma morbidity. Some studies have shown poorer asthma control, increased airway hyperresponsiveness, and a decline in lung function associated with regular use of β-agonists (65–68). In other studies (33,69–72), the deleterious effect of regular β-agonist use has not been seen. Nonetheless, the current recommendation is to use short-acting β-agonists "as needed" for relief of symptoms (1,60).

Route of Administration

The mode of administration of β-adrenergic agents is extremely important, particularly in the elderly patient. Because β_2-adrenergic receptors are found not only in the lung but also distributed throughout the body, adverse side effects result primarily from the β_2-agonist that is present in the systemic circulation (11). Administration of β-agonists by inhalation decreases the plasma concentration and reduces side effects (73). Thus, although β-agonists can be administered orally, parenterally, or by inhalation, the inhaled route is preferred. When the oral route of administration was compared to the inhaled, the inhaled route produced more rapid and more effective bronchodilation with fewer systemic side effects such as tremor, nervousness, and palpitations (74). Oral sustained-release preparations have been used to treat nocturnal symptoms, but these oral agents are not as effective as the newer long-acting inhaled agents, which are associated with fewer side effects (75). Although parenteral administration produces rapid onset of action, it is associated with marked tachycardia and tremor (76). A theoretical problem with the inhaled route of administration is that the bronchodilating agent may not reach the peripheral airways, especially if acute bronchospasm is present. In fact, in studies of patients with acute asthma, there is no difference in effectiveness between inhaled and intravenous terbutaline (77).

Inhaled β-agonists are most commonly given by using an MDI. A major problem with the use of MDIs is improper inhalation technique, a problem that is a particularly important in the elderly (78). A study of MDI and use of in 30 elderly patients found that only 60% used appropriate technique and only 10% ideal technique (79). Frequent errors were failure to breath-hold after inhalation, not continuing to inhale after actuation of the canister, lack of any coordination whatsoever between inhalation and actuation, and inhalation through the nose. In 595 patients who attended a chest clinic, elderly patients were less likely to use correct MDI technique (29% of elderly versus 45% of young adults) and more likely to be unteachable (80). In a test of the ability of elderly patients to trigger a variety of MDIs, over one-third were unable to generate sufficient force to trigger any of the inhalers tested and less than one-third could trigger all of the inhalers (80).

The elderly patient must be instructed carefully in the use of the MDI (81). Observation of the MDI technique is essential to ensure correct procedure. The MDI should be shaken prior to each activation. The patient should breathe out slowly to a volume just below normal resting volume but should not exhale forcibly. The mouthpiece should be placed in the mouth with the opening between the teeth and directed over the tongue with the head tilted back slightly. The patient should begin to inhale slowly through the mouth and then activate the inhaler. Inhalation should continue to total lung capacity and breath should be held for at least 10 sec. Improper MDI technique is a major reason for the failure of therapy in older patients, and ongoing education in the proper MDI technique is necessary (82). Spacer devices are helpful for elderly patients who have difficulty coordinating triggering and inhalation with MDIs (83). Use of spacers improved MDI technique, and they were preferred by 70% of the patients. Also, the use of a spacer when inhaling β-adrenergic agonist from an MDI produced a greater bronchodilating effect in a group of elderly patients with obstructive lung disease (84).

For patients with poor coordination of canister actuation and inspiration, breath-actuated inhalers have been developed. In a study of inhaler technique and patient preference in elderly subjects, breath-actuated inhalers were used correctly and preferred by patients more often than conventional MDIs (85). Also, dry-powder inhalers may be easier for patients who have difficulty synchronizing activation and inhalation to use. Medication delivery with dry-powder inhalers is activated by patient inhalation, and synchronization of activation and inhalation is unnecessary. Although the elderly had more difficulty than younger patients with correct use in a patient trial with a multidose dry-powder inhaler, only 3% of older patients had difficulty after being taught at the initial visit and 90% retained correct technique at 2-week follow-up (86).

Adverse Effects

Tremor and palpitations are the most common side effects of β_2-adrenergic agonists (4). Tremor results from stimulation of β_2-adrenergic receptors in skeletal muscle, and palpitations occur primarily from stimulation of β_2-adrenergic receptors in the peripheral vasculature, resulting in vasodilation with reflex increase in the force and rate of cardiac contraction (87–89). Although cardiac side effects are decreased with the use of the newer, more selective β_2-agonists, some of the β-adrenergic receptors in the heart are the β_2-subtype and have been shown to mediate an increase in heart rate when activated (90). As described above, there may be β-adrenergic receptor hyporesponsiveness in the heart and skeletal muscle in the elderly (20). However, when electrocardiographic, hemodynamic, and hypokalemic responses to inhaled albuterol were compared in young and elderly subjects, no differences were found except that the elderly demonstrated greater hemodynamic changes (91). Cardiac arrhythmias secondary to β_2-adrenergic agonist therapy are thought to be rare, especially when the drug is given by the inhaled route; but this question has not been extensively studied in the elderly. There are isolated reports of arrhythmias in elderly patients following inhaled β_2-agonist administration (92). In addition, an increased incidence of arrhythmias has been reported in patients who were treated with a combination of theophylline and β-agonists (93–95).

β_2-agonists, through stimulation of extrapulmonary β_2-adrenergic receptors, also produce a number of metabolic effects, including hypokalemia, hypomagnesemia, hyperglycemia, lipolysis, and lactic acidosis (96). Hypokalemia is a potentially serious effect of β_2-agonist therapy because it is associated with arrhythmias, particularly in the elderly patient with an increased risk of heart disease (97,98). Catecholamines stimulate potassium uptake by skeletal muscle, the largest pool of body potassium, via muscle Na^+,K^+-ATPase coupled to β_2-adrenergic receptors (99,100). The hypokalemic effects of inhaled albuterol have been shown to be associated with S-T depression, Q-T prolongation, and T-wave flattening (101). In addition, these electrocardiographic changes associated with inhaled albuterol are augmented by diuretic therapy (102)—therapy common in the elderly patient. In addition, the β_2-agonist–induced hypokalemia can be influenced by other drugs commonly used in the elderly asthmatic patient, such as corticosteroids, theophylline, and digoxin. The well-described mineralocorticoid effect of corticosteroids may aggravate β_2-agonist–induced hypokalemia (103). Theophylline accentuates β_2-agonist–induced hypokalemia (104), and potassium competes with digoxin for the same binding site on Na^+,K^+-ATPase (96), so that

β_2-agonist–induced hypokalemia could produce digitalis toxicity. Significant increases in plasma glucose can occur with inhaled β_2-agonist, especially after higher doses, and may be of importance clinically in the elderly asthmatic patient with concomitant diabetes mellitus (105). This effect could be especially severe if superimposed on preexisting hypokalemia secondary to diuretic or corticosteroid therapy or associated with hypoxemia during an acute exacerbation of airways obstruction.

Tolerance to tremor and the cardiovascular and metabolic side effects usually develops within weeks with regular use (105,106), and these changes have not been considered to be clinically important in asthmatics in general (4). Although tolerance does develop to these systemic effects of inhaled β_2-agonist, the effects diminish but do not disappear (105,106). Lipworth and coworkers found significant development of tolerance to chronotropic and hypokalemic effects of inhaled albuterol when given in extremely high doses (4000 μg daily), but not at the usual maximal daily dose (800 μg) (105). Although there was no objective evidence of tolerance to tremor, there was subjective tolerance to both tremor and palpitations. The possibility that tolerance to the systemic side effects may not be consistent clinically is emphasized by a study of patients with exacerbations of asthma seen in an emergency department setting (107). In these patients, nebulized albuterol according to emergency department protocol produced a significant decrease in potassium (0.8 mEq/L) within 75 min of initiation of treatment. Thus, although patients may develop a degree of tolerance to the systemic adverse effects of inhaled β_2-agonists with regular use, these effects may be of clinical importance in the elderly, particularly in the patient with underlying ischemic heart disease, preexisting hypokalemia secondary to diuretic or corticosteroid therapy, or hypoxemia during an acute exacerbation of airways obstruction. In patients with acute bronchospasm, inhaled β_2-agonists may cause a decrease in arterial oxygen tension by aggravating ventilation/perfusion abnormalities in the lung (108). This could be a serious problem in the older asthmatic patient with an age-related lower baseline pO_2. The risk of adverse effects with β_2-agonist use in the elderly patient merits further study.

B. Theophylline

The use of theophylline, particularly in the United States, has varied tremendously over the past 25 years. Beginning in the 1970s, theophylline use increased dramatically, and by the 1980s, most patients with airways obstruction were treated with oral theophylline (109). The introduction of slow-release theophylline preparations led to the use of theophylline as first-line monotherapy for asthma by many physicians. However, concern about toxicity, the introduction of newer agents, and recommendations in national and international guidelines have contributed to a decrease in theophylline use over the past decade (110,111). At present, guidelines recommend that theophylline be added to the regimen after inhaled steroids have failed to control symptoms (60). With the recent recognition that theophylline has anti-inflammatory properties (112), the pendulum of theophylline use may swing again.

Mechanism of Action

Although theophylline has been in use for over fifty years, the mechanism of action remains unclear (113). The generally accepted pharmacological effects in asthma are airways smooth muscle relaxation, improved diaphragmatic contraction, and increased mucociliary clearance (114). There is now evidence that theophylline has anti-inflammatory, immunodulatory, and bronchoprotective effects. In vitro, theophylline blocks histamine release from mast cells (115), inhibits the alveolar macrophage respiratory burst (116), and inhibits some eosinophil functions (117,118). In humans, theophylline therapy appears to regulate cell trafficking into the airways (119), and there is also evidence that it inhibits the late-phase asthmatic response (120,121). Immunomodulation in asthma by theophylline has been demonstrated by withdrawal of therapy, even in patients receiving inhaled corticosteroids (122). Withdrawal of theophylline produced clinical deterioration with increased symptoms and decreased pulmonary function, which was associated with an increase in activated T cells in the airways mucosa and a fall in these cells in the blood. These data suggest a role for theophylline in regulation of trafficking of activated lymphocyte in the airways of asthmatic patients.

At the molecular level, it is not clear how theophylline produces bronchodilation and its other antiasthma effects. Theophylline can relax airways smooth muscle by inhibiting phosphodiesterase and increasing the cellular concentration of cyclic nucleotides (114). But, at serum theophylline concentrations of 5–20 μg/ml, there is little inhibition of phosphodiesterase (112). It has also been proposed that the action of theophylline is the result of antagonism of adenosine receptors, but this does not appear to be the mechanism of bronchodilation. Although antagonism of adenosine receptors occurs at theophylline levels in the therapeutic range, a related drug that is a potent bronchodilator, enprofylline, is not an adenosine-receptor antagonist. Also, 8-phenyltheophylline, which does not inhibit phosphodiesterase but does antagonize adenosine receptors, has no bronchodilator activity (123). Nevertheless, antagonism of adenosine receptors may be responsible for some of the other effects of theophylline, such as the increase in ventilatory drive, diuresis, and increased psychomotor activity (114).

Pharmacokinetics

Theophylline is well absorbed from the gastrointestinal tract, and bioavailability is not altered in the elderly patient (124,125). The volume of distribution for

Table 2 Conditions and Drugs Modifying Theophylline Elimination

Decreased elimination	Increased elimination
Congestive heart failure	Cigarette smoking
Liver disease	Charcoal-broiled meats
Cor pulmonale	Hyperthyroidism
Hypothyroidism	Low-carbohydrate,
Sustained fever	high-protein diet
Flu vaccine	Carbamazepine
High-carbohydrate,	Phenobarbital
low-protein diet	Phenytoin
Allopurinol (high dose)	Rifampin
Cimetidine	
Ciprofloxacin	
Clarithromycin	
Enoxacin	
Erythromycin	
Methotrexate	
Propranolol	
Tacrine	
Thiabendazole	
Ticlopidine	
Troleandomycin	
Verapamil	

Source: Refs. 110 and 128.

theophylline is relatively constant between individuals at 0.5 L/kg so that 1 mg/kg theophylline will raise the serum level 2 μg/ml (126). Thus, 5 mg/kg of theophylline will result in a serum concentration of approximately 10 μg/ml. Although the volume of distribution is relatively constant among individuals resulting in a standardized loading dose, the clearance of theophylline varies markedly between individuals and may also vary in the same individual over time (114). Only about 10% of theophylline is excreted unchanged through the kidneys. The major route of clearance is metabolism by the cytochrome microsomal enzyme system in the liver (127). Thus, any of several drugs or related conditions that affect hepatic metabolism may alter theophylline clearance (Table 2) (110,128). Factors that decrease theophylline clearance are especially important, because they may result in toxic serum concentrations. The physician must be particularly careful not to give an antibiotic that reduces theophylline clearance (e.g., erythromycin or ciprofloxacin) during an exacerbation of symptoms without checking serum theophylline levels and adjusting the dose appropriately.

Whether theophylline clearance is reduced in the elderly is unclear. Equal numbers of studies demonstrate either decreased clearance in the elderly or no effect of age (129–133). Interpretation of these studies is difficult because of confounding factors such as associated illnesses, cigarette smoking, and the presence of other medications (134,135). Certainly, associated illnesses and medication interactions may explain the widespread clinical impression that theophylline clearance is decreased by approximately one-third in the elderly population. Although obesity does not affect theophylline metabolism directly, it must be taken into account when maintenance dose calculations are made. Dose calculations should be made on the basis of ideal body weight (136,137).

Toxicity

The major drawback to theophylline therapy is the high incidence of toxic effects. There is evidence, outlined below, that the risk of theophylline toxicity is heightened in the elderly. Common side effects are nausea, tremor, headache, agitation, and insomnia. These side effects are especially common when therapy is started and may be reduced by gradually increasing the dose when initiating therapy. Although the results are controversial (138), such studies have demonstrated that asthmatic children treated with theophylline may have learning and behavior problems (139,140). These studies raise the possibility that theophylline may have similar adverse effects in the elderly, especially in those who are neurologically compromised (141).

Of particular concern are severe toxic effects, including seizures and cardiac arrhythmias that may be life-threatening (142). Although seizures are usually associated with higher serum concentrations, theophylline-associated arrhythmias may occur at serum concentrations of 15–25 μg/ml (143). In 15 older patients (mean age, 66 years) with chronic airways obstruction, oral theophylline administration was associated with a significant increase in ventricular ectopic beats from 43 to 72 per hr (144). In another study of arrthythmias in 16 elderly patients, multifocal atrial tachycardia (MAT) was found to be a toxic effect of theophylline at serum levels of less than 20 μg/ml (145). When theophylline was discontinued, the atrial rate decreased and MAT resolved. In five patients who were rechallenged with intravenous aminophylline, MAT recurred at serum levels between 16 and 25 μg/ml. Similarly, in a recent study of 100 hospitalized patients with airways obstruction, the authors concluded that theophylline causes tachycardia and serious arrhythmias even at relatively low serum theophylline concentrations (146). Elderly patients in this study were more likely to develop theophylline-associated arrhythmias. In another study of patients referred with chronic theophylline intoxication, life-threatening events, seizures, and ventricular arrhythmias occurred in 39% of patients (147). Interestingly, the risk of a life-threatening event

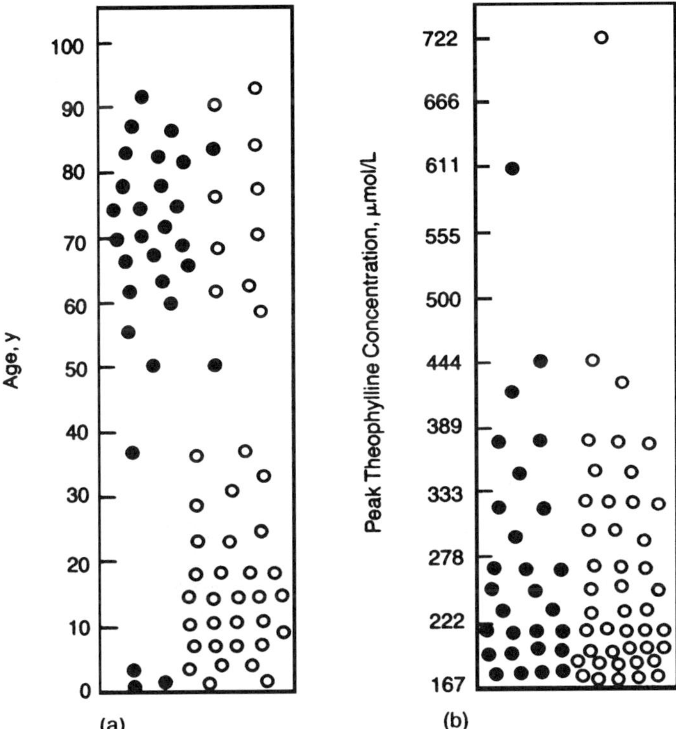

Figure 2 Distribution of life-threatening events by (a) age and (b) peak serum theophylline concentration. Solid circles indicate patients with life-threatening events; open circles, those without life-threatening events. (From Ref. 147.)

correlated with the age of the patient but not with the peak serum theophylline concentration (Fig. 2). Elderly patients were found to have an inordinately greater risk; patients more than 75 years old had a 16.7-fold greater risk of a life-threatening event than patients less than 25 years old. In addition to an increased risk of serious toxic effects, the elderly appear to be more prone to overmedication with theophylline. In a review of cases of theophylline toxicity due to overmedication through patient or physician error (142), over half of those toxic due to chronic overmedication were in the over-60 age group (Fig. 3). Other studies have demonstrated that the over-60 age groups accounts for only about 20% of the patients taking theophylline. Thus, this finding is not a function of increased use of theophylline in the older patient (148). Hospitalization for theophylline toxic-

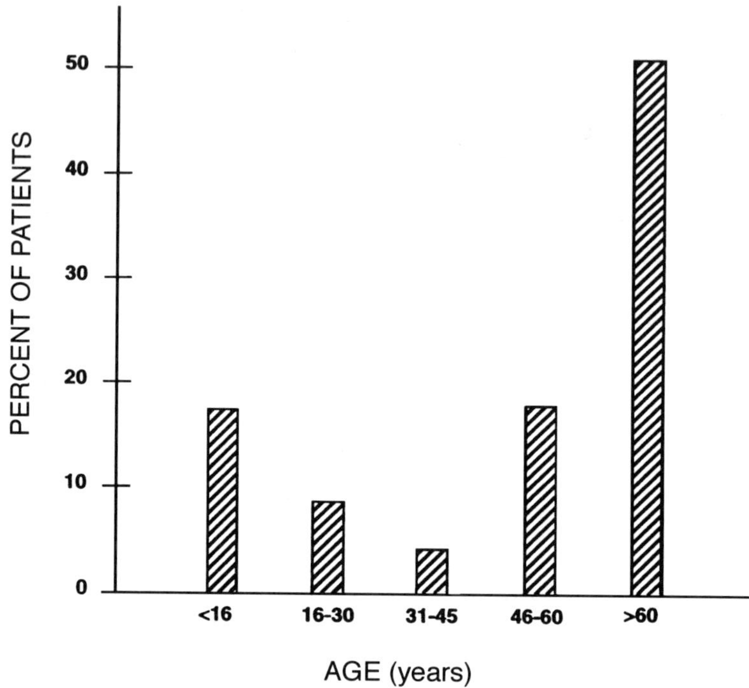

Figure 3 Percentage of patients with acute overdose and patients with chronic over-medication in specific age groups. (From Ref. 142.)

ity in patients over 70 years of age was 10-fold more frequent than in the 20–49 age group (148).

In the National Asthma Education Program (NAEP) guidelines for therapy, the recommended therapeutic range for serum theophylline levels was 8–15 μg/ml (60). The recent NHLBI recommendations for management of asthma in the elderly suggest an even lower range of 8–12 μg/ml (1). These recommended therapeutic ranges are lower than the traditional range of 10–20 μg/ml (113). The traditional range of 10–20 μg/ml was first challenged by Rogers and coworkers (109). The traditional approach was based on the belief that the dose response curve for theophylline is linear over the range of serum concentrations of 5–20 μg/ml. This belief is derived from data obtained from a study of six young asthmatics (149). In this study, the data from the six asthmatic patients were plotted on a log scale. If these data are plotted on a linear scale as shown in Fig. 4, it is clear that the improvement in FEV_1 reaches a plateau in the range of 10 μg/ml with relatively little improvement between 10 and 20 μg/ml. This finding was

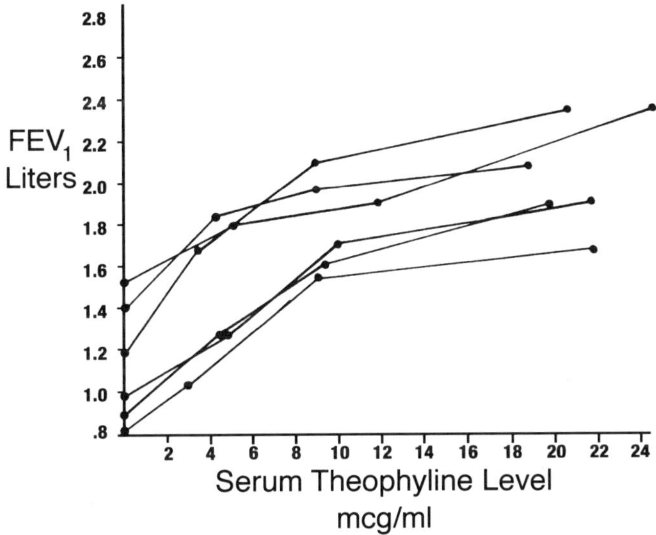

Figure 4 Improvement in FEV$_1$ with increasing theophylline level. (From Ref. 109.)

confirmed by Klein and coworkers in a study of nine stable adult asthmatic patients (150). In these patients, the FEV$_1$ increased significantly as the mean theophyline level increased from 6.4 to 12.8 μg/ml, but there was no further significant improvement at a mean value of 19.2 μg/ml. Furthermore, it appears that the immunomodulatory effects of theophylline occur at serum theophylline concentrations of >5 μg/ml (122). Thus, because of the increased risk of toxicity at theophylline levels of 15–20 μg/ml and the recognition of efficacy at lower levels, the use of theophylline at reduced serum levels is rational, particularly in the elderly patient. The NAEP guidelines recommend monitoring serum theophylline levels at a minimum of every 6–12 months (60). In the elderly patient, more frequent monitoring may be indicated, especially in the presence of one of the conditions or drugs noted in Table 2.

Indications

For acute exacerbations of asthma, intravenous aminophylline is commonly given. Siegel and coworkers evaluated the efficacy of intravenous aminophylline in patients seen in the emergency department with acute asthma (94). All patients were treated with the β-adrenergic agonist metaproterenol by inhalation from a small-volume nebulizer (15 mg hourly for 3 hr) and were randomly assigned to receive intravenous aminophylline or placebo. Pulmonary function improved to a similar degree in the placebo and aminophylline groups. There was no additional benefit of aminophylline even in asthmatics with more severe obstruction. Furthermore, there were significantly more side effects in the aminophylline-treated patients than those receiving only β-adrenergic agonists. A recent meta-analysis evaluated the efficacy of intravenous aminophylline therapy for acute exacerbations of asthma (151). Analysis of 13 clinical trials, judged to be of acceptable design, demonstrated no benefit of adding aminophylline to sympathomimetic bronchodilators. Again, toxic effects were more common in aminophylline-treated patients. Therefore, the routine use of intravenous aminophylline in acute exacerbations of asthma generally is associated with an increased risk of toxicity but no therapeutic benefit. In the elderly asthmatic patient, the risk of toxicity, particularly arrhythmias, may be especially important due to underlying cardiovascular disease, hypoxemia, or hypokalemia secondary to therapy for coexisting medical problems.

Despite its decline in use of recent years, theophylline continues to be recommended for the treatment of chronic asthma (110). Theophylline has been shown to be more effective in controlling symptoms than inhaled albuterol given four times a day (152) but less effective than the long-acting β_2-agonist salmeterol (153). When compared with inhaled glucocorticoids in the control of asthma, the addition of theophylline to regimens of systemic or inhaled steroids provides significant clinical benefit, including decreased symptoms, improved pulmonary function, and increased excersie tolerance (122,154–156). In the elderly patient, theophylline may be a less effective bronchodilator than in younger asthmatics. The bronchodilator effect of increasing serum theophylline concentrations was less in the elderly as compared with younger subjects (157), but this result may be the consequence of less reversibility of airways obstruction in the older subjects (158).

C. Anticholinergics

Anticholinergic agents have been used to treat respiratory disorders for centuries (159). These drugs were derived from the *Atropa belladonna* and *Datura stramonium* plants and consisted primarily of the alkaloid atropine. The therapeutic usefulness of atropine was limited by side effects. Because atropine was well absorbed, even when administered by inhalation, it produced systemic effects such as trachycardia, blurred vision, dry mouth, and urinary retention due to blockade of muscarinic receptors outside the lung (160). Development of quaternary ammonium analogs of atropine, such as ipratropium bromide, has resolved the problem of side effects associated with inhaled anticholinergic therapy (161). Because of the positive charge on the quaternary ammonium group, ipratropium is poorly absorbed into the systemic circulation and therefore produces no significant side effects.

Cholinergic control of airways smooth muscle tone is mediated by nerves that travel in the vagus. Cholinergic nerves release acetylcholine, which acts on muscarinic receptors in the airways to produce cholinergic effects. At least three subtypes of muscarinic receptors have been identified in airways (162). The M3 muscarinic receptor subtype located on airway smooth muscle mediates bronchoconstriction (163). This pathway can be activated through reflex mechanisms by stimulation of irritant receptors in the airway lumen. Anticholinergic agents produce bronchodilation by directing antagonizing the effects of acetylcholine on the M3 muscarinic receptor in airway smooth muscle. Because anticholinergics block only bronchoconstriction mediated through cholinergics nerves, they are not very protective against some bronchoconstrictor stimuli. There is evidence that anticholinergic therapy may be effective in a subset of patients with nocturnal asthma (164), but the effectiveness is limited by the duration of action of the presently available agents (165). They provide only partial protection against allergen challenge, do not block mediator release from mast cells, and are not useful in preventing exercise-induced bronchoconstriction. Anticholinergics do not block the direct effects of various allergic mediators, such as histamine, on airway smooth muscle. In contrast, β-adrenergic agonists directly stimulate β_2-adrenergic receptors in airways smooth muscle to produce bronchodilation regardless of the bronchospastic stimulus (166). Thus, although anticholinergic agents have been shown to be effective in patients with COPD, β-agonists are more effective in patients with asthma. In addition, the onset of bronchodilation with the presently available quaternary anticholinergic agent ipratropium bromide is relatively slow (requiring 15–30 min, with peak effect at 1–2 hr) but long-lasting (6–8 hr) (161). Therefore, β-agonists are the bronchodilators of choice in patients with asthma, and anticholinergic therapy has received little consideration in recent guidelines (60,167). Nonetheless, anticholinergic therapy may be beneficial in elderly asthmatic patients (1). In a comparison of the bronchodilator response of ipratropium to albuterol, nonallergic and older patients (over 60 years) were more likely to have a beneficial response to ipratropium (30). Also, the response to albuterol has been shown to decline with age, whereas the response to ipratropium does not (27). In contrast, Kradjan and coworkers found no effect of age on bronchodilator response in the study comparing young and elderly asthmatic subjects (28). In comparison to chronic asthma therapy, anticholinergics may have a more important role in acute asthma regardless of age. Several studies of bronchodilator therapy in acute exacerbations of asthma demonstrate improved bronchodilation when anticholinergics are used in combination with β-agonists (168–171).

Thus, anticholinergics may be particularly beneficial in the elderly patient, particularly in the patient with a marked bronchitic component or mixed asthma and COPD. Also, the relative lack of side effects associated with inhaled ipratropium therapy makes it a good choice as a bronchodilator in the elderly patient. In addition, no drug interactions have been reported with inhaled ipratropium (161). In acute exacerbations, the use of ipratropium in combination with β-agonists for treatment of bronchospasm may limit the total amount of β-agonist required and decrease adverse effects in the elderly patient. Interestingly, cholinergic mechanisms appear to be involved in β-blocker–induced bronchoconstriction in asthmatics, because anticholinergic agents effectively inhibit bronchospasm due to propranolol (172). Management of elderly asthmatic patients who develop bronchospasm due to the inadvertent use of beta blockers, such as timolol eyedrops for glaucoma, should include anticholinergic therapy.

III. Anti-Inflammatory Agents

Anti-inflammatory drugs—such as glucocorticoids, cromolyn sodium, and nedocromil sodium—do not have an immediate bronchodilator effects and are not useful for rapid relief of symptoms. Anti-inflammatory agents must be given on a long-term basis as prophylactic therapy with the goal of suppressing the chronic inflammation thought to be involved in the pathogenesis of asthma.

A. Glucocorticoids

Glucocorticoids are the most effective agents for the treatment of chronic asthma (173). With the recognition that airways inflammation is present even in mild disease (174) and the development of safer inhaled preparations, glucocorticoids have become first-line therapy for persistent asthma. They are extremely effective for suppressing the inflammation that appears to play a key role in producing the bronchial hyperresponsiveness of asthma (175).

Mechanism of Action

At a molecular level, glucocorticoid effects are mediated in responsive cells by binding and activating specific cytosolic glucocorticoid receptors, which are ligand-dependent transcription factors. After binding by glucocorticoid, the glucocorticoid receptor enters the nucleus of the cell and binds regulatory elements in glucocorticoid-responsive genes or interacts with other transcription factors to increase or decrease gene transcription (176).

Although glucocorticoids decrease the inflammatory response in asthma, the exact mechanism of action is unknown. Glucocorticoids not only have direct inhibitory effects on the inflammatory cells involved in airway inflammation—such as lymphocytes, eosinophils, and bronchial epithelial cells (177)–but also decrease the inflammatory cell infiltrate in the airways (178,179). Also, they reduce sputum and blood eosinophilia and block the release of mediators from eosinophils and macrophages, but not from mast cells (180). Glucocorticoids may have a direct effect on vascular endothelial cells to reduce the effects of inflammatory mediators, which produce microvascular leakage in the airways (181). They do not block the immediate response to allergen challenge but inhibit the influx of inflammatory cells into the lung after exposure to allergen (180). In studies of asthmatic patients, glucocorticoid therapy consistently decreases bronchial hyperresponsiveness (175). Glucocorticoids appear to reverse the desensitization of β_2-adrenergic receptors in airways smooth muscle and may prevent the development of tachyphylaxis to β_2-adrenergic agents (54).

Pharmacokinetics in the Elderly

There is evidence in the elderly for a decreased clearance of exogenous steroid (182,183). After oral prednisone, elderly subjects were able to convert prednisone to prednisolone as well as younger subjects, reflecting normal 11β-hydroxy-dehydrogenase activity. However, the metabolic clearance of prednisolone was decreased, indicating that 6β-hydroxylase activity is impaired in the elderly (183). A similar increased half-life in the elderly has also been demonstrated for methylprednisolone given intravenously (182). Interestingly, despite higher plasma prednisolone concentrations after an oral dose of prednisone, the endogenous cortisol concentrations were less suppressed in the elderly than in younger subjects (183). Thus, the effect of the prolonged prednisolone kinetics in the elderly may be offset by reduced adrenal gland responsiveness to steroid. This apparent diminished end-organ responsiveness may be the result of a decline in glucocorticoid receptor number with aging (184,185). It is unclear whether the decreased responsiveness of target organs to glucocorticoids with aging is of any clinical importance (186).

Adverse Effects of Systemic Therapy

Systemic glucocorticoid therapy, either oral or parenteral, is recommended for treatment of acute, severe exacerbations of asthma and as chronic therapy in some severe asthmatic patients (60). The multiple adverse effects associated with chronic oral corticosteroid therapy have been well documented (Table 3) (187–189). There is evidence that the risk and magnitude of several of the glucocorticoid-related side effects are greater in the elderly patient. In a study of elderly patients (mean age, 77 years) with airways obstruction receiving oral corticosteroid therapy (prednisolone 2.5–12.5 mg/day), the incidence of serious side effects was increased 40% over those in a matched control group and appeared to be dose-related (190).

Osteoporosis increases in incidence and severity with age and is a major problem in the elderly population. Two phases of bone loss have been identified (191): a slow, age-dependent phase and an accelerated postmenopausal phase. Because of the rapid bone loss after menopause, elderly women are at greater risk

Table 3 Potential Adverse Effects of Chronic
Systemic Glucocorticoid Therapy in the Elderly Patient

Endocrine	Cutaneous
HPA axis dysfunction	Atrophy/Fragility
Diabetes mellitus	Purpura
Musculoskeletal	Hirsutism
Osteoporosis	Acne
Myopathy	Delayed wound healing
Osteonecrosis	Gastrointestinal
Ophthalmological	Pancreatitis
Cataracts	Diverticular rupture
Glaucoma	General
Cardiovascular	Cushingoid appearance
Hypertension	Obesity
Lipoprotein abnormalities	Infection
Atherosclerosis	Hypokalemia
Psychiatric	
Psychosis	
Depression	
Mania	

for fractures than male counterparts who have undergone only the slower age-related loss. One-third of white women over age 65 will have vertebral fractures (192). Oral glucocorticoid therapy accelerates the rate of bone loss (193,194). Although it has been shown that men are as susceptible as women to the effects of glucocorticoids on bone, elderly women are at greater risk for fractures because they have menopause-related bone loss in addition to age-related loss. Also, postmenopausal women are especially at risk, since any dose of glucocorticoid that suppresses the morning plasma cortisol also suppresses adrenocortical production of androgens (195). Postmenopausal women derive their estrogen entirely from conversion of adrenocortical androgen precursors (196). Glucocorticoids increase bone resorption and reduce bone formation, resulting in the loss of bone mass (194). In addition, decreased intestinal absorption of calcium and increased calcium loss in the urine are associated with glucocorticoid therapy (193). Trabecular or spongy bone is metabolically more active than cortical bone and more susceptible to the adverse effects of glucocorticoid therapy (192). Although trabecular bone makes up only about 20% of the skeleton, it is a major component of much of the weight-bearing axial skeleton. Thus, spine and rib fractures are common in glucocorticoid-induced osteoporosis. A large amount of steroid-induced bone loss may occur relatively soon, within 6 months after beginning glucocorticoid therapy, but the magnitude of the effects are dose- and duration-dependent (197,198). Cumulative doses of greater than 10 g of prednisone are a risk factor for osteoporosis (197), and 30–50% of patients treated long-term with doses of prednisone in excess of 7.5–10 mg/day develop fractures (199). No protective effect was seen with alternate-day versus daily therapy (200).

Estrogen replacement therapy is recommended for the postmenopausal woman receiving glucocorticoid therapy (194,201). In addition, therapy with the disphosphonate alendronate decreases the incidence of fractures in postmeno-pausal osteoporosis and increases vertebral bone mass (202). Prophylactic therapy with calcitriol and calcium, with or without calcitonin, prevented glucocorticoid-induced bone loss in the lumbar spine (203). Also, the combination of the diphosphonate calcium and vitamin D has been useful for the management of steroid-induced bone loss in adult asthmatics, mean age 55 years (204). Nonetheless, although several regimens have shown some benefits for the prevention and therapy of osteoporosis, the optimal regimen has not been found (205).

In addition to glucocorticoid-induced osteoporosis, the elderly patient may be at increased risk for several other complications of systemic glucocorticoid therapy. Hypertension is a well-documented side effect of glucocorticoid administration (206) and is more common in the elderly age group (207). In elderly patients, hypertension was noted after only 1 week of therapy with 20 mg of prednisolone daily (207).

The posterior subcapsular cataracts associated with glucocorticoid therapy differ from the senile cataracts of the elderly. Although there is no evidence indicating that the elderly patient is at increased risk of developing glucocorticoid-induced cataracts, the development of posterior subcapsular cataracts could have a more important effect on vision in the patient with preexisting retinal disease or cataracts (1). The prevalence of posterior subcapsular cataracts in 10 survey studies ranged as high as 60% (208,209) and, not surprisingly, was influenced by daily and cumulative doses of glucocorticoid (210). The elderly asthmatic patient on oral glucocorticoid therapy may be at a particular risk of developing glaucoma. Intraocular pressure increases with age, and the prevalence is higher in the elderly population (211). Because glucocorticoid therapy increases intraocular pressure (212), it is not surprising that glucocorticoid therapy increases the risk for glaucoma. Routine measurements of intraocular pressure are especially important in the patient on glucocorticoid therapy, particularly the older patient.

There is extensive clinical evidence that the mineralocorticoid effects associated with steroid therapy may produce hypokalemia (206). Although there is no evidence to demonstrate that this effect is accentuated in the elderly, the greater use of associated diuretic and digoxin therapy in the elderly patient increases the risk of this adverse effect (1).

Systemic glucocorticoid therapy produces hyperglycemia and aggravates diabetes mellitus (206). Glucose tolerance decreases with age, and there is an increased risk of diabetes mellitus in the elderly population (213,214). As a result, the elderly asthmatic on systemic glucocorticoid therapy is at an increased risk for the development of the hyperglycemic complications (215,216). Even low doses of glucocorticoid can produce glucose intolerance, and older patients with a history of glucose intolerance or elevated fasting blood glucose should be monitored closely.

Serious infectious complications have also been reported in elderly patients treated with oral glucocorticoid therapy for airways obstructive diseases (217). These included invasive pulmonary aspergillosis, septicemia, cryptococcal meningitis, and cytomegalovirus pneumonia. In a recent meta-analysis, the risk of steroid-associated infectious complications in patients of all ages increased with doses of prednisone greater than 10 mg/day or a cumulative dose of greater than 700 mg (218). Although the elderly are more likely to have had previous tuberculosis infection, reactivation of tuberculosis associated with glucocorticoid therapy has not been documented in the elderly population. Isoniazid chemoprophylaxis is controversial in patients with positive tuberculin skin tests receiving chronic oral glucocorticoid therapy, but most data suggest that chemoprophylaxis is not necessary (219,220).

There is a well-established association between glucocorticoid therapy and muscle atrophy (206). The elderly patient may be at particular risk for myopathy because muscle strength declines with age (221). In addition, there is evidence from animal studies that glucocorticoid-induced muscle wasting occurs more rapidly in older animals (222). This finding is supported by a clinical study of leg muscle strength in older patients taking low-dose prednisone (223). Glucocorticoid-induced myopathy may also involve the respiratory muscles (224–226).

In a study of 25,947 medical inpatients, the most common drugs associated with psychosis were glucocorticoids (227). Elderly patients are more likely than younger patients to develop drug-related psychiatric problems (228). In one study, the mean age of patients developing drug-related psychiatric disturbances was 65 years (227). Steroid-induced psychosis has usually been reported associated with high-dose glucocorticoid therapy (>40 mg prednisone/day) (229,230). Depression, which is especially prevalent in the elderly population with chronic medical problems (231), is associated with glucocorticoid therapy (232), and the elderly asthmatic patient may be at greater risk for this adverse effect. Thus, the elderly asthmatic patient appears to be at increased risk for multiple complications of systemic glucocorticoid therapy.

Inhaled Glucocorticoid Therapy

The introduction of inhaled glucocorticoid therapy for asthma has decreased the necessity for the use of oral glucocorticoids. Studies have demonstrated that, in many patients, inhaled glucocorticoids can be substituted for oral therapy with comparable efficacy (233–236). When compared with regular β_2-agonist therapy in patients with newly diagnosed mild asthma, inhaled corticosteroids reduced symptoms, improved lung function, and decreased bronchial hyperresponsiveness during a 2-year study (237). In the third year of study, the investigators determined whether the steroid dose could be reduced or discontinued and what effect crossover of patients from regularly administered β_2-agonist to glucocorticoid therapy would have (238). They found that maintenance glucocorticoid therapy could be given at a reduced dose, but discontinuation of treatment was typically accompanied by exacerbation of disease. Also, although the patients who were crossed over from β_2-agonist to inhaled glucocorticoid improved, the degree of improvement was less than among those who were treated with inhaled glucocorticoid from the beginning of the study, suggesting that early use of inhaled glucocorticoid therapy might have beneficial effects. Although there are no prospective trials demonstrating a reduction in mortality, treatment with inhaled glucocorticoids may decrease asthma morbidity and mortality (239). Inhaled glucocorticoid therapy has not been studied specifically in an elderly population, but there is no experimental evidence to suggest a loss of effect with aging. There is evidence that the elderly patient with chronic asthma is at increased risk of developing irreversible airflow obstruction (158). The pathophysiological explanation for the fixed obstruction is unclear, but it may be the result of chronic inflammation that could be prevented by anti-inflammatory treatment.

Pharmacokinetic Properties of Inhaled Glucocorticoids

Various inhaled glucocorticoid preparations are available (Table 4). In addition to excellent topical activity, important pharmacokinetic properties that limit adverse effects include low oral bioavailability and swift clearance of drug that reaches the systemic circulation. Following inhalation, 80% or more of the inhaled puff is deposited in the oropharynx and swallowed (73,240). The amount deposited in the oropharynx can be reduced significantly by use of a spacer or by rinsing the mouth after inhalation (241). The swallowed glucocorticoid can be absorbed, but the amount reaching the systemic circulation is determined by the extent of first-pass inactivation in the liver (Fig. 5) (178). Up to 20% of the drug reaches the respiratory tract and can be absorbed into the systemic circulation. The systemic glucocorticoid, which is eliminated over time by continuous recirculation and inactivation in the liver, produces the systemic side effects. Beclomethasone dipropionate, triamcinolone, and flunisolide have been available in the United States for several years and do not appear to have major differences (242,243). Fluticasone, which has recently become available in the United States, has very low oral bioavailability (244).

Initially, the recommendation was to give inhaled corticosteroid four times a

Table 4 Topical Potency of Inhaled
Glucocorticoid Preparations

Glucocorticoid	Blanching potency[a]
Dexamethasone	1
BDP/BMP[b]	0.4/13.5
Flunisolide	330
Triamcinolone acetonide	330
Fluticasone propionate	1200
Budesonide[c]	980

[a]Blanching potency on human skin is an indication of
topical potency.
[b]Beclomethasone dipropionate (BDP) is converted in
the liver to the more active beclomethasone monopro-
pionate (BMP).
[c]Not currently available in the United States.
Source: Ref. 178.

day. Subsequent studies have shown no significant differences in respiratory symptoms or pulmonary function between dosing regimens of two and four times daily in patients with moderate asthma (245). Because compliance in the elderly patient is better on a twice-daily schedule (246), this regimen is recommended.

Adverse Effects of Inhaled Therapy

Use of inhaled glucocorticoids is associated with local oropharyngeal side effects, which may be a particular problem in the elderly (242). These include oropharyngeal candidiasis and dysphonia. Oropharyngeal candidiasis usually occurs only at higher doses or when the drug is given more than twice daily, but the incidence may be reduced by use of a spacer, which reduces the amount of drug reaching the oropharynx (241). Dysphonia appears to be due to myopathy of the laryngeal muscles; although usually not a serious problem, it resolves with discontinuation of inhaled glucocorticoid.

Although the systemic side effects associated with inhaled glucocorticoid therapy are unquestionably of less significance than with oral glucocorticoid therapy, there has been concern regarding adverse systemic effects with inhaled glucocorticoid therapy. As described above, part of the inhaled dose of glucocorticoids reaches the systemic circulation and is capable of producing systemic side effects (Fig. 5). There is evidence in healthy volunteers that inhaled glucocorticoids raise the blood glucose concentration (247), but this effect on blood glucose is probably not of significance. In elderly diabetic subjects, high doses of

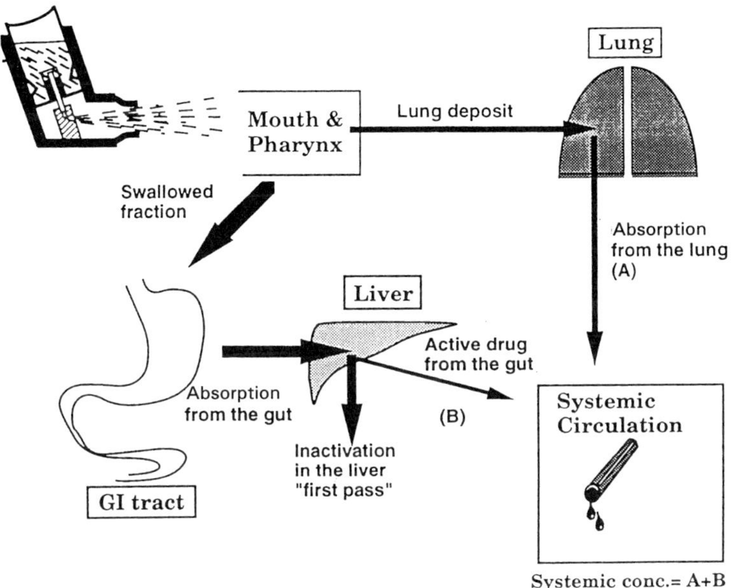

Figure 5 Disposition of inhaled glucocorticoids. (From Ref. 178.)

inhaled beclomethasone have no adverse effect on glucose tolerance (248). Oral glucocorticoid therapy clearly suppresses the function of the HPA axis by reducing ACTH secretion and can reduce adrenal responses to stress if it is prolonged (206). Whether inhaled glucocorticoid therapy has important effects on the adrenal response to stress is unclear. There is evidence that high doses ($>$1600 μg/day of beclomethasone dipropionate) of inhaled glucocorticoids do affect basal adrenal function, but whether the adrenal response to stress is affected significantly is not clear (242). In adults, doses of less than 1600 μg/day do not appear to have any important effects on adrenal function, and there is consensus that in doses of less than 800 μg/day, no significant systemic effects occur (249). Although inhaled glucocorticoids do not appear to have significant affects on the HPA axis in the population in general, there are reports of adrenal atrophy associated with inhaled glucocorticoid therapy (250). Thus, some individuals may be at increased risk, perhaps because they metabolize glucocorticoids more slowly. Whether the elderly patient is more susceptible to effects on the HPA axis than the younger adult is unknown.

As described previously in this review, the elderly patient is at greater risk of the glucocorticoid effects on bone metabolism. There is evidence that inhaled glucocorticoids are capable of interfering with bone turnover, but the extent of the effect is much less than with oral therapy (251–254). Also, interpretation of studies of the effects of inhaled glucocorticoids on bone is complicated by previous oral glucocorticoid therapy and the lack of appropriate controls. Nonetheless, sensitive biochemical indices of bone metabolism suggest that higher doses of inhaled glucocorticoids may have effects on bone metabolism (195,252,255). Recently, bone mineral density and the risk of fracture have been examined in a group of older asthmatics (average age 60 years) taking long-term inhaled glucocorticoids (256). The results of this study suggest that long-term use of inhaled glucocorticoids had little or no effect on bone density and risk of fracture. In fact, in patients with prednisone-dependent asthma, inhaled glucocorticoid therapy was associated with increased bone density and a reduced risk of fracture. Also, supplemental estrogen therapy appeared to protect bone density in postmenopausal women receiving prolonged oral or inhaled glucocorticoids (256). Thus, although higher doses of inhaled glucocorticoids may pose some risk of osteoporosis in the elderly asthmatic patient, the risks are markedly reduced as compared to those with oral therapy and are probably not significant at lower doses.

Skin thinning and bruising, commonly associated with oral glucocorticoid therapy, may result from high doses of inhaled glucocorticoids in some patients (257,258). Easy bruising associated with inhaled therapy appears to be more common in the older patient (257). Although there are reports of a possible association between inhaled glucocorticoid therapy and posterior subcapsular cataracts (259,260), there is no well-documented association (247). Also, there are only case reports of psychiatric disturbances associated with inhaled glucocorticoids (178) and no reports of a relationship between inhaled glucocorticoids and an increased risk of systemic infection.

Because of the possibility of adverse effects with inhaled glucocorticoids, particularly at higher doses, the dose should be tapered to the minimal effective daily dose after optimal control has been achieved by an initial higher daily dose. In the elderly patient with established osteoporosis and vertebral fractures, it may be more prudent to add a long-acting bronchodilator to the regimen rather than increasing the dose of inhaled glucocorticoid to achieve better control of symptoms (261).

B. Cromolyn Sodium and Nedocromil Sodium

Cromolyn sodium and nedocromil sodium have anti-inflammatory effects and improve bronchial hyperresponsiveness with chronic therapy (262,263). They can also protect against bronchoconstrictive stimuli such as exercise and both the early and late response to allergen challenge (264, 265). The mechanisms of action for both cromolyn and nedocromil are not well defined. These agents prevent release of preformed mediators and arachidonic acid metabolites from a number of cells, including mast cells, T-lymphocytes, eosinophils, and macrophages (266–270). There may be effects on sensory nerves in the airways by these agents, preventing irritant induced bronchospasm (271). There is also evidence that nedocromil inhibits immunoglubulin E synthesis by human B-lymphocytes (272).

Although studies comparing cromolyn or nedocromil with inhaled glucocorticoids have demonstrated varying results (265,273–276), the consensus is that inhaled glucocorticoids are the anti-inflammatory therapy of choice in the adult patient (242). Nonetheless, cromolyn and nedocromil have been demonstrated to have beneficial effects in adult asthmatics (265,277–279). Whether cromolyn and nedocromil can have steroid-sparing effects has been investigated, but study results vary, suggesting that the steroid-sparing effect, if any, is small (280–282). Cromolyn is often used as first-line anti-inflammatory therapy in children because of the lack of adverse effects associated with the drug. Because cromolyn and nedocromil have virtually no important side effects, a trial of one of these agents might be reasonable in the elderly patient with severe asthma in the hope that the steroid-sparing effect would minimize the adverse effects associated with high doses of glucocorticoids. However, the general consensus is that cromolyn and nedocromil are not as effective in the elderly asthmatic patient as in the younger patient (1).

C. Other Agents

Several alternative therapies—including methotrexate, gold salts, troleandromycin, cyclosporine, hydroxychloroquine, dapsone, and intravenous immunoglubulin (IVIG)—have been used primarily in attempts to reduce the dose of glucocorticoids in patients with severe asthma (283). The use of methotrexate has been in vogue since Mullarkey and coworkers showed that a low dose allowed a reduction in the dose of oral corticosteroids in patients with severe asthma without deterioration in pulmonary function (284,285). Subsequent studies have yielded conflicting results (284,286–290). This discordance suggests that the steroid-sparing effect of methotrexate is at best small. As with methotrexate, the benefits achieved using the other agents listed above have produced only small reductions in glucocorticoid requirements (283). In addition, the potential clinical effects of these agents were often associated with the risk of significant drug toxicity, which could be particularly devastating in the elderly patient. At present, the value of any of these agents in the elderly asthmatic patient is questionable.

Recently, a number of drugs, termed antileukotriene agents or leukotriene modifiers, have been studied for the treatment of asthma. These agents act by preventing the synthesis or action of cysteinyl leukotrienes (291). Cysteinyl leukotrienes, which are potent mediators produced by inflammatory cells, can cause bronchoconstriction, mucous secretion, and edema in the airways. Antileukotriene drugs are effective in blunting the response to a variety of airways challenges, particularly aspirin challenge in asthmatics with aspirin-induced asthma (292–295). These agents are also somewhat effective in producing acute bronchodilation and in asthma control when administered chronically (296,297). The antileukotriene agents are currently in clinical trials in the United States.

IV. Approach to Therapy

The patient should be educated concerning the nature of the disease and the goals of therapy. Management should include frequent monitoring of symptoms, bronchodilator requirements, and objective measures of lung function both to assess the effectiveness of therapy and to identify deterioration (1). The frequency of follow-up by the clinician depends on the severity of the asthma and the ability of the patient to monitor asthma at home. The capability of the patient to monitor the disease will vary considerably, particularly in the elderly asthmatic patient. Because elderly patients are more likely to have a poor perception of symptoms (298), objective measures of lung function are particularly important. Written asthma management plans are an important part of successful management. In general, elderly patients have greater difficulty with MDI technique and require observed review of technique with feedback. Education in avoidance of environmental triggers may be helpful for some elderly asthmatic patients.

Pneumococcal vaccine should be given every 5–7 years in patients ages 60–75 years and every 3–4 years in the over 75 age group (1); influenza vaccine is given on a yearly basis. Medications that aggravate bronchospasm should be avoided, especially β-adrenergic blocking agents. Oral beta blockers, regardless of their selectivity, should not be used for the treatment of hypertension or angina in patients with airways obstruction. Many elderly patients are treated with β-adrenergic-blocker eyedrops for glaucoma, and the use of nonselective beta-blocker eyedrops, such as timolol, may cause acute bronchospasm or an insidious decline in lung function (299,300). The elderly patient appears to be at an increased risk of deterioration in lung function with the use of timolol eyedrops (301). There is evidence that the cardioselective beta blocker betaxolol is better tolerated by those asthmatics who require a beta blocker eyedrop for treatment of glaucoma (302,303). Some patients with asthma are sensitive to aspirin and other nonsteroidal anti-inflammatory drugs (NSAIDs) (304). These agents may cause life-threatening bronchospasm in these patients. Because arthritis is the most common medical problem in the elderly patient (305), the physician must be alert to the possibility of worsening asthma due to the use of aspirin or other NSAIDs.

Over the past several years, guidelines, both national and international, have been developed for the management of asthma (60,167). Although there is not total consensus between the various guidelines, they are basically similar in classifying asthma according to symptoms and pulmonary function as mild, moderate, and severe. It is important to note that for many details of the guidelines, evidence from controlled trials is lacking (306). Thus, many of the recommendations are based on clinical experience and do not represent a strict protocol for asthma management.

Recently, specific guidelines have been developed for the management of the elderly asthmatic patient (1). As with the previous guidelines, asthma is classified by severity and treatment is stepped up or stepped down as necessary. The therapeutic approach in the elderly patient is basically the same as that recommended for younger adults with asthma (60), but there are important management distinctions. In the elderly, it is essential to consider the possibility of coexisting disease. As outlined previously in this chapter, the potential for adverse effects of therapy and the risk of drug and disease interactions are both greater in the elderly patient. In regard to guidelines for pulmonary function, it is essential to remember that there is an increased prevalence of irreversible obstruction in the elderly asthmatic patient (158). Thus, achieving normal lung function may either be impossible or require drug doses associated with hazardous adverse effects.

In the elderly patient, the guidelines define mild, intermittent asthma as symptoms or exacerbations less than twice a week, nocturnal symptoms less than twice a month, and absence of symptoms between exacerbations. No pulmonary function guidelines are given, but in previous NAEP guidelines for younger adults, peak expiratory flow (PEF) or forced expiratory volume in 1 sec (FEV_1) of $\geq$80% of baseline with $\geq$20% variability when symptomatic were the function parameters for mild asthma. For the elderly asthmatic patient with milid asthma, the recommended treatment is a short-acting inhaled β_2-agonist, as necessary. The need for a step-up in therapy is signaled by an increasing need for β-agonist, such as use more than three to four times a week or use of more than one canister a month.

Moderate asthma is defined as exacerbations more than twice a week that affect sleep and activity; nighttime awakenings due to asthma more than twice a month; and chronic asthma symptoms that require a short-acting inhaled β_2-agonist daily or every other day. Pulmonary function for moderate asthma is 60–80% of predicted, with variability of 20–30%. Severe asthma is defined as the presence of continuous symptoms, frequent exacerbations, frequent nighttime awakenings due to asthma, and limitation of activities. Pulmonary function in severe asthma is defined as PEF or FEV_1 baseline less than 60% of predicted and PEF variability of 20–30%. In the guidelines created for younger adults with asthma, anti-inflammatory therapy (e.g., inhaled glucocorticoids, cromolyn sodium, or nedocromil) is recommended for the patient with moderate asthma. If symptoms are not controlled, the recommendation is to increase the inhaled glucocorticoids or add a long-acting bronchodilator (theophylline or long-acting

β_2-agonist). For the patient with severe asthma, consideration of daily or alternate-day oral glucocorticoid therapy is recommended. In the guidelines, there are several recommendations specific for the elderly asthmatic patient as compared with the younger adult (1). Management of the elderly patient with moderate or severe asthma may be influenced by the presence of a significant irreversible component of airways obstruction. In some cases, it may be necessary to administer a short course of oral glucocorticoids (1–2 weeks) to assess reversibility. In patients with significant reversibility of obstruction, inhaled anti-inflammatory therapy should be initiated. The guidelines state that inhaled glucocorticoids may be preferable to cromolyn or nedocromil in the older patient. Cromolyn and nedocromil have been studied primarily in younger, allergic patients, but they have shown some efficacy in adults with airways obstruction (227,307). However, in the adult patient, the benefits of inhaled glucocorticoids clearly outweigh the risks when compared with those of cromolyn or nedocromil. Short-acting inhaled β_2-agonists should be administered as needed for acute symptoms, and, as in mild asthma, increasing use is an indication for a step-up in therapy. Therapy can be stepped up by raising the dose of inhaled glucocorticoids or adding a long-acting bronchodilator, such as a long-acting inhaled β_2-agonist, ipratropium, or sustained-release theophylline. The long-acting β_2-agonist salmeterol has been shown to be as effective in controlling symptoms and preventing exacerbations as increasing the dose of inhaled glucocorticoid (261). Because of the narrow therapeutic window and the increased risk of serious toxicity with theophylline in the elderly, theophylline should be used cautiously in these patients. Another approach would be a trial of anticholinergic therapy with inhaled ipratropium bromide. In contrast to oral theophylline, inhaled ipratropium has essentially no important side effects. Ipratropium may be more effective in the elderly patient than in the younger adult, but, as noted below, it is particularly recommended for the asthmatic patient without a significant reversible component or coexisting COPD.

For the patient without a significant reversible component, especially the patient with coexisting COPD, bronchodilator therapy may play an important role. Inhaled ipratropium is recommended earlier in the course of therapy in these patients. However, increasing use of inhaled β_2-agonist therapy continues to be evidence of worsening asthma and an indication for increased anti-inflammatory therapy, although the benefits of inhaled glucocorticoids may be less apparent in these asthmatic patients with more fixed obstruction.

For patients who continue to have symptoms on the regimen outlined above, oral corticosteroids are necessary. Oral corticosteroids are recommended last because of the serious side effects associated with long-term administration. As described in this chapter, the elderly are especially susceptible to the adverse side effects of chronic oral corticosteroid therapy. When the patient is stable, a switch to alternate-day therapy should be attempted; if the patient does well, attempts should be made on an intermittent basis to eliminate the oral corticosteroid from the regimen.

Although chronic administration of oral corticosteroids should be avoided if possible, a short course of oral corticosteroid therapy is recommended for an acute exacerbation of asthma and should not be delayed. This is especially important in the elderly, who are at a greater risk of death from asthma than younger adults (308–310). The adverse effects of a short course of oral prednisone are less dangerous than the frequent use of β_2-adrenergic agonist inhalers in the elderly patient who may be hypoxemic in the setting of severe bronchospasm and may have underlying ischemic heart disease. A comprehensive approach to the management of acute exacerbation in the elderly asthmatic patient is described in Chap. 8.

V. Conclusions

Although pharmacological management of asthma is similiar for all ages, there are special considerations in the elderly. The risk of adverse effects from asthma medications is greater in the elderly patient, particularly with systemic glucocorticoid and theophylline therapy. The potential for drug interactions is enhanced in elderly asthmatic patients because of the increased likelihood that they may be taking multiple medications for coexisting diseases. As in the younger adult with asthma, inhaled therapy is the cornerstone of management. Unfortunately, older patients experience greater difficulty using inhaler devices correctly. Evidence from clinical studies to support the recommendations for asthma management is especially lacking for care of the elderly patient. The benefits of newer asthma therapies for the elderly patient must be confirmed in clinical trials.

Abbreviations

COMT	catechol-O-methyltransferase
MDI	metered-dose inhaler
MAT	multifocal atrial tachycardia
NAEP	National Asthma Education Program
PEF	peak expiratory flow
FEV_1	forced expiratory volume in 1 sec

References

1. National Heart, Lung and Blood Institute. Considerations for Diagnosing and Managing Asthma in the Elderly. U.S. Department of Health and Human Services, National Institutes of Health, 1996.

2. Nijkamp FP, Engels F, Henricks PA, Van Oosterhout AJ. Mechanisms of beta-adrenergic receptor regulation in lungs and its implications for physiological responses. Physiol Rev 1992; 72:323–367.
3. Carstairs JR, Nimmo AJ, Barnes PJ. Autoradiographic visualization of beta-adrenoceptor subtypes in human lung. Am Rev Respir Dis 1985; 132:541–547.
4. Nelson HS. Beta-adrenergic bronchodilators. N Engl J Med 1995: 333:499–506.
5. Torphy TJ. Beta-adrenoceptors, cAMP and airway smooth muscle relaxation: Challenges to the dogma. Trends Pharmacol Sci 1994; 15:370–374.
6. Jiang H, Shabb JB, Corbin JD. Cross-activation: Overriding cAMP/cGMP selectivities of protein kinases in tissues. Biochem Cell Biol 1992; 70:1283–1289.
7. Roger DF. Scorpion venoms: Taking the sting out of lung disease. Thorax 1996; 51:546–548.
8. Kume H, Mikawa K, Takagi K, Kotlikoff MI. Role of G proteins and KCa channels in the muscarinic and beta-adrenergic regulation of airway smooth muscle. Am J Physiol 1995: 268:L221–L229.
9. Kume H, Hall IP, Washabau RJ, et al. Beta-adrenergic agonists regulate Kca channels in airway smooth muscle by cAMP-dependent and -independent mechanisms. J Clin Invest 1994; 93:371–379.
10. Kotlikoff MI. Potassium channels in airway smooth muscle: A tale of two channels. Pharmacol Ther 1993; 58:1–12.
11. Barnes PJ. Beta-adrenergic receptors and their regulation. American Respir Crit Care Med 1995; 152:838–860.
12. Church MK, Hiroi J. Inhibition of IgE-dependent histamine release from human dispersed lung mast cells by anti-allergic drugs and salbutamol. Br J Pharmacol 1987; 90:421–429.
13. Butchers PR, Skidmore IF, Vardey CJ, Wheeldon A. Characterization of the receptor mediating the antianaphylactic effects of beta-adrenoceptor agonists in human lung tissue in vitro. Br J Pharmacol 1980; 71:663–667.
14. Rhoden KJ, Meldrum LA, Barnes PJ. Inhibition of cholinergic neurotransmission in human airways by beta 2-adrenoceptors. J Appl Physiol 1988; 65:700–705.
15. Mortensen J, Groth S, Lange P, Hermansen F. Effect of terbutaline on mucociliary clearance in asthmatic and healthy subjects after inhalation from a pressurised inhaler and a dry powder inhaler. Thorax 1991; 46:817–823.
16. Isawa T, Teshima T, Hirano T, et al. Does a beta 2-stimulator really facilitate mucociliary transport in the human lungs in vitro? A study with procaterol. Am Rev Respir Dis 1990; 141:715–720.
17. Greiff L, Erjefalt I, Svensson C, et al. Plasma exudation and solute absorption across the airway mucosa. Clin Physiol 1993; 13:219–233.
18. Erjefalt I, Persson CG. Pharmacologic control of plasma exudation into tracheobronchial airways. Am Rev Respir Dis 1991; 143:1008–1014.
19. Barnes PJ. Anti-inflammatory therapy for asthma. Annu Rev Med 1993; 44:229–242.
20. Scarpace PJ, Tumer N, Mader SL. Beta-adrenergic function in aging: Basic mechanisms and clinical implications. Drugs Aging 1991; 1:116–129.

21. Conolly MJ. Ageing, late-onset asthma and the beta-adrenoceptor. Pharmacol Ther 1993; 60:389–404.
22. Feldman RD, Limbird LE, Nadeau J, et al. Alterations in leukocyte beta-receptor affinity with aging: A potential explanation for altered beta-adrenergic sensitivity in the elderly. N Engl J Med 1984; 310:815–819.
23. Krall JF, Connelly-Fittingoff M, Tuck ML. Lymphocyte adenylate cyclase and human aging. Proc Soc Exp Biol Med 1983; 173:475–480.
24. Scarpace PJ, Abrass IB. Decreased beta-adrenergic agonist affinity and adenylate cyclase activity in senescent rat lung. J Gerontol 1983; 38:143–147.
25. O'Connor SW, Scarpace PJ, Abrass IB. Age-associated decrease in the catalytic unit activity of rat myocardial adenylate cyclase. Mech Ageing Dev 1983; 21: 357–363.
26. Connolly MJ, Crowley JJ, Charan NB, et al. Impaired bronchodilator response to albuterol in healthy elderly men and women. Chest 1995; 108:401–406.
27. Ullah MI, Newman GB, Saunders KB. Influence of age on response to ipratropium and salbutamol in asthma. Thorax 1981; 36:523–529.
28. Kradjan WA, Driesner NK, Abuan TH, et al. Effect of age on bronchodilator response. Chest 1992; 101:1545–1551.
29. Hamelin BA, Blouin RA, Wolf KM, et al. In vivo and in vitro beta 2-adrenergic receptor responsiveness in young and elderly asthmatics. Pharmacotherapy 1992; 12:376–382.
30. van Schayck CP, Folgering H, Harbers H, et al. Effects of allergy and age on responses to salbutamol and ipratropium bromide in moderate asthma and chronic bronchitis. Thorax 1991; 46:355–359.
31. Hoffman BB, Lefkowitz RJ. Catecholamines, sympathomimetic drugs, and adrenergic receptor antagonists. In: Hardman JG, Limbird LE, eds. The Pharmacological Basis of Therapeutics, 9th ed. New York: McGraw-Hill, 1996:199–248.
32. Rabe KF, Jorres R, Nowak D, et al. Comparison of the effects of salmeterol and formoterol on airway tone and responsiveness over 24 hours in bronchial asthma. Am Rev Respir Dis 1993; 147:1436–1441.
33. Pearlman DS, Chervinsky P, LaForce C, et al. A comparison of salmeterol with albuterol in the treatment of mild-to-moderate asthma. N Engl J Med 1992; 327: 1420–1425.
34. Anderson GP, Linden A, Rabe KF. Why are long-acting beta-adrenoceptor agonists long-acting? Eur Respir J 1994; 7:569–578.
35. Repsher LH, Anderson JA, Bush RK, et al. Assessment of tachyphylaxis following prolonged therapy of asthma with inhaled albuterol aerosol. Chest 1984; 85:34–38.
36. Weber RW, Smith JA, Nelson HS. Aerosolized terbutaline in asthmatics: Development of subsensitivity with long-term administration. J Allergy Clin Immuno 1982; 70:417–422.
37. Nelson HS, Raine D Jr, Doner HC, Posey WC. Subsensitivity to the bronchodilator action of albuterol produced by chronic administration. Am Rev Respir Dis 1977; 116:871–878.
38. Tashkin DP, Conolly ME, Deutsch RI, et al. Subsensitization of beta-adrenoceptors

in airways and lymphocytes of healthy and asthmatic subjects. Am Rev Respir Dis 1982; 125:185–193.

39. Repsher LH, Miller TD, Smith S. The lack of tachyphylaxis following prolonged therapy of asthma with inhaled albuterol aerosol. Ann Allergy 1981; 47:405–409.

40. Larsson S, Svedmyr N, Thiringer G. Lack of bronchial beta adrenoceptor resistance in asthmatics during long-term treatment with terbutaline. J Allergy Clin Immunol 1977; 59:93–100.

41. Cockcroft DW, McParland CP, Britto SA, et al. Regular inhaled salbutamol and airway responsiveness to allergen. Lancet 1993; 342:833–837.

42. O'Connor BJ, Aikman SL, Barnes PJ. Tolerance to the nonbronchodilator effects of inhaled beta 2-agonists in asthma. N Engl J Med 1992; 327:1204–1208.

43. Cheung D, Timmers MC, Zwinderman AH, et al. Long-term effects of a long-acting beta 2-adrenoceptor agonist, salmeterol, on airway hyperresponsiveness in patients with mild asthma. N Engl J Med 1992; 327:1198–1203.

44. Ullman A, Hedner J, Svedmyr N. Inhaled salmeterol and salbutamol in asthmatic patients: An evaluation of asthma symptoms and the possible development of tachyphylaxis. Am Rev Respir Dis 1990: 142:571–575.

45. Ramage L, Lipworth BJ, Ingram CG, et al. Reduced protection against exercise induced bronchoconstriction after chronic dosing with salmeterol. Respir Med 1994; 88:363–368.

46. Newnham DM, McDevitt DG, Lipworth BJ. Bronchodilator subsensitivity after chronic dosing with eformoterol in patients with asthma. Am J Med 1994; 97:29–37.

47. Newnham DM, Grove A, McDevitt DG, Lipworth BJ. Subsensitivity of bronchodilator and systemic beta 2 adrenoceptor responses after regular twice daily treatment with eformoterol dry powder in asthmatic patients. Thorax 1995; 50:497–504.

48. Lipworth BJ, Newnham DM, Clark RA, et al. Comparison of the relative airways and systemic potencies of inhaled fenoterol and salbutamol in asthmatic patients. Thorax 1995; 50:54–61.

49. Grove A, Lipworth BJ. Tolerance with beta 2-adrenoceptor agonists: Time for reappraisal. Br J Clin Pharmacol 1995; 39:109–118.

50. Mak JC, Nishikawa M, Shirasaki H, et al. Protective effects of a glucocorticoid on downregulation of pulmonary beta 2-adrenergic receptors in vivo. J Clin Invest 1995; 96:99–106.

51. Collins S, Caron MG, Lefkowitz RJ. Regulation of adrenergic receptor responsiveness through modulation of receptor gene expresion. Annu Rev Physiol 1991; 53:497–508.

52. Davies AO, Lefkowitz RJ. Regulation of beta-adrenergic receptors by steroid hormones. Annu Rev Physiol 1984; 46:119–130.

53. Ellul-Micallef R, Fenech FF. Effect of intravenous prednisolone in asthmatics with diminished adrenergic responsiveness. Lancet 1975; 2:1269–1271.

54. Kerstjens HA, Brand PL, Quanjer PH, et al. Variability of bronchodilator response and effects of inhaled corticosteroid treatment in obstructive airway disease: Dutch CNSLD Study Group. Thorax 1993; 48:722–729.

55. Stolley PD, Schinnar R. Association between asthma mortality and isoproterenol aerosols: A review. Prev Med 1978; 7:519–538.

56. Pearce N, Beasley R, Crane J, et al. End of the New Zealand asthma mortality epidemic. Lancet 1995; 345:41–44.

57. Crane J, Pearce N, Flatt A, et al. Prescribed fenoterol and death from asthma in New Zealand, 1981–83: Case-control study. Lancet 1989; 1:917–922.

58. Spitzer WO, Suissa S, Ernst P, et al. The use of beta-agonists and the risk of death and near death from asthma. N Engl J Med 1992; 326:501–506.

59. Suissa S, Ernst P, Boivin JF, et al. A cohort analysis of excess mortality in asthma and the use of inhaled beta-agonists. Am J Respir Crit Care Med 1994; 149:604–610.

60. National Heart, Lung and Blood Institute. Guidelines for the Diagnosis and Management of Asthma. Bethesda, MD: U.S. Department of Health and Human Services, National Institute of Health, 1991.

61. Wanner A. Is the routine use of inhaled beta-adrenergic agonists appropriate in asthma treatment? Yes (editorial). Am J Respir Crit Care Med 1995; 151:597–599.

62. van Schayck CP, Cloosterman SG, Hofland ID, et al. How detrimental is chronic use of bronchodilators in asthma and chronic obstructive pulmonary disease? Am J Respir Crit Care Med 1995; 151:1317–1319.

63. Nelson HS, Szefler SJ, Martin RJ. Regular inhaled beta-adrenergic agonists in the treatment of bronchial asthma: beneficial or detrimental (editorial)? Am Rev Respir Dis 1991; 144:249–250.

64. Sears MR. Is the routine use of inhaled beta-adrenergic agonists appropriate in asthma treatment? No (editorial). Am J Respir Crit Care Med 1995; 151:600–601.

65. de Jong JW, Teengs JP, Postma DS, et al. Nedocromil sodium versus albuterol in the management of allergic asthma. Am J Respir Crit Care Med 1994; 149:91–97.

66. Taylor DR, Sears MR, Herbison GP, et al. Regular inhaled beta agonist in asthma: Effects on exacerbations and lung function. Thorax 1993; 48:134–138.

67. Sears MR, Taylor DR, Print CG, et al. Regular inhaled beta-agonist treatment in bronchial asthma. Lancet 1990; 336:1391–1396.

68. van Schayck CP, Dompeling E, van Herwaarden CLA, et al. Bronchodilator treatment in moderate asthma or chronic bronchitis: Continuous or on demand? A randomised controlled study. Br Med J 1991; 303:1426–1431.

69. Chapman KR, Kesten S, Szalai JP. Regular vs as-needed inhaled salbutamol in asthma control. Lancet 1994; 343:1379–1382.

70. D'Alonzo GE, Nathan RA, Henochowicz S, et al. Salmeterol xinafoate as maintenance therapy compared with albuterol in patients with asthma. JAMA 1994; 271:1412–1416.

71. Vandewalker ML, Kray KT, Weber RW, Nelson HS. Addition of terbutaline to optimal theophylline therapy: Double blind crossover study in asthmatic patients. Chest 1986; 90:198–203.

72. Drazen JM, Israel E, Boushey HA, et al. Comparison of regularly scheduled with as-needed use of albuterol in mild asthma. N Engl J Med 1996; 335:841–847.

73. Newhouse MT, Dolovich MB. Control of asthma by aerosols. N Engl J Med 1986; 315:870–874.

74. Shim C, Williams MH, Jr. Bronchial response to oral versus aerosol metaproterenol in asthma. Ann Intern Med 1980; 93:428–431.

75. Brambilla C, Chastang C, Georges D, Bertin L. Salmeterol compared with slow-release terbutaline in nocturnal asthma: A multicenter, randomized, double-blind,

double-dummy, sequential clinical trial. French Multicenter Study Group. Allergy 1994; 49:421–426.

76. Thiringer G, Svedmyr N. Comparison of infused and inhaled terbutaline in patients with asthma. Scand J Respir Dis 1976; 57:17–24.

77. Williams SJ, Winner SJ, Clark TJ. Comparison of inhaled and intravenous terbutaline in acute severe asthma. Thorax 1981; 36:629–632.

78. Bloom JW, Barreuther AD. Drug therapy of airways obstructive diseases. In: Bressler R, Katz MD, eds. Geriatric Pharmacology. New York: McGraw-Hill, 1993:507–533.

79. Allen SC, Prior A. What determines whether an elderly patient can use a metered dose inhaler correctly? Br J Dis Chest 1986; 80:45–49.

80. Armitage JM, Williams SJ. Inhaler technique in the elderly. Age Ageing 1988; 17:275–278.

81. Dow I, Holgate ST. Assessment and treatment of obstructive airways disease in the elderly. Br Med Bull 1990; 46:230–245.

82. Traver GA, Tremper-Mitchell J, Flodquist-Priestly G. Respiratory Care—A Clinical Approach. Gaithersburg, MD: Aspen, 1991:87–93.

83. Connolly MJ. Inhaler technique of elderly patients: Comparison of metered-dose inhalers and large volume spacer devices. Age Ageing 1995; 24:190–192.

84. Thompson A, Traver GA. Comparison of three methods of administering a self-propelled bronchodilator. Am Rev Respir Dis 1982; 125:140.

85. Chapman KR, Love L, Brubaker H. A comparison of breath-acutated and conventional metered-dose inhaler inhalation techniques in elderly subjects. Chest 1993; 104:1332–1337.

86. Kesten S, Elias M, Cartier A, Chapman KR. Patient handling of a multidose dry powder inhalation device for albuterol. Chest 1994; 105:1077–1081.

87. Lofdahl CG, Svedmyr K, Svedmyr N, et al. Comparison of beta 2-adrenoceptor stimulation in bronchial and skeletal muscle in experimental and clinical studies. Eur J Respir Dis Suppl 1984; 135:124–127.

88. Bengtsson B. Plasma concentration and side-effects of terbutaline. Eur J Respir Dis Suppl 1984; 134:231–235.

89. Teule GJ, Majid PA. Haemodynamic effects of terbutaline in chronic obstructive airways disease. Thorax 1980; 35:536–542.

90. Levine MA, Leenen FH. Role of beta 1-receptors and vagal tone in cardiac inotropic and chronotropic responses to a beta 2-agonist in humans. Circulation 1989; 79: 107–115.

91. Lipworth BJ, Tregaskis BF, McDevitt DG. Comparison of hypokalaemic, electrocardiographic and haemodynamic responses to inhaled isoprenaline and salbutamol in young and elderly subjects. Eur J Clin Pharmacol 1991; 40:255–260.

92. Kinney EL, Trautlein JJ, Harbaugh CV, et al. Ventricular tachycardia after terbulatine (letter). JAMA 1978; 240:2247.

93. Eidelman DH, Sami MH, McGregor M, Cosio MG. Combination of theophylline and salbutamol for arrhythmias in severe COPD. Chest 1987; 91:808–812.

94. Siegel D, Sheppard D, Gelb A, Weinberg PF. Aminophylline increases the toxicity but not the efficacy of an inhaled beta-adrenergic agonist in the treatment of acute exacerbations of asthma. Am Rev Respir Dis 1985; 132:283–286.

95. Josephson GW, Kennedy HL, MacKenzie EJ, Gibson G. Cardiac dysrhythmias during the treatment of acute asthma: A comparison of two treatment regimens by a double blind protocol. Chest 1980; 78:429–435.

96. Haffner CA, Kendall MJ. Metabolic effects of beta 2-agonists. J Clin Pharm Ther 1992; 17:155–164.

97. Scher DL, Arsura EL. Multifocal atrial tachycardia: Mechanisms, clinical correlates, and treatment. Am Heart J 1989; 118:574–580.

98. Ikram H. Arrhythmias, electrolytes, and ACE inhibitor therapy in the elderly. Gerontology 1987; 33(suppl 1):42–47.

99. Brown MJ, Brown DC, Murphy MB. Hypokalemia from beta2-receptor stimulation by circulating epinephrine. N Engl J Med 1983; 309:1414–1419.

100. Struthers AD, Reid JL. The role of adrenal medullary catecholamines in potassium homoeostasis. Clin Sci 1984; 66:377–382.

101. Lipworth BJ, McDevitt DG, Struthers AD. Systemic beta-adrenoceptor responses to salbutamol given by metered-dose inhaler alone and with pear shaped spacer attachment: Comparison of electrocardiographic, hypokalaemic and haemodynamic effects. Br J Clin Pharmacol 1989; 27:837–842.

102. Lipworth BJ, McDevitt DG, Struthers AD. Prior treatment with diuretic augments the hypokalemic and electrocardiographic effects of inhaled albuterol. Am J Med 1989; 86:653–657.

103. Taylor DR, Wilkins GT, Herbison GP, Flannery EM. Interaction between corticosteroid and beta-agonist drugs: Biochemical and cardiovascular effects in normal subjects. Chest 1992; 102:519–524.

104. Flack JM, Ryder KW, Strickland D, Whang R. Metabolic correlates of theophylline therapy: A concentration-related phenomenon. Ann Pharmacother 1994; 28:175–179.

105. Lipworth BJ, Struthers AD, McDevitt DG. Tachyphylaxis to systemic but not to airway responses during prolonged therapy with high dose inhaled salbutamol in asthmatics. Am Rev Respir Dis 1989; 140:586–592.

106. Harvey JE, Baldwin CJ, Wood PJ, et al. Airway and metabolic responsiveness to intravenous salbutamol in asthma: Effect of regular inhaled salbutamol. Clin Sci 1981; 60:579–585.

107. Dickens GR, McCoy RA, West R, et al. Effect of nebulized albuterol on serum potassiuim and cardiac rhythm in patients with asthma or chronic obstructive pulmonary disease. Pharmacotherapy 1994; 14:729–733.

108. Knudson RJ, Constantine HP. An effect of isoproterenol on ventilation-perfusion in asthmatic versus normal subjects. J Appl Physiol 1967; 22:402–406.

109. Rogers RM, Owens GR, Pennock BE. The pendulum swings again: Toward a rational use of theophylline (editorial). Chest 1985; 87:280–282.

110. Weinberger M, Hendeles L. Theophylline in asthma. N Engl J Med 1996; 334: 1380–1388.

111. Lam A, Newhouse MT. Management of asthma and chronic airflow limitation: Are methylxanthines obsolete? Chest 1990; 98:44–52.

112. Aubier M, Barnes PJ. Theophylline and phosphodiesterase inhibitors (editorial, comment). Eur Respir J 1995; 8:347–348.

113. Bukowskyj M, Nakatsu K, Munt PW. Theophylline reassessed. Ann Intern Med 1984; 101:63–73.

114. Persson CG. Overview of effects of theophylline. J Allergy Clin Immunol 1986; 78:780–787.

115. Louis RE, Radermecker MF. Substance P-induced histamine release from human basophils, skin and lung fragments: effect of nedocromil sodium and theophylline. Int Arch Allergy Appl Immunol 1990; 92:329–333.

116. Dent G, Giembycz MA, Rabe KF, et al. Theophylline suppresses human alveolar macrophage respiratory burst through phosphodiesterase inhibition. Am J Respir Cell Mol Biol 1994; 10:565–572.

117. Dent G, Giembycz MA, Evans PM, et al. Suppression of human eosinophil respiratory burst and cyclic AMP hydrolysis by inhibitors of type IV phosphodiesterase: interaction with the beta adrenoceptor agonist albuterol. J Pharmacol Exp Ther 1994; 271:1167–1174.

118. Yukawa T, Kroegel C, Chanez P, et al. Effect of theophylline and adenosine on eosinophil function. Am Rev Respir Dis 1989; 140:327–333.

119. Sullivan P, Bekir S, Jaffar Z, et al. Anti-inflammatory effects of low-dose oral theophylline in atopic asthma. Lancet 1994; 343:1006–1008.

120. Ward AJ, McKenniff M, Evans JM, et al. Theophylline—An immunomodulatory role in asthma? Am Rev Respir Dis 1993; 147:518–523.

121. Hendeles L, Harman E, Huang D, et al. Theophylline attenuation of airway responses to allergen: Comparison with cromolyn metered-dose inhaler. J Allergy Clin Immunol 1995; 95:505–514.

122. Kidney J, Dominguez M, Taylor PM, et al. Immunomodulation by theophylline in asthma: Demonstration by withdrawal of therapy. Am J Respir Crit Care Med 1995; 151:1907–1914.

123. Howell RE. Multiple mechanisms of xanthine actions on airway reactivity. J Pharmacol Exp Ther 1990; 255:1008–1014.

124. Vestal RE, Cusack BJ, Mercer GD, et al. Aging and drug interactions: I. Effect of cimetidine and smoking on the oxidation of theophylline and cortisol in healthy men. J Pharmacol Exp Ther 1987; 241:488–500.

125. Weinberger M, Hendeles L, Bighley L. The relation of product formulation to absorption of oral theophylline. N Engl J Med 1978; 299:852–857.

126. Jusko WJ, Koup JR, Vance JW, et al. Intravenous theophylline therapy: Nomogram guidelines. Ann Intern Med 1977; 86:400–404.

127. Sarkar MA, Hunt C, Guzelian PS, Karnes HT. Characterization of human liver cytochromes P-450 involved in theophylline metabolism. Drug Metab Disp 1992; 20:31–37.

128. Kamada AK, Szelfer SJ. Pharmacological management of severe asthma. In: Szefler SJ, Leung DYM, eds. Severe Asthma: Pathogenesis and Clinical Management. New York: Marcel Dekker, 1996:165–205.

129. Au WY, Dutt AK, DeSoyza N. Theophylline kinetics in chronic obstructive airway disease in the elderly. Clin Pharmacol Ther 1985; 37:472–478.

130. Antal EJ, Kramer PA, Mercik SA, et al. Theophylline pharmacokinetics in advanced age. Br J Clin Pharmacol 1981; 12:637–645.

131. Talseth T, Kornstad S, Boye NP, Bredesen JE. Individualization of oral theophylline dosage in elderly patients. Acta Med Scand 1981; 210:489–492.

132. Bauer LA, Blouin RA. Influence of age on theophylline clearance in patients with chronic obstructive pulmonary disease. Clin Pharm 1981; 6:469–474.

133. Cusack B, Kelly JG, Lavan J. Theophylline kinetics in relation to age: The importance of smoking. Br J Clin Pharmacol 1980; 10:109–114.

134. Ramsay LE, Mackay A, Eppel ML, Oliver JS. Oral sustained-release aminophylline in medical inpatients: Factors related to toxicity and plasma theophylline concentrations. Br J Clin Pharmacol 1980; 10:101–107.

135. Powell JR, Vozeh S, Hopewell P, et al. Theophylline disposition in acutely ill hospitalized patients: The effect of smoking, heart failure, severe airway obstruction, and pneumonia. Am Rev Respir Dis 1978; 118:229–238.

136. Jewesson PJ, Ensom RJ. Influence of body fat on the volume of distribution of theophylline. Ther Drug Mon 1985; 7:197–201.

137. Zell M, Curtis RA, Troyer WG Jr, Fischer JH. Volume of distribution of theophylline in acute exacerbations of reversible airway disease: Effect of body weight. Chest 1985; 87:212–216.

138. Lindgren S, Lokshin B, Stromquist A, et al. Does asthma or treatment with theophylline limit children's academic performance? N Engl J Med 1992; 327:926–930.

139. Rachelefsky GS, Wo J, Adelson J, et al. Behavior abnormalities and poor school performance due to oral theophylline use. Pediatrics 1986; 78:1133–1138.

140. Furukawa CT, Shapiro GG, DuHamel T, et al. Learning and behaviour problems associated with theophylline therapy (letter). Lancet 1984; 1:621.

141. Fanta CH. Asthma in the elderly. Asthma 1989; 26:87–97.

142. Sessler CN. Theophylline toxicity: Clinical features of 116 consecutive cases. Am J Med 1990; 88:567–576.

143. Zwillich CW, Sutton FD, Neff TA, et al. Theophylline-induced seizures in adults: Correlation with serum concentrations. Ann Intern Med 1975; 82:784–787.

144. Patel AK, Skatrud JB, Thomsen JH. Cardiac arrhythmias due to oral aminophylline in patients with chronic obstructive pulmonary disease. Chest 1981; 80:661–665.

145. Levine JH, Michael JR, Guarnieri T. Multifocal atrial tachycardia: A toxic effect of theophylline. Lancet 1985; 1:12–14.

146. Bittar G, Friedman HS. The arrhythmogenicity of theophylline: A multivariate analysis of clinical determinants. Chest 1991; 99:1415–1420.

147. Shannon M, Lovejoy FJ Jr. The influence of age vs peak serum concentration on life-threatening events after chronic theophylline intoxication. Arch Intern Med 1990; 150:2045–2048.

148. Derby LE, Jick SS, Langlois JC, et al. Hospital admission for xanthine toxicity. Pharmacotherapy 1990; 10:112–114.

149. Mitenko PA, Ogilvie RI. Rational intravenous doses of theophylline. N Eng J Med 1973; 289:600–603.

150. Klein JJ, Lefkowitz MS, Spector SL, Cherniack RM. Relationship between serum theophylline levels and pulmonary function before and after inhaled beta-agonist in "stable' asthmatics. Am Rev Respir Dis 1983; 127:413–416.

151. Littenberg B. Aminophylline treatment in severe, acute asthma: A meta-analysis. JAMA 1988; 259:1678–1684.

152. Joad JP, Ahrens RC, Lindgren SD, Weinberger MM. Relative efficacy of maintenance therapy with theophylline, inhaled albuterol, and the combination for chronic asthma. J Allergy Clin Immunol 1987; 79:78–85.

153. Fjellbirkeland L, Gulsvik A, Palmer JB. The efficacy and tolerability of inhaled salmeterol and individually dose-titrated, sustained-release theophylline in patients with reversible airways disease. Respir Med 1994; 88:599–607.

154. Rivington RN, Boulet LP, Cote J, et al. Efficacy of uniphyl, salbutamol, and their combination in asthmatic patients on high-dose inhaled steroids. Am J Respir Crit Care Med 1995; 151:325–332.

155. Brenner M, Berkowitz R, Marshall N, Strunk RC. Need for theophylline in severe steroid-requiring asthmatics. Clin Allergy 1988; 18:143–150.

156. Nassif EG, Weinberger M, Thompson R, Huntley W. The value of maintenance theophylline in steroid-dependent asthma. N Engl J Med 1981; 304:71–75.

157. Chandler MH, Clifton GD, Burki NK, et al. Pulmonary function in the elderly: Response to theophylline bronchodilation. J Clin Pharmacol 1990; 30:330–335.

158. Braman SS, Kaemmerlen JT, Davis SM. Asthma in the elderly: A comparison between patients with recently acquired and long-standing disease. Am Rev Respir Dis 1991; 143:336–340.

159. Gandevia B. Historical review of the use of parasympatholytic agents in the treatment of respiratory disorders. Postgrad Med J 1975; 51:13–20.

160. Gross NJ, Skorodin MS. Anticholinergic, antimuscarinic bronchodilators. Am Rev Respir Dis 1984; 129:856–870.

161. Gross NJ. Ipratropium bromide. N Engl J Med 1988; 319:486–494.

162. Barnes PJ. Muscarinic receptors in airways: Recent developments. J Appl Physiol 1990; 68:1777–1785.

163. Mahesh VK, Nunan LM, Halonen M, et al. A minority of muscarinic receptors mediate rabbit tracheal smooth muscle contraction. Am J Respir Cell Mol Biol 1992; 6:279–286.

164. Coe CI, Barnes PJ. Reduction of nocturnal asthma by an inhaled anticholinergic drug. Chest 1986; 90:485–488.

165. Martin RJ. Nocturnal asthma: circadian rhythms and therapeutic interventions. Am Rev Respir Dis 1993; 147:S25–S28.

166. Gross NJ. The use of anticholinergic agents in the treatment of airways disease. Clin Chest Med 1988; 9:591–598.

167. National Heart, Lung and Blood Institute. International Consensus Report on Diagnosis and Management of Asthma. Bethesda, MD: National Institutes of Health, 1992.

168. Rebuck AS, Chapman KR, Abboud R, et al. Nebulized anticholinergic and sympathomimetic treatment of asthma and chronic obstructive airways disease in the emergency room. Am J Med 1987; 82:59–64.

169. Bryant DH. Nebulized ipratropium bromide in the treatment of acute asthma. Chest 1985; 88:24–29.

170. Leahy BC, Gomm SA, Allen SC. Comparison of nebulized salbutamol with nebulized ipratropium bromide in acute asthma. Br J Dis Chest 1983; 77:159–163.

171. Ward MJ, Fentem PH, Smith WH, Davies D. Ipratropium bromide in acute asthma. Br Med J Clin Res 1981; 282:598–600.

172. Ind PW, Dixon CM, Fuller RW, Barnes PJ. Anticholinergic blockade of beta-blocker-induced bronchoconstriction. Am Rev Respir Dis 1989; 139:1390–1394.

173. Barnes PJ. A new approach to the treatment of asthma. N Engl J Med 1989; 321:1517–1527.

174. Laitinen LA, Laitinen A, Haahtela T. Airway mucosal inflammation even in patients with newly diagnosed asthma. Am Rev Respir Dis 1993; 147:697–704.

175. Barnes PJ. Effect of corticosteroids on airways hyperresponsiveness. Am Rev Respir Dis 1990; 141:S70–S76.

176. Bloom JW, Miesfeld RL. Molecular mechanisms of glucocorticoid action. In: Szefler SJ, Leung DYM, eds. Severe Asthma: Pathogenesis and Clinical Management. New York: Marcel Dekker, 1996:255–284.

177. Schleimer RP. Effects of glucocorticosteroids on inflammatory cells relevant to their therapeutic applications in asthma. Am Rev Respir Dis 1990; 141:S59–S69.

178. Barnes PJ, Pedersen S. Efficacy and safety of inhaled corticosteroids in asthma: Report of a workshop held in Eze, France, October 1992. Am Rev Respir Dis 1993; 148:S1–S6.

179. Laitinen LA, Laitinen A, Haahtela T. A comparative study of the effects of an inhaled corticosteroid, budesonide, and a beta 2-agonist, terbutaline, on airway inflammation in newly diagnosed asthma: A randomized, double-blind, parallel-group controlled trial. J Allergy Clin Immunol 1992; 90:32–42.

180. Morris HG. Mechanisms of action and therapeutic role of corticosteroids in asthma. J Allergy Clin Immunol 1985; 75:1–13.

181. Boschetto P, Rogers DF, Fabbri LM, Barnes PJ. Corticosteroid inhibition of airway microvascular leakage. Am Rev Respir Dis 1991; 143:605–609.

182. Tornatore KM, Logue G, Venuto RC, Davis PJ. Pharmacokinetics of methylprednisolone in elderly and young healthy males. J Am Geriatr Soc 1994; 42:1118–1122.

183. Stuck AE, Frey BM, Frey FJ. Kinetics of prednisolone and endogenous cortisol suppression in the elderly. Clin Pharmacol Ther 1988; 43:354–362.

184. Armanini D, Scali M, Vittadello G, et al. Corticosteroid receptors and aging. J Steroid Biochem Mol Biol 1993; 45:191–194.

185. Armanini D, Karbowiak I, Scali M, et al. Corticosteroid receptors and lymphocyte subsets in mononuclear leukocytes in aging. Am J Physiol 1992; 262:E464–E466.

186. Thakur MK. Molecular mechanism of steroid hormone action during aging: A review. Mech Ageing Dev 1988; 45:93–110.

187. Saag KG, Koehnke R, Caldwell JR, et al. Low dose long-term corticosteroid therapy in rheumatoid arthritis: An analysis of serious adverse events. Am J Med 1994; 96:115–123.

188. Ellis EF. Adverse effects of corticosteroid therapy. J Allergy Clin Immunol 1987; 80:515–517.

189. Kwong FK, Sue MA, Klaustermeyer WB. Corticosteroid complications in respiratory disease. Ann Allergy 1987; 58:326–330.

190. Thomas TP. The complications of systemic corticosteroid therapy in the elderly: A retrospective study. Gerontology 1984; 30:60–65.

191. Riggs BL, Wahner HW, Seeman E, et al. Changes in bone mineral density of the proximal femur and spine with aging: Differences between the postmenopausal and senile osteoporosis syndromes. J Clin Invest 1982; 70:716–723.

192. Edwards BJ, Perry HM. Age-related osteoporosis. Clin Geriatr Med 1994; 10: 575–588.

193. Bohannon AD, Lyles KW. Drug-induced bone disease. Clin Geriatr Med 1994; 10: 611–623.

194. Joseph JC. Corticosteroid-induced osteoporosis. Am J Hosp Pharm 1994; 51: 188–197.

195. Toogood JH, Crilly RG, Jones G, et al. Effect of high-dose inhaled budesonide on calcium and phosphate metabolism and the risk of osteoporosis. Am Rev Respir Dis 1988; 138:57–61.

196. Crilly RG, Marshall DH, Nordin BE. Metabolic effects of corticosteroid therapy in post-menopausal women. J Steroid Biochem 1979; 11:429–433.

197. Dykman TR, Gluck OS, Murphy WA, et al. Evaluation of factors associated with glucocorticoid-induced osteopenia in patients with rheumatic diseases. Arthritis Rheum 1985; 28:361–368.

198. Ruegsegger P, Medici TC, Anliker M. Corticosteroid-induced bone loss: A longitudinal study of alternate date therapy in patients with bronchial asthma using quantitative computed tomography. Eur J Clin Pharmacol 1983; 25:615–620.

199. Lukert BP, Raisz LG. Glucocorticoid-induced osteoporosis: Pathogenesis and management. Ann Intern Med 1990; 112:352–364.

200. Gluck OS, Murphy WA, Hahn TJ, Hahn B. Bone loss in adults receiving alternate day glucocorticoid therapy: A comparison with daily therapy. Arthritis Rheum 1981; 24:892–898.

201. Toogood JH, Hodsman AB. Effects of inhaled and oral corticosteroids on bone (editorial). Ann Allergy 1991; 67:87–90.

202. Liberman UA, Weiss SR, Broll J, et al. Effect of oral alendronate on bone mineral density and the incidence of fractures in postmenopausal osteoporosis: The Alendronate Phase III Osteoporosis Treatment Study Group. N Engl J Med 1995; 333: 1437–1443.

203. Sambrook P, Birmingham J, Kelly P, et al. Prevention of corticosteroid osteoporosis: A comparison of calcium, calcitriol, and calcitonin. N Engl J Med 1993; 328: 1747–1752.

204. Worth H, Stammen D, Keck E. Therapy of steroid-induced bone loss in adult asthmatics with calcium, vitamin D, and a diphosphonate. Am J Respir Crit Care Med 1994; 150:394–397.

205. Meunier PJ. Is steroid-induced osteoporosis preventable (editorial)? N Engl J Med 1993; 328:1781–1782.

206. Haynes RC Jr. Adrenocorticotropic hormones, adrenocortical steroids and their synthetic analogs: Inhibitors of the synthesis and actions of adrenocortical hormones. In: Gilman AG, Rall TW, Nies AS, Taylor P, eds. The Pharmacological Basis of Therapeutics, 8th ed. New York: Pergamon Press, 1990:1431–1462.

207. Sato A, Funder JW, Okubo M, et al. Glucocorticoid-induced hypertension in the elderly. Relation to serum calcium and family history of essential hypertension. Am J Hypertens 1995; 8:823–828.

208. Urban RC Jr, Cotlier E. Corticosteroid-induced cataracts. Survey Ophthalmol 1986; 31:102–110.

209. Williamson J, Paterson RW, McGavin DD, et al. Posterior subcapsular cataracts and glaucoma associated with long-term oral corticosteroid therapy: In patients with rheumatoid arthritis and related conditions. Br J Ophthalmol 1969; 53:361–372.

210. David DS, Berkowitz JS. Ocular effects of topical and systemic corticosteroids. Lancet 1969; 2:149–151.

211. Rich LF. Ophthalmology. In: Cassel CK, Riesenberg DE, Sorensen LB, Walsh JR, eds. Geriatric Medicine, 2d ed. New York: Springer-Verlag, 1990:394–404.

212. Francois J. Corticosteroid glaucoma. Ann Ophthalmol 1977; 9:1075–1980.

213. Bourey RE, Kohrt WM. Kirwan JP, et al. Relationship between glucose tolerance and glucose-stimulated insulin response in 65-year-olds. J Gerontol 1993; 48:M122–M127.

214. Harris MI. Epidemiology of diabetes mellitus among the elderly in the United States. Clin Geriatr Med 1990; 6:703–719.

215. Watters JM, Moulton SB, Clancey SM. Aging exaggerates glucose intolerance following injury. J Trauma 1994; 37:786–791.

216. Caldwell JR, Furst DE. The efficacy and safety of low-dose corticosteroids for rheumatoid arthritis. Semin Arthritis Rheum 1991; 21:1–11.

217. Wiest PM, Flanigan T, Salata RA, et al. Serious infectious complications of corticosteroid therapy for COPD. Chest 1989; 95:1180–1184.

218. Stuck AE, Minder CE, Frey FJ. Risk of infectious complications in patients taking glucocorticosteroids. Rev Infect Dis 1989; 11:954–963.

219. Alhashimi MM, Citron ML, Fossieck BE Jr, et al. Lung cancer, tuberculin reactivity, and isoniazid. South Med J 1988; 81:337–340.

220. Schatz M, Patterson R, Kloner R, Falk J. The prevalence of tuberculosis and positive tuberculin skin tests in a steroid-treated asthmatic population. Ann Intern Med 1976; 84:261–265.

221. Forbes GB, Halloran E. The adult decline in lean body mass. Hum Biol 1976; 48:162–173.

222. Dardevet D, Sornet C, Taillandier D, et al. Sensitivity and protein turnover response to glucocorticoids are different in skeletal muscle from adult and old rats: Lack of regulation of the ubiquitin-proteasome proteolytic pathway in aging. J Clin Invest 1995; 96:2113–2119.

223. Danneskiold-Samsoe B, Grimby G. The relationship between the leg muscle strength and physical capacity in patients with rheumatoid arthritis, with reference to the influence of corticosteroids. Clin Rheumatol 1986; 5:468–474.

224. Decramer M, Lacquet LM, Fagard R, Rogiers P. Corticosteroids contribute to muscle weakness in chronic airflow obstruction. Am J Respir Crit Care Med 1994; 150: 11–16.

225. Decramer M, Stas KJ. Corticosteroid-induced myopathy involving respiratory muscles in patients with chronic obstructive pulmonary disease or asthma. Am Rev Respir Dis 1992; 146:800–802.

226. Picado C, Fiz JA, Montserrat JM, et al. Respiratory and skeletal muscle function in steroid-dependent bronchial asthma. Am Rev Respir Dis 1990; 141:14–20.

227. Danielson DA, Porter JB, Lawson DH, et al. Drug-associated psychiatric disturbances in medical inpatients. Psychopharmacology 1981; 74:105–108.

228. Wood KA, Harris MJ, Morreale A, Rizos AL. Drug-induced psychosis and depression in the elderly. Psychiat Clin North Am 198; 11:167–193.

229. Kaufmann M, Kahaner K, Peselow ED, Gershon S. Steroid psychoses: Case report and brief overview. J Clin Psychiatry 1982; 43:75–76.

230. Hall RC, Popkin MK, Stickney SK, Gardner ER. Presentation of the steroid psychoses. J Nerv Men Dis 1979; 167:229–236.

231. Koenig HG, Blazer DG. Depression and other affective disorders. In: Cassel CK, Riesenberg DE, Sorensen LB, Walsh JR, eds. Geriatric Medicine, 2d ed. New York: Springer-Verlag, 1990:473–490.

232. Mitchell DM, Collins JV. Do corticosteroids really alter mood? Postgrad Med J 1984; 60:467–470.

233. Toogood JH. High-dose inhaled steroid therapy for asthma. J Allergy Clin Immunol 1989; 83:528–536.

234. Noonan M, Chervinsky P, Busse WW, et al. Fluticasone propionate reduces oral prednisone use while it improves asthma control and quality of life. Am J Respir Crit Care Med 1995; 152:1467–1473.

235. Lacronique J, Renon D, Georges D, et al. High-dose beclomethasone: oral steroid-sparing effect in severe asthmatic patients. Eur Respir J 1991; 4:807–812.

236. Jenkins CR, Woolcock AJ. Effect of prednisone and beclomethasone dipropionate on airway responsiveness in asthma: A comparative study. Thorax 1988; 43: 378–384.

237. Haahtela T, Jarvinen M, Kava T, et al. Comparison of a beta 2-agonist, terbutaline, with an inhaled corticosteroid, budesonide, in newly detected asthma. N Engl J Med 1991; 325:388–392.

238. Haahtela T, Jarvinen M, Kava T, et al. Effects of reducing or discontinuing inhaled budesonide in patients with mild asthma. N Engl J Med 1994; 331:700–705.

239. Ernst P, Spitzer WO, Suissa S, et al. Risk of fatal and near-fatal asthma in relation to inhaled corticosteroid use. JAMA 1992; 268:3462–3464.

240. Szefler SJ. Glucocorticoid therapy for asthma: Clinical pharmacology. J Allergy Clin Immunol 1991; 88:147–165.

241. Toogood JH. Complications of topical steroid therapy for asthma. Am Rev Respir Dis 1990; 141:S89–S96.

242. Barnes PJ. Inhaled glucocorticoids for asthma. N Engl J Med 1995; 332:868–875.

243. Lipworth BJ. Clinical pharmacology of corticosteroids in bronchial asthma. Pharmacol Ther 1993; 58:173–209.

244. Harding SM. The human pharmacology of fluticasone propionate. Respir Med 1990; 84(suppl A):25–29.

245. Meltzer EO, Kemp JP, Welch MJ, Orgel HA. Effect of dosing schedule on efficacy of beclomethasone dipropionate aerosol in chronic asthma. Am Rev Respir Dis 1985; 131:732–736.

246. Murray MD, Birt JA, Manatunga AK, Darnell JC. Medication compliance in elderly outpatients using twice-daily dosing and unit-of-use packaging. Ann Pharmacother 1993; 27:616–621.

247. Geddes DM. Inhaled corticosteroids: benefits and risks (editorial). Thorax 1992; 47:404–407.

248. Ebden P, McNally P, Samanta A, Fancourt GJ. The effects of high dose inhaled beclomethasone dipropionate on glucose and lipid profiles in normal and diet controlled diabetic subjects. Respir Med 1989; 83:289–291.

249. Robinson DS, Geddes DM. Inhaled corticosteroids: Benefits and risks. J Asthma 1996; 33:5–16.

250. Toogood JH. Inhaled glucocorticoids—Benefits and risks. In: Szefler SJ, Leung DYM, eds. Severe Asthma: Pathogenesis and Clinical Management. New York: Marcel Dekker, 1996:207–242.

251. Hodsman AB, Toogood JH, Jennings B, et al. Differential effects of inhaled budesonide and oral prednisolone on serum osteocalcin. J Clin Endocrinol Metab 1991; 72:530–540.

252. Ali NJ, Capewell S, Ward MJ. Bone turnover during high dose inhaled corticosteroid treatment. Thorax 1991; 46:160–164.

253. Packe GE, Douglas JG, McDonald AF, et al. Bone density in asthmatic patients taking high dose inhaled beclomethasone dipropionate and intermittent systemic corticosteroids. Thorax 1992; 47:414–417.

254. Jennings BH, Andersson KE, Johansson SA. Assessment of systemic effects of inhaled glucocorticosteroids: Comparison of the effects of inhaled budesonide and oral prednisolone on adrenal function and markers of bone turnover. Eur J Clin Pharmacol 1991; 40:77–82.

255. Puolijoki H, Liippo K, Herrala J, et al. Inhaled beclomethasone decreases serum osteocalcin in postmenopausal asthmatic women. Bone 1992; 13:285–288.

256. Toogood JH, Baskerville JC, Markov AE, et al. Bone mineral density and the risk of fracture in patients receiving long-term inhaled steroid therapy for asthma. J Allergy Clin Immunol 1995; 96:157–166.

257. Mak VH, Melchor R, Spiro SG. Easy bruising as a side-effect of inhaled corticosteroids. Eur Respir J 1992; 5:1068–1074.

258. Capewell S, Reynolds S, Shuttleworth D, et al. Purpura and dermal thinning associated with high dose inhaled corticosteroids. Br Med J 1990; 300:1548–1551.

259. Fraunfelder FT, Meyer SM. Posterior subcapsular cataracts associated with nasal or inhalation corticosteroids. Am J Ophthalmol 1990; 109:489–490.

260. Kewley GD. Possible association between beclomethasone dipropionate aerosol and cataracts. Aus Paediatr J 1980; 16:117–118.

261. Greening AP, Ind PW, Northfield M, Shaw G. Added salmeterol versus higher-dose corticosteroid in asthma patients with symptoms on existing inhaled corticosteroid: Allen & Hanburys Limited UK Study Group. Lancet 1994; 344:219–224.

262. Wasserman SI, Furukawa CT, Henochowicz SI, et al. Asthma symptoms and airway hyperresponsiveness are lower during treatment with nedocromil sodium than during treatment with regular inhaled albuterol. J Allergy Clin Immunol 1995; 95:541–547.

263. Barnes PJ. Effect of nedocromil sodium on platelet-activating factor-induced airway responses. J Allergy Clin Immunol 1993; 92:187–189.

264. Pelikan Z, Knottnerus I. Inhibition of the late asthmatic response by nedocromil sodium administered more than two hours after allergen challenge. J Allergy Clin Immunol 1993; 92:19–28.

265. Bernstein IL. Cromolyn sodium in the treatment of asthma: Coming of age in the United States. J Allergy Clin Immunol 1985; 76:381–388.

266. Warringa RA, Mengelers HJ, Maikoe T, et al. Inhibition of cytokine-primed eosinophil chemotaxis by nedocromil sodium. J Allergy Clin Immunol 1993; 91:802–809.

267. Pearce FL. Effect of nedocromil sodium on mediator release from mast cells. J Allergy Clin Immunol 1993; 92:155–158.

268. Joseph M, Tsicopoulos A, Tonnel AB, Capron A. Modulation by nedocromil sodium of immunologic and nonimmunologic activation of monocytes, macrophages, and platelets. J Allergy Clin Immunol 1993; 92:165–170.

269. Bruijnzeel PL, Warringa RA, Kok PT, et al. Effects of nedocromil sodium on in vitro induced migration, activation, and mediator release from human granulocytes. J Allergy Clin Immunol 1993; 92:159–164.

270. Mekori YA, Baram D, Goldberg A, et al. Nedocromil sodium inhibits T-cell function in vitro and in vivo. J Allergy Clin Immunol 1993; 91:817–824.

271. Barnes PJ. Effect of nedocromil sodium on airway sensory nerves. J Allergy Clin Immunol 1993; 92:182–186.

272. Loh RK, Jabara HH, Geha RS. Mechanisms of inhibition of IgE synthesis by nedocromil sodium: Nedocromil sodium inhibits deletional switch recombination in human B cells. J Allergy Clin Immunol 1996; 97:1141–1150.

273. Cockcroft DW, McParland CP, O'Byrne PM, et al. Beclomethasone given after the early asthmatic response inhibits the late response and the increased methacholine responsiveness and cromolyn does not. J Allergy Clin Immunol 1993; 91:1163–1168.

274. Harper GD, Neill P, Vathenen AS, et al. A comparison of inhaled beclomethasone dipropionate and nedocromil sodium as additional therapy in asthma. Respir Med 1990; 84:463–469.

275. Bel EH, Timmers MC, Hermans J, et al. The long-term effects of nedocromil sodium and beclomethasone dipropionate on bronchial responsiveness to methacholine in nonatopic asthmatic subjects. Am Rev Respir Dis 1990; 141:21–28.

276. Cockcroft DW, Murdock KY. Comparative effects of inhaled salbutamol, sodium cromoglycate, and beclomethasone dipropionate on allergen-induced early asthmatic responses, late asthmatic responses, and increased bronchial responsiveness to histamine. J Allergy Clin Immunol 1987; 79:734–740.

277. Wasserman SI. A review of some recent clinical studies with nedocromil sodium. J Allergy Clin Immunol 1993; 92:210–215.

278. Marin JM, Carrizo SJ, Garcia R, Ejea MV. Effects of nedocromil sodium in steroid-resistant asthma: A randomized controlled trial. J Allergy Clin Immunol 1996; 97:602–610.

279. Creticos P, Burk J, Smith L, et al. The use of twice daily nedocromil sodium in the treatment of asthma. J Allergy Clin Immunol 1995; 95:829–836.

280. Wong CS, Cooper S, Britton JR, Tattersfield AE. Steroid sparing effect of nedocromil sodium in asthmatic patients on high doses of inhaled steroids. Clin Exp Allergy 1993; 23:370–376.

281. Boulet LP, Cartier A, Cockcroft DW, et al. Tolerance to reduction of oral steroid dosage in severely asthmatic patients receiving nedocromil soldium. Respir Med 1990; 84:317–323.

282. Goldin JG, Bateman ED. Does nedocromil sodium have a steroid sparing effect in adult asthmatic patients requiring maintenance oral corticosteroids? Thorax 1988; 43:982–986.
283. Jarjor N, Gelfand E, McGill K, Busse WW. Alternative anti-inflammatory and immunomodulatory therapy. In: Szefler SJ, Leung DYM, eds. Severe Asthma: Pathogenesis and Clinical Management. New York: Marcel Dekker, 1996:333–369.
284. Mullarkey MF, Lammert JK, Blumenstein BA. Long-term methotrexate treatment in corticosteroid-dependent asthma. Ann Intern Med 1990; 112:577–581.
285. Mullarkey MF, Blumenstein BA, Andrade WP, et al. Methotrexate in the treatment of corticosteroid-dependent asthma: A double-blind crossover study. N Engl J Med 1988; 318:603–607.
286. Shiner RJ, Katz I, Shulimzon T, et al. Methotrexate in steroid-dependent asthma: Long-term results. Allergy 1994; 49:565–568.
287. Coffey MJ, Sanders G, Eschenbacher WL, et al. The role of methotrexate in the management of steroid-dependent asthma. Chest 1994; 105:117–121.
288. Dyer PD, Vaughan TR, Weber RW. Methotrexate in the treatment of steroid-dependent asthma. J Allergy Clin Immunol 1991; 88:208–212.
289. Erzurum SC, Leff JA, Cochran JE, et al. Lack of benefit of methotrexate in severe, steroid-dependent asthma: A double-blind, placebo-controlled study. Ann Intern Med 1991; 114:353–360.
290. Shiner RJ, Nunn AJ, Chung KF, Geddes DM. Randomised, double-blind, placebo-controlled trial of methotrexate in steroid-dependent asthma. Lancet 1990; 336: 137–140.
291. Henderson WR Jr. The role of leukotrienes in inflammation. Ann Intern Med 1994; 121:684–697.
292. Meltzer SS, Hasday JD, Cohn J, Bleecker ER. Inhibition of exercise-induced bronchospasm by zileuton: a 5-lipoxygenase inhibitor. Am J Respir Crit Care Med 1996; 153:931–935.
293. Israel E, Fischer AR, Rosenberg MA, et al. The pivotal role of 5-lipoxygenase products in the reaction of aspirin-sensitive asthmatics to aspirin. Am Rev Respir Dis 1993; 148:1447–1451.
294. Findlay SR, Barden JM, Easley CB, Glass M. Effect of the oral leukotriene antagonist, ICI 204,219, on antigen-induced bronchoconstriction in subjects with asthma. J Allergy Clin Immunol 1992; 89:1040–1045.
295. Israel E, Dermarkarian R, Rosenberg M, et al. The effects of a 5-lipoxygenase inhibitor on asthma induced by cold, dry air. N Engl J Med 1990; 323:1740–1744.
296. Spector SL, Smith LJ, Glass M. Effects of 6 weeks of therapy with oral doses of ICI 204,219, a leukotriene D4 receptor antagonist, in subjects with bronchial asthma: ACCOLATE Asthma Trialists Group. Am J Respir Crit Care Med 1994; 150: 618–623.
297. Hui KP, Barnes NC. Lung function improvement in asthma with a cysteinyl-leukotriene receptor antagonist. Lancet 1991; 337:1062–1063.
298. Connolly MJ, Crowley JJ, Charan NB, et al. Reduced subjective awareness of bronchoconstriction provoked by methacholine in elderly asthmatic and normal subjects as measured on a simple awareness scale. Thorax 1992; 47:410–413.
299. Diggory P, Heyworth P, Chau G, et al. Improved lung function tests on changing

from topical timolol: Non-selective beta-blockade impairs lung function tests in elderly patients. Eye 1993; 7:661–663.

300. Munroe WP, Rindone JP, Kershner RM. Systemic side effects associated with the ophthalmic administration of timolol. Drug Intell Clin Pharm 1985; 19:85–89.

301. Vuori ML, Kaila T. Plasma kinetics and antagonist activity of topical ocular timolol in elderly patients. Graefes Arch Clin Exp Ophthalmol 1995; 233:131–134.

302. Diggory P, Cassels-Brown A, Vail A, et al. Avoiding unsuspected respiratory side-effects of topical timolol with cardioselective or sympathomimetic agents. Lancet 1995; 345:1604–1606.

303. Diggory P, Heyworth P, Chau G, et al. Unsuspected bronchospasm in association with topical timolol—a common problem in elderly people: Can we easily identify those affected and do cardioselective agents lead to improvement? Age Ageing 1994; 23:17–21.

304. Insel PA. Analgesic-antipyretics and anti-inflammatory agents: Drugs employed in the treatment of rheumatoid arthritis and gout. In: Gillman AG, Rall TW, Nies AS, Taylor P, eds. The Pharmacological Basis of Therapeutics, 8th ed. New York: Pergamon Press, 1990:638–681.

305. Cassel CK, Brody JA. Demography, epidemiology, and aging. In: Cassel CK, Riesenberg DE, Sorensen LB, Walsh JR, eds. Geriatric Medicine, 2d ed. New York: Springer-Verlag, 1990:16–27.

306. Pearson MG. Asthma guidelines: who is guiding whom and where to (editorial)? Thorax 1993; 48:197–198.

307. Petty TL, Rollins DR, Christopher K, et al. Cromolyn sodium is effective in adult chronic asthmatics. Am Rev Respir Dis 1989; 139:694–701.

308. Robin ED. Death from bronchial asthma. Chest 1988; 93:614–618.

309. Buist AS. Is asthma mortality increasing (editorial)? Chest 1988; 93:449–450.

310. Sly RM. Increases in deaths from asthma. Ann Allergy 1984; 53:20–25.

8

Management of Acute Exacerbations in the Elderly Asthmatic

SUSAN K. PINGLETON

University of Kansas Medical Center
Kansas City, Kansas

I. Introduction

Fundamentals of asthma management at any age include knowledge of and expertise in pathophysiology, common etiologies, as well as diagnosis and treatment of the basic disease. Likewise basic goals of asthma management include maintenance of normal pulmonary function and return to baseline function whenever exacerbations of the disease occur. These fundamentals and basic goals are not different in the elderly as compared with the younger asthma patient. However, aspects of care of elderly asthmatics may differ because of their age and its associated effects. This chapter reviews management issues when acute exacerbations of asthma occur in elderly asthmatics, taking into account those areas of care that are common to all asthmatics as well as those that differ from the care of the younger asthmatic.

The term elderly in the context of this chapter includes patients aged 65 or older, while recognizing that a precise definition may be somewhat arbitrary. Pathophysiology, etiology, differential diagnosis, and assessment of an exacerbation in the elderly asthmatic are addressed. Management is discussed in relation to routine office or emergency department care as well as the inpatient and intensive care unit for those with acute respiratory failure.

II. Pathophysiology

Bronchial asthma is classically defined as recurrent episodes of airflow obstruction that are usually reversible either spontaneously or with appropriate treatment (1). In elderly patients, however, incomplete reversibility is more common. Nevertheless, airflow limitation results in symptoms of breathlessness or wheezing. An important pathogenetic component of airflow limitation is airway hyperresponsiveness. One primary mechanism of airway hyperresponsiveness is airway inflammation.

Airway inflammation is described pathologically by mucosal infiltration by eosinophils, mast cell degranulation, and epithelial damage. These changes are found in bronchial biopsies even in mild asthma (2,3). Eosinophilic bronchitis is characterized by pronounced areas of mucosal edema, epithelial desquamation, and thickening beneath the basement membrane as well as by hypertrophy and hyperplasia of the bronchial smooth muscle. Macroscopically, the lung in severe asthma is hyperinflated, with thick tenacious mucus filling the airways (4).

The causes of airway inflammation are multiple. Inhaled allergens, pollutants, smoke, and viral infections all may play a role in establishing or augmenting airway inflammation (5–7). In patients with allergy as an etiology, exposure to the inciting allergen causes inflammation by binding to IgE on the mast cells, with the subsequent release of inflammatory mediators such as histamine, platelet activating factor, leukotrienes, and thromboxanes (5). Other inflammatory cells such as eosinophils are attracted to the airway by these mediators, resulting in further inflammation. Inflammatory mediators alter smooth muscle cell function, cause microvascular leakage, participate in neural regulation of the airways, and stimulate glands to secrete. Histamine in particular causes bronchial smooth muscle contraction, vasodilation and increased permeability of pulmonary vessels, as well as enhanced production of mucus. Eosinophils release cell toxins that cause epithelial cell damage.

Multiple causes of airways obstruction, including airways inflammation, are found in asthma. Smooth muscle contraction, mucosal edema, and airways narrowing by intraluminal mucus all contribute to the obstruction that is the primary feature of asthma. Another consequence of airways inflammation is bronchial hyperreactivity, the hallmark of asthma and the basis for methacholine challenge testing (8). Inflammatory mediator release causes the airways smooth muscle to be abnormally sensitive to contractile stimuli such as inhaled allergens, smoke, pollutants, cold air, exercise, dusts, and irritant fumes. These stimuli result in the contraction of airways smooth muscle, narrowing of airway caliber, and increased obstruction to expiratory airflow. Airways smooth muscle contraction is generally rapidly reversed by beta-adrenergic stimulation. However, reversing the underlying state of bronchial hyperreactivity is achieved more slowly with anti-inflammatory therapy in the form of corticosteroids or cromolyn. The airways edema and inflammation that cause the underlying bronchial hyperreactivity are not readily reversed with beta-adrenergic therapy and therefore require anti-inflammatory treatment.

The pathophysiology of asthma in the elderly patient does not appreciably differ from that of the younger patient. Smooth muscle hypertrophy, bronchial gland hyperplasia, and mucus plugging—common findings in all patients with asthma—were found in six elderly asthmatics dying of other causes (9). These pathological changes, however, were not more pronounced in the elderly as compared with controls.

Physiological changes do, however, occur with aging. Some sympathetic and parasympathetic nervous system functions diminish with age, consistent with the general diminution of peripheral somatic nerve function (10). The protective laryngeal gag reflex appears diminished in elderly subjects, although the cough reflex is probably not affected (11,12). Cholinergic bronchoconstricting reflexes, such as bronchial reactivity to methacholine, are not lessened and indeed may be increased with age (13). Beta-receptor function or number does appear to diminish with age as response to beta agonists is lessened (14). The response to anticholinergic therapy is not affected by age; thus anticholinergics should be strongly considered in bronchodilator therapy in the aged. Elderly asthmatic patients may also have a decreased subjective awareness of moderate acute bronchial obstruction. In elderly asthmatics greater than 60 years old, awareness scores were significantly less despite greater bronchoconstriction than in young normal subjects (15). The precise influence of age alone has not yet been determined, as young asthmatics with a history of near fatal asthma have also been shown to exhibit diminished subjective awareness of increased bronchoconstriction as compared with normals (16).

Atopy is also an age-related phenomenon. The peak prevalence of immediate skin-test reactivity occurs during the third decade and falls dramatically after age 50 (17). The significance of atopy in the pathogenesis of asthma in the elderly is controversial. None of 25 nonsmoking elderly asthmatics had immediate skin-test positivity as compared with elderly controls (18). When these 25 patients were divided into groups with early-onset and late-onset asthma, more differences were apparent. Of early-onset asthmatics (mean age 42 years), 63% reported some form of symptoms of eczema or seasonal allergic rhinitis, while none of the late-onset asthmatic patients had this history. In contrast, positive allergy skin-test reactivity and blood eosinophilia were found to be high risk factors for asthma in patients greater than 60 years old (19). Although this issue may be somewhat contentious, it appears that a small percentage of elderly patients may have either a history of allergies or positive skin-test reactivity. Nevertheless, it is rare to find clinical provocation of asthma by aeroallergens to be a dominant feature in this age group.

The pathophysiological sequence of events in asthma is similar for both elderly and younger patients. Airways inflammation from whatever cause leads to airways narrowing, obstruction to expiratory airflow, increased airways resistance, hyperinflation, and therefore increased work of breathing, causing the symptom of dyspnea. Classically, this sequence of pathophysiological events is thought to be reversible either spontaneously or with treatment (1). Several difficulties exist with this definition in the elderly asthmatic. Asthma, chronic bronchitis, and emphysema share similar features of expiratory airflow obstruction, making clinical distinction at times difficult despite the different pathophysiology and natural history (20). Some patients with chronic bronchitis show partial reversibility of airflow obstruction after treatment. Likewise, long-standing asthma in the elderly may be associated with fixed airflow obstruction even after maximum therapeutic intervention with bronchodilators and corticosteriods. Percent predicted FEV_1 (forced expiratory volume in 1 sec) was 58% in long-standing elderly asthmatics compared to 75% in patients with asthma for less than 5 years (18). Airways hyperreactivity may be increased due to smoking or age alone. Smoking history is not uncommon in elderly patients, thus making the distinction of persistent asthma from chronic obstructive pulmonary disease (COPD) difficult. Elderly asthmatics may have relatively low ventilatory function throughout life but can have increasing symptoms associated with an accelerated loss of function that leads them to seek medical care (19). These variations of asthma in the elderly are important to understand, as they influence the therapeutic approach, especially during acute exacerbations.

III. Etiology of Acute Exacerbation

As in younger asthmatics, multiple etiologies can cause an acute exacerbation in the elderly (Table 1). Although allergy and/or an allergic diathesis in the form of eczema or rhinitis can accompany asthma in the elderly, aeroallergens are probably less important in causing asthma symptoms (18). The most important provocative factors include viral respiratory infections, irritants such as cigarette smoke, paints, varnish, and household aerosols, as well as pharmacological agents that are often prescribed for concomitant illnesses. Other drugs and disease may also precipitate asthma in the elderly. Beta-adrenoreceptor antagonists (beta blockers) commonly used for hypertension and ischemic heart disease in the elderly may precipitate bronchospasm (21). These include both noncardioselective (propranolol, pindolol, and timolol) and, to a lesser degree, cardioselective agents (metoprolol and acebutolol) (22). Although topical beta blockers used for wide-angle glaucoma are thought to be less risky, systemic absorption can occur and result in an asthma exacerbation (23). Arthritis often coexists with asthma in the elderly. Drug treatment for arthritis, with aspirin and other nonsteroidal anti-inflammatory agents (NSAIDs), may precipitate an asthma exacerbation in susceptible asthmatics. Gastroesophageal reflux can also increase or precipitate

Table 1 Etiology of Acute Asthma
Exacerbation in the Elderly

Viral respiratory infection
Irritants (smoke, paints, household aerosols)
Aeroallergens
Pharmacological agents
  Beta blockers
  Nonsteroidal anti-inflammatory agents
Gastroesophageal reflux

asthma symptoms in the elderly. The association of gastroesophageal reflux and asthma increases with age (24).

IV. Differential Diagnosis

Symptoms of an acute exacerbation of asthma are not different in the elderly than in younger patients. Dyspnea, wheezing, cough, and chest tightness are common symptoms. Despite the commonality of symptoms, the subjective response to bronchoconstriction may be diminished in elderly patients (15). For a given level of physiological bronchoconstriction, an elderly asthmatic may not complain of dyspnea to the same degree as a younger patient. Associated symptoms of an exacerbation may include rhinitis, sinusitis, sputum production, or atopic dermatitis.

Physicians caring for elderly asthmatic should focus on two important issues regarding the assessment (25). First, other diseases causing the well-known symptoms of asthma are common in the elderly. Congestive heart failure, for example, may produce symptoms identical to those of asthma and therefore may be particularly difficult to distinguish in an elderly patient with known risk factors for heart disease. Indeed, in the past, symptoms of heart failure mimicking asthma have been described as "cardiac asthma." Thus, symptoms of chest tightness and nocturnal dyspnea may be present in both congestive heart failure and asthma. The timing of nocturnal dyspnea may be helpful in distinguishing etiology. Symptoms associated with asthma usually occur between the hours of 4 and 6 A.M., while those associated with congestive heart failure usually occur 1–2 hr after retiring. Cardiac abnormalities on physical examination and radiographic changes in the cardiac silhouette and lung fields distinguish congestive heart failure from asthma in many instances. Signs and symptoms that are more likely to indicate cardiac disease include lower extremity edema, neck vein distention, gallop rhythm, inspiratory crackles, and vascular congestion on the chest radiograph. At other times specific tests of cardiac function are required to assess left ventricular function.

One of the most difficult diseases to differentiate from asthma in the elderly is COPD. Several signs and symptoms help distinguish one disease from the other. Chronic cough and sputum production are typical for chronic bronchitis, but they can occur in some patients with asthma. Cyanosis, ankle edema, and distended neck veins indicate right heart failure as a result of cor pulmonale from chronic bronchitis. Marked weight loss, spontaneous pursed-lip breathing, hyperinflation, radiographic bullous changes, and a quiet chest on auscultation characterize emphysema. Dyspnea can be exertional or nonexertional in both asthma and chronic bronchitis, although the acute development of dyspnea and bronchospasm suggest the diagnosis of asthma.

Acute pulmonary thromboembolism can also masquerade as an exacerbation of asthma. Chest pain, dyspnea, wheezing, and hypoxemia are also seen in asthma exacerbation, as are pulmonary thromboemboli. Pleuritic chest pain and radiographic pleural effusions are rare in asthma. Pulmonary emboli can cause similar symptoms as asthma because the mediators released by platelets in thromboemboli cause bronchoconstriction and wheezing. Many elderly patients may be at increased risk for lower extremity thrombosis because of diminished activity levels. Radiographic assessment of the deep venous system as well as ventilation/perfusion examination may be required.

Foreign body aspiration results in wheezing, although typically the wheezing is localized rather than diffuse. Factors contributing to aspiration in the elderly are a diminished gag reflex and diminished mental status caused by sedatives, alcohol, and neuropsychiatric disorders.

Inspiratory wheezing (stridor) is sometimes confused with asthma. Encroaching tumors, vocal cord paralysis, and thyroid enlargement also produce airflow obstruction and wheezing. Due to the extrathoracic location of these conditions, inspiratory obstruction is common and causes stridor in some patients.

As many elderly patients have hypertension and/or coronary artery disease, treatment with beta blockers and angiotensin converting enzyme (ACE) inhibitors is common. Cough and at times wheezing may be associated with these drugs. Older patients with asthma appear to run a similar risk from beta-blocking drugs as younger patients with these conditions, although there are no direct comparisons.

Gastroesophageal reflux can increase symptoms of asthma. In the elderly person with frequent exacerbations who is unusually resistant to routine therapy, and who has heartburn, cough, and nocturnal symptoms that occur early in the night, gastroesophageal reflux should be considered.

V. Assessment

Assessment of asthma involves combining evaluations of symptoms and physical findings, in conjunction with measurements of lung function, to yield a useful

Table 2 Historical and Physical Examination Features Suggestive of Severe Asthma

History
  Severe dyspnea
  Frequent or recent emergency department visits or hospitalization for asthma
  Current or recent use of corticosteroids
  History of syncope or seizure during prior asthma exacerbation
Physical examination
  Tachypnea, tachycardia, diaphoresis
  Pulsus paradoxus
  Use of accessory muscles of inspiration
  Respiratory muscle fatigue
    Respiratory alternans
    Abdominal paradox
    Depressed mental status

characterization of the severity of the illness. Assessment of an acute asthmatic exacerbation in patients of any age requires knowledge of the historical and physical details suggesting that a patient is at high risk for severe, life-threatening obstruction. Little specific data are available for elderly asthmatics in exacerbation. For purposes of this discussion, however, it may be assumed that there are no essential differences in determining high-risk disease between elderly patients and younger patients with asthma (26) (Table 2). It should be noted that while definitions for high-risk asthma may not be different, elderly patients would be expected to tolerate severe physiological disturbances less well than younger patients. Elderly patients are more likely to have comorbid conditions—such as cardiac disease, obesity, or neurological disease—that limit pulmonary reserve.

The severity of an acute exacerbation of asthma is often underestimated by patients, their relatives, and sometimes their health care professionals. It is important to recognize that any patient with asthma may have an acute, severe asthma exacerbation. To avoid the complications and the consequences of acute, severe asthma, an approach to assessment should include historical details, physical findings, laboratory tests of lung function, and gas exchange.

Patient complaints of severe breathlessness, chest tightness, or difficulty in walking more than 100 ft suggest severe asthmatic obstruction (27). Prior endotracheal intubation for asthma, frequent or recent emergency department visits or hospitalizations for asthma, current or recent use of systemic corticosteroids, and a history of syncope or seizure during prior asthma exacerbations should suggest the patient's tendency to severe airflow obstruction (28).

The physical examination is important for excluding other causes of dyspnea and wheezing as well as assessing the degree of airway obstruction. Tachycardia (>120 beats per min), tachypnea (>30 breaths per min), diaphoresis, bolt upright posture in bed, pulsus paradoxus greater than 10 mmHg, and accessory muscle use should all be regarded as signs of severe airways obstruction (29). The absence of these signs does not rule out severe asthma, and the physical examination should not be relied upon exclusively to assess the degree of airflow obstruction. Wheezing, for example, is not only a function of airways obstruction but also of the volume of air exhaled. Patients with severe obstruction and hyperinflation may have minimal wheezing on auscultation (30). Relief of symptoms may not correlate with significant increase in pulmonary function tests. Cyanosis is a very late and insensitive marker of hypoxemia. Respiratory alternans, abdominal paradox, and depressed mental status are ominous indicators of muscle fatigue and often herald the necessity for consideration of intubation and mechanical ventilation (31).

An objective measure of airflow obstruction is required in all acute exacerbations of asthma (27). Symptoms or physical findings alone are not reliable indicators of the degree of airflow obstruction (30). Pulmonary function tests such as the peak expiratory flow rate (PEFR) or forced FEV_1 are equally good bedside tools for evaluation. These tests are necessary not only for diagnostic evaluation but also to objectively follow treatment response. In some elderly patients, age-related factors such as increased rigidity of the chest wall or muscle weakness may more easily affect measurement of peak flows. Generally tests of < 40% predicted PEFR or FEV_1 indicate severe obstruction. Improvement of diminished PEFR to >70% of baseline likewise indicates significant reversibility (27,32). While these are generally accepted signs of reversibility, elderly asthmatics are recognized to have less reversibility with treatment or a persistent degree of airflow obstruction even with optimal treatment (19).

Arterial blood gas analysis is important for diagnosing and managing acute asthma in those cases where the assessment suggests severe airflow obstruction (33). Also, arterial blood gas levels aid in the management of severely obstructed patients because the degree of hypoxemia and hypercapnia is important in deciding when to institute mechanical ventilation. Changes in arterial blood gases, especially the $Paco_2$, correlate with the degree of airflow obstruction and are important for recognizing a deteriorating clinical course (Table 3) (34). With modest airways obstruction, dyspnea develops, resulting in a stimulation of minute ventilation and a mild drop in the $Paco_2$ (stage 1). As airways obstruction worsens, dyspnea is more severe and minute ventilation increases further. At this stage, patients with moderate to severe obstruction have lower than normal $Paco_2$ and respiratory alkalosis (stage 2). As airways obstruction becomes even more severe or prolonged enough to cause fatigue of the respiratory muscles, high minute ventilation can no longer be maintained and alveolar ventilation decreases. The $Paco_2$ rises to normal levels (stage 3) or exceeds normal levels (stage 4). A normal or high $Paco_2$ in a patient with severe airways obstruction signifies fatigue,

Table 3 Arterial Blood Gas Analysis in Severe Asthma

Stage of asthma	Pa_{O_2}	Pa_{CO_2}	pH
I. Mild	↓	↓	↑
II. Moderate	↓	↓↓	↑↑
III. Severe	↓↓	Normal	Normal
IV. Very severe	↓↓	↑	↓

impending respiratory failure, and a need for prompt attention. Any other associated condition (malnutrition, advanced age) resulting in deconditioning or muscle fatigue can lead to hypercapnic respiratory failure with a lesser degree of airways obstruction (35). Elderly patients would be expected to have a lower arterial oxygen gas tension secondary to their advancing age.

Other laboratory tests that are important in elderly patients include the chest radiograph and the electrocardiogram. Chest radiography is useful primarily to include or exclude other causes of symptoms (36). For example, radiographic evidence suggestive of pneumonia, congestive heart failure, or pulmonary emboli would lead to changes in diagnostic and therapeutic plans. In addition, chest radiography allows for the early detection of some complications of severe asthma, including pneumothorax, pneumomediastinum, and atelectasis. An electrocardiogram should always be performed in an elderly patient with severe asthma exacerbation or hypoxemia. Cardiac disease as a cause of symptoms should be excluded. Likewise, hypoxemia due to severe asthma can cause myocardial ischemia or infarction. Sinus tachycardia is common during acute exacerbations (37). Other less common findings include right axis deviation, P pulmonale, S-T wave abnormalities, right bundle branch block, and ventricular ectopic beats, the etiology of which may be very difficult to ascribe to asthma in the setting of the elderly patient with coronary artery or chronic obstructive pulmonary disease (38).

VI. Management

A. General Principles

The National Asthma Education and Prevention Program (NAEPP) of the National Heart, Lung and Blood Institute recently published guidelines for the assessment and management of patients with chronic asthma and acute exacerbation of asthma (27). Even more recently, the Global Initiatives for Asthma (GINA) guidelines were also published (39). Initial management in either scenario is based on the physician's assessment of the degree of airways obstruction. General treatment principles are based on diagnosis of mild, moderate, or severe asthma with the NAEPP guidelines or intermittent, mild, moderate, or severe persistent asthma in the GINA guidelines. While elderly asthmatics may fit into any of the criteria, the data do suggest that many suffer from severe persistent asthma, where continuous symptoms and frequent exacerbations are common (18). Fixed airways obstruction is also common, thereby requiring continuous treatment programs to control the disease. Thus an exacerbation in many elderly asthmatics has the potential to be more severe in that moderate to severe fixed airways obstruction is a chronic baseline from which further deterioration is likely to cause severe symptoms and physiological derangements.

As many elderly asthmatics have severe asthma chronically, they often require complicated and frequent dosing with multiple expensive drugs, often with significant toxicity. This can lead to a significant degree of noncompliance. Attempts to identify specific risk factors for noncompliance, however, have failed (40). Elderly asthmatics also frequently live alone, producing an additional barrier to appropriate care. Such patients may also suffer from inadequate nutrition and lack of immediate physical and emotional comfort. Finally, older patients with asthma may deteriorate for longer periods of time before hospital admission than younger patients. In one study, 65% of elderly patients had worsening symptoms for more than 14 days before admission compared with 29% for the younger group (41). One reason for this delay may be the blunted perception of breathlessness found in elderly as compared with younger asthmatics. All these psychosocial issues are important in the evaluation and management of an acute exacerbation in the elderly patient.

The clinical spectrum of an asthma exacerbation in the elderly ranges from a mild increase in dyspnea and/or wheezing documented in an ambulatory setting to a life-threatening asthma attack necessitating mechanical ventilation in an intensive care unit. The following discussion describes management of an acute asthma exacerbation in a physician's office or emergency department, routine inpatient therapy, and management of acute respiratory failure in the intensive care unit.

Therapeutic decision analysis in an exacerbation of asthma in any setting requires the assessment of the degree of airways obstruction and the patient's response to initial bronchodilatory therapy using inhaled bronchodilators (27). Unfortunately few specific data regarding asthma therapy of acute exacerbation in the elderly exist. The following guidelines to therapy are appropriate for patients of all ages.

B. Ambulatory Care

When patients present either to the doctor's office or the emergency department with an exacerbation, initial therapy should always depend on assessment of the patient's severity of disease. Many patients present with symptoms of increasing dyspnea and wheezing, especially after an upper respiratory tract infection. Generally the diagnosis of asthma is known and the patient is already receiving inhaled beta agonist bronchodilators and perhaps inhaled corticosteroids. Spirometry may reveal worsened flow rates or airways obstruction. Without evidence of other common etiologies of dyspnea or wheezing in this population, therapy often consists of initiating or increasing systemic corticosteroid therapy (40). Inhaled beta-agonist therapy may need to be intensified or nebulized therapy begun. If a short-acting beta$_2$-agonist has been prescribed and taken every 4 hr, consideration should be given to the addition of a spacer or the institution of nebulization of the beta agonist with a powered machine. Broad-spectrum antibiotic therapy can be administered when acute bronchitis is suspected. Additional medications such as theophylline and ipratropium bromide can also be considered. Theophylline has been used in the treatment of chronic asthma and acute, severe asthma. However, a narrow therapeutic range and an increased susceptibility of elderly patients to adverse side effects makes theophylline less attractive in all but the most severe clinical situations. Response to the therapy initiated should be reevaluated in 1–2 weeks.

Often the patient presents to the emergency department with more severe symptoms. If the patient is in extreme respiratory distress or has evidence of fatigue, impaired consciousness, or hypercapnia, respiratory arrest is a distinct possibility and endotracheal intubation and mechanical ventilation should be the first priority provided that both patient and family are in agreement with this extent of therapy (42).

Fortunately many patients present with less severe symptoms and therapy is less dramatic. Spirometry measuring the PEFR or FEV$_1$ should be instituted initially and repeated frequently after therapy. Supplemental oxygen at 2–3 L/min should be initiated and beta-adrenergic agonists delivered by aerosol. For mild to moderate exacerbations, repetitive administration of an inhaled short-acting beta agonist delivered by aerosol every 20 min for three doses is usually the best way to achieve rapid relief of airways obstruction. Repeated doses are generally safe in most elderly patients with asthma. However, attention should be given to changes in the cardiac rhythm. Continuous electrocardiographic monitoring may be needed, particularly in those patients with comorbid cardiac conditions or those with a history of arrhythmia. After these initial treatments are administered, more thorough history, physical, and laboratory examination can be completed.

Response to initial bronchodilator therapy is helpful in guiding the following therapeutic decision, especially the indications and need for hospitalization (31). When symptoms resolve and PEFR or FEV$_1$ increases to 70% of baseline and is maintained for at least 1 hr, a good response is obtained. Generally this suggests that airways obstruction was primarily due to bronchial smooth muscle contraction. Hospitalization is generally not required except when patients have other risk factors for mortality from asthma. If the patient is discharged from the emergency department, strong consideration should be given to initiation of oral corticosteroid therapy that can decrease recurrent emergency visits and improve asthma symptoms (43). In those elderly patients already receiving chronic oral corticosteroid therapy, hospitalization should be strongly considered even when symptoms are improved with aerosol bronchodilators, as symptom relapse is likely in patients with severe chronic disease.

If symptoms persist or the PEFR or FEV_1 is less than 70% of predicted after initial inhaled bronchodilator therapy, further treatment is required. In these instances, which represent the most likely scenario in severe chronic asthma, the patient's asthma is usually related to active airways inflammation. Frequent, as much as hourly, or continuous nebulized beta-adrenergic therapy should be begun and systemic corticosteroids administered (44). Metered-dose inhalers are generally not as helpful during acute exacerbations as nebulized beta-agonists (37). During the next 4 hr, the patient's symptoms, physical findings, and spirometry should be monitored frequently and a decision to hospitalize or not hospitalize made. Patients with resolution of symptoms and improvement of spirometry to 70% of predicted may be discharged with close medical follow-up and a course of oral corticosteroids. Patients with an incomplete response (40–70% of predicted) after 4 hr of therapy represent a difficult therapeutic decision. Some patients may do well without hospitalization. Others may not. The current recommendations include hospital admission for those asthmatics with a poor response to initial therapy and other clinical risk factors for asthma mortality (27). These include severe symptoms, severe airflow obstruction, past history of severe asthma, prior history of intubation for asthma, prolonged duration of symptoms before presentation, chronic oral corticosteroid use, poor home situation, inadequate access to care, or other physical or mental conditions that impair adherence to the medical regimen prescribed. Many elderly asthmatics may fall into one or more of these categories.

C. Inpatient Care

Many asthmatics admitted to hospital can be safely monitored and managed on a hospital ward. However, patients with severe airways obstruction with increased risk of asthma mortality should be admitted to the intensive care unit. Patients who remain hypercapnic despite intensive therapy are at increased risk for asthma death and should be intensively monitored and managed, probably in the intensive care unit. Even if the patient is admitted to a hospital ward, repeated history, physical examination, and measures of airflow obstruction should be made on a timely regular basis to guide any adjustments in therapy (27).

Pharmacotherapy of hospitalized patients includes inhaled, usually nebulized, beta-agonist therapy and systemic corticosteroids (45). Antibiotic therapy is considered in those cases where infection can be demonstrated or is thought to be clinically important. Empiric broad-spectrum antibiotics are generally prescribed in the setting of acute bronchitis. The role of systemic methylxanthine is more controversial (46,47). While many authors include theophylline as a basic therapy in severe asthma, it is important to recognize the multiple problems associated with its use, especially in the elderly (48). Many diseases and treatment for those diseases change theophylline metabolism in the elderly. Heart failure or hepatic cirrhosis depresses degradation and increases drug levels, while medications such as erythromycin, allopurinol, and cimetidine reduce clearance and increase blood levels (48). High blood levels place the patient at risk for seizures, cardiac dysrhythmias, and death (49). The efficacy and safety of theophylline use in elderly asthmatics with a severe exacerbation has not been studied. Therefore, very careful consideration should be given to the institution of theophylline. If begun, it should be monitored very closely. If drug levels are found to be elevated, the drug should be stopped. Inhaled anticholinergics also have not been studied in the elderly asthmatic in exacerbation. However, inhaled ipratropium bromide may be an important additive therapy in the elderly, as the response to anticholinergic therapy has no known negative correlation with age (13). It may also be beneficial in older patients with a bronchitic component or those with long-standing asthmatic with chronic, fixed obstruction (50). Ipratropium bromide has an additive effect when nebulized with a short-acting beta agonist (51).

The duration of hospital therapy varies widely in patients with asthma. However, many adult asthmatics and those elderly patients with poor baseline lung function may require many days of intensive bronchodilator therapy before return to baseline function. As the elderly asthmatic recovers, the intensity of therapy decreases. Periodic episodes of bronchospasm are not uncommon, especially at night or with exercise. These usually respond to inhaled beta-agonist therapy. Hospital discharge should be considered only when the patient has returned to baseline symptom function, has minimal or no bronchospasm, tolerates activity without wheezing, and whose spirometry is 70% or greater of baseline function.

Discharge planning is very important in the elderly asthmatic. Patients should be educated or reeducated about their disease as well as their medications. The use of the metered-dose inhaler (MDI) is especially crucial as many elderly patients have been found to use the MDI incorrectly (52). Most or all elderly asthmatics should be provided with a spacer to ensure accurate drug delivery. Monitoring of pulmonary function on a daily outpatient basis should also be recommended and the patient provided with a simple device for peak flow measurements at home (27). The patient is usually discharged on oral prednisone, 20–40 mg, with instructions to taper in 2.5- or 5-mg increments over a predetermined period of time. Written instructions in the form of a prednisone "calendar" are very important for patient understanding and compliance. Attempts to eliminate oral prednisone entirely should be undertaken, as side effects of chronic steroid therapy are particularly troublesome in the elderly population. Osteoporosis, diabetes mellitus, hypertension, and cataracts are important common problems in this patient population that are associated with chronic steroid use. Unfortunately many elderly asthmatics may require chronic steroids even with maximum inhaled bronchodilator therapy (18). Institution or reinstitution of inhaled corticosteroid therapy should begin at this time. Maximum doses of inhaled corticosteroids that minimize or eliminate oral corticosteroids should be prescribed. In the steroid-dependent elderly asthmatic, this may be as much as 1000–2000 μ g/day of inhaled steroid. The patient should be reevaluated on an outpatient basis within 1–2 weeks after hospital discharge.

D. Management of Acute Respiratory Failure in the Intensive Care Unit

Admission to the intensive care unit should be considered in the elderly asthmatic when alveolar ventilation is severely compromised and hypercapnic respiratory failure ensues or when intensive bronchodilator therapy is required that cannot be administered in a ward situation. It is hoped that a frank patient-physician discussion will occur in every elderly asthmatic with severe asthma prior to an ICU admission. Goals of such a discussion should include a realistic appraisal of the patient's disease severity, response to therapy, and prognosis. With this information, the physician and patient should discuss the patient's wishes regarding intensity of therapy, especially endotracheal intubation and mechanical ventilation.

Very few data specific to the intensive care of the critically ill elderly asthmatic are available. However, principles of asthma care in the ICU are not too different from those for younger patients. Patients with severe airways obstruction but without evidence of alveolar hypoventilation (i.e., hypercapnia) should receive frequent or continuous inhaled beta-adrenergic therapy. Although not specifically studied in elderly patients, beta agonists nebulized as often as every 30 min in severe cases may be required to avoid mechanical ventilation (42). Continuous nebulization of beta agonists may afford smoother action and relief of symptoms. Intravenous or subcutaneous beta agonists play no role in elderly asthmatics because of the concern for systemic toxicity, especially myocardial ischemia. Inhaled ipratropium bromide should be strongly considered. Intravenous corticosteroids should be administered. All medical therapy should be administered with a background of intensive nursing and respiratory therapy support.

Despite intensive therapy, some asthmatics may not improve or may continue to deteriorate. Indications for endotracheal intubation and mechanical ventilation include respiratory arrest or the clinical judgment that respiratory arrest is imminent or likely (53). The development or worsening of hypercapnia, signs of respiratory muscle fatigue as evidenced by paradoxical abdominal wall motion during inspiration, or deteriorating mental status despite intensive bronchodilator therapy suggest that respiratory arrest is likely and that intubation is indicated. Oral rather than nasal intubation is preferred because sinusitis is a common complication with nasoendotracheal tubes, especially in a patient population where sinusitis is common (54). The oral route also allows for larger endotracheal tubes and preserves the option of bronchoscopy.

Before specific ventilatory recommendations can be given for any disease, standard ventilatory goals must be outlined. Such goals for asthmatics include relief of hypoxemia and respiratory muscle fatigue. General ventilatory goals in the asthmatic, in contrast to other patients, also include minimization of barotrauma and dynamic hyperinflation. Pulmonary barotrauma is a common and potential deadly complication in ventilated asthmatics. It is defined as the presence of extra-alveolar air where it is not expected (55). Clinical examples of pulmonary barotrauma include pneumothorax, pneumomediastinum, and subcutaneous emphysema. Barotrauma is related to the high airways pressures needed to ventilate patients who have high airways resistance. High inspiratory airways pressures are associated with overdistended alveoli that rupture. Air then dissects along the bronchovascular interstitium, where it can dissect centrally with the formation of mediastinal and/or subcutaneous emphysema. Alternatively, air from ruptured alveoli may dissect through the pleural surface into the pleural space to create a pneumothorax. Ventilated patients who develop pneumothorax are at risk for the development of tension pneumothorax.

Another standard ventilatory goal in asthmatics is minimization of dynamic hyperinflation. A consequence of the high airways pressures needed to ventilate asthmatics with increased airways resistance is dynamic hyperinflation or end-expiratory alveolar pressure above set positive end-expiratory pressure (PEEP), called auto-PEEP (56,57). Dynamic hyperinflation occurs during the ventilatory circumstances of tachypnea and increased inspiratory time due to the increased inspiratory resistances found in severe asthma. In this situation, expiration is simply not long enough and air trapping ensues. Therefore, dynamic hyperinflation is associated with an increase in functional residual capacity (FRC) at the end of expiration. This has been termed auto-PEEP or intrinsic PEEP. Hyperinflation can cause significant patient discomfort by increasing the work of breathing (58). Other significant clinical consequences of auto-PEEP include effects on gas exchange and cardiac output similar to applied or extrinsic PEEP. Gas exchange may worsen and cardiac output decreases with the application of PEEP. Because of these complications, ventilatory goals in asthmatics include not only providing adequate oxygenation but also minimizing barotrauma and dynamic hyperinflation. Therefore standard ventilatory strategies are different from conventional strategies utilized in patients with other types of lung disease.

To decrease barotrauma and dynamic hyperinflation, specific ventilatory goals in asthmatics include minimizing lung volumes and airways pressures. With conventional mechanical ventilation, a high tidal volume (10–15 ml/kg) is delivered to normalize the $Paco_2$. The resultant high minute ventilation with decreased expiratory time may cause air trapping (dynamic hyperinflation) with an increased potential for barotrauma. Therefore current ventilatory strategy in asthmatics is controlled hypoventilation or permissive hypercapnia (59,60). With this strategy, normalized $Paco_2$ is not the goal. Rather, an elevated $Paco_2$ is tolerated as one means to maintain lower minute ventilation, improved tidal volumes, and, as a result, lower airway pressures. While somewhat controversial, a reasonable goal for setting the ventilator is to adjust the tidal volume so that maximum inspiratory pressure does not exceed 50 cmH_2O, a level that corresponds to a tidal volume of 5–10 ml/kg. The degree of auto-PEEP should be monitored. Maintaining a respiratory rate less than 10 breaths per minute will tend to decrease the incidence and severity of auto-PEEP by allowing for increased expiratory time.

Respiratory acidosis may continue or result with the use of permissive hypercapnia. The minimum safe level of pH is not known with certainty; however, a level of 7.2 is regarded as acceptable. Generally sodium bicarbonate is infused when pH is < 7.2, although this remains somewhat controversial.

The use of permissive hypercapnia as a ventilatory strategy usually requires the use of neuromuscular blocking agents such as pancuronium and vecuronium to help maintain low airway pressures during the delivery of mechanical ventilation (61). Limiting inspiratory pressures can be uncomfortable for the patient and paralysis is usually required to avoid having the patient fight the ventilator. As with almost every aspect of treatment in the critically ill, complications can result. The use of neuromuscular blockade, even for a short period of time, in association with the use of corticosteroids can result in a significant myopathic illness manifest clinically by severe muscle weakness (62). In an attempt to avoid this complication, paralytic agents should be used only if absolutely necessary and the use limited to intermittent as versus continuous administration if at all possible.

Many other complications of critical illness and mechanical ventilation are possible (63). Most are preventable or treatable if recognized early. Complications can include thromboembolism and gastrointestinal hemorrhage from stress ulcers, nosocomial pneumonia, dysrhythmias, and renal insufficiency. None of these are specific to the asthmatic.

The duration of mechanical ventilation varies with the individual patient. Most patients can be extubated after several days, but some require ventilatory support for as long as several weeks, especially if complications of mechanical ventilation such as pneumonia ensue. Patients should be extubated only after weaning parameters are met (62).

VII. Summary

Management of acute exacerbations in elderly asthmatics requires knowledge and expertise not only of asthma but also of how age influences pathophysiology, diagnosis, and treatment. While general fundamentals of managing an acute exacerbation are similar, age increases the complexity level of management needed to treat these patients successfully in any care setting. In the acutely ill elderly asthmatic, special attention should be paid to the differential diagnosis of dyspnea and wheezing, which is clearly more complicated in an older patient than a younger one. Therapy of an exacerbation should routinely encompass a larger psychosocial spectrum of concerns in addition to the standard medical care issues. Patient education on disease and drugs, compliance with therapy, and the influence of other medical comorbidities assumes greater importance in asthmatics who are elderly.

Abbreviations

ACE	angiotensin converting enzyme
Auto-PEEP	auto-positive end-expiratory pressure
COPD	chronic obstructive pulmonary disease
FEV_1	forced expiratory volume in 1 second
MDI	metered-dose inhaler
PEEP	positive end-expiratory pressure
PEFR	peak expiratory flow rate

References

1. American Thoracic Society. Chronic bronchitis, asthma, and pulmonary emphysema: A statement by the Committee on Diagnostic Standards for Nontuberculous Respiratory Diseases. Am Rev Respir Dis 1962; 85:762–768.
2. Beasley R, Roche WR, Roberts JA, Holgate ST. Cellular events in the bronchi in mild asthma and after bronchial provocation. Am Rev Respir Dis 1989; 139:806–817.
3. Bousquet J, Chanez P, Lacoste JY, et al. Eosinophilic inflammation in asthma. N Engl J Med 1990; 323:1033–1039.
4. Dunnill MS. The pathology of asthma, with special reference to changes in the bronchial mucosa. J Clin Pathol 1960; 13:27–40.
5. Barnes PJ. New concepts in the pathogenesis of bronchial hyperresponsiveness and asthma. J Allergy Clin Immunol 1989; 83:1013–1026.
6. Golden JA, Nadel JA, Boushey HA. Bronchial hyperirritability in health subjects after exposure to ozone. Am Rev Respir Dis 1978; 118:287–295.
7. Empey DW, Laitinen LA, Jacobs L, et al. Mechanisms of bronchial hyperreactivity in

normal subjects after upper respiratory tract infection. Am Rev Respir Dis 1976; 113: 131–139.

8. Boushey HA, Holtzman MJ, Sheller JR, Nadel JM. Bronchial hyperreactivity. Am Rev Respir Dis 1980; 121:389–413.

9. Sobonya RE. Quantitative structural alterations in long-standing allergic asthma. Am Rev Respir Dis 1984; 130:289–292.

10. Pfeifer MA, Weinberg CR, Cook D, et al. Differential changes of autonomic nervous system function with age in man. Am J Med 1983; 75:249–258.

11. Pontoppidan H, Beecher HK. Progressive loss of protective reflexes in the airway with the advance of age. JAMA 1960; 174:2210–2218.

12. Braman SS, Amico CA, Steigman D, et al. Cough and bronchoconstrictive reflexes in normal elderly subject. Am Rev Respir Dis 1987;135(suppl):476.

13. vanSchayck CP, Folgering H, Harbers H. Effects of allergy and age on responses to salbutamol and ipratropium bromide in moderate asthma and chronic bronchitis. Thorax 1991; 46:355–361.

14. Ullah MI, Newman GB, Saunders KB. Influence of age on response to ipratropium and salbutamol in asthma. Thorax 1981; 36:523–529.

15. Connolly MF, Crowley JJ, Charan NB, et al. Reduced subjective awareness of bronchoconstriction provoked by methacholine in elderly asthmatic and normal subjects as measured on a simple awareness scale. Thorax 1992; 47:410–413.

16. Kikuchi Y, Okabe S, Tamura G, et al. Chemosensitivity and perception of dyspnea in patients with a history of near-fatal asthma. N Engl J Med 1994; 330:1329–1334.

17. Barbee RA, Lebowitz MD, Thompson HC, Burrows B. Immediate skin-test reactivity in a general population sample. Ann Intern Med 1976; 84:129–133.

18. Braman SS, Kaemmerlen JT, Davis SM. Asthma in the elderly: A comparison between patients with recently acquired and long-standing disease. Am Rev Respir Dis 1991; 143:336–340.

19. Burrows B, Lebowitz MD, Barbee RA, Cline MG. Findings before diagnoses of asthma among elderly in a longitudinal study of a general population sample. J Allergy Clin Immunol 1991; 88:870–877.

20. America Thoracic Society. Standards for the diagnosis and care of patients with chronic obstructive pulmonary disease: Definitions, epidemiology, pathophysiology, diagnosis, and staging. Am J Respir Crit Care Med 1995; 152:S77–S83.

21. Declamer PBS, Chatterjee SS, Cruickshank JM. Beta-blocker and asthma. Br Hear J 1978; 40:184–186.

22. Tattersfield AE, Harrison RN. Effect of beta-blocker therapy on airway function. Drugs 1983; 25:227–231.

23. Fraunfeder FT, Barker AF. Respiratory effects of timolol. N Engl J Med 1984; 311:1441–1444.

24. Gurevitch MJ, Valenzuela JE. Lung and gastroesophageal disorders. Semin Respir Med 1988; 9:254–261.

25. FitzGerald JM, Hargreave FE. The assessment and management of acute life-threatening asthma. Chest 1989; 95:888–893.

26. Kallenbach JM, Frankel AH, Lapinsky SE, et al. Determinants of near fatality in acute severe asthma. Am J Med 1993; 95:265–272.

27. U.S. Department of Health and Human Services, Public Health Service, National

Institutes of Health: Expert Panel Report: *Guidelines for the Diagnosis and Management of Asthma*. Publication No. 91-3042, August 1991.

28. Scoggin CH, Sahn SA, Petty TL. Status asthmaticus: A nine year experience. JAMA 1977; 238:1158–1162.

29. Sahn SA, Mountina RD. Clinical features and outcome in patients with acute asthma presenting with hypercapnia. Am Rev Respir Dis 1988; 138:535–539.

30. Shin CS, Willians HM. Relationship of wheezing to the severity of obstruction in asthma. Arch Intern Med 1983; 143:890–895.

31. Cohen CA, Zagelbaum G, Cross D, et al. Clinical manifestations of inspiratory muscle fatigue. Am J Med 1982; 73:308–316.

32. Fischl MA, Pitchenik A, Gardner LB. An index predicting relapse and need for hospitalization in patients with acute bronchial asthma. N Engl J Med 1981; 305: 783–789.

33. Fanta CH, Rossing TH, McFadden ER. Emergency room treatment of asthma. Am J Med 1982; 72:416–422.

34. McFadden ER, Lyons HA. Arterial blood gas tensions in asthma. N Engl J Med 1968; 278:1027–1032.

35. Palmer KNV, Diament ML. Spirometry and blood gas tension in bronchial asthma and chronic bronchitis. Lancet 1967; 2:383–384.

36. Findley LJ, Sahn SA. The value of chest roentgenograms in acute asthma in adults. Chest 1981; 80:535–538.

37. Siegler D. Reversible electrocardiographic changes in severe acute asthma. Thorax 1977; 32:328–332.

38. Gelb AF, Lyons HA, Fairshter RD, et al. P pulmonale in status asthmaticus. J Allergy Clin Immunol 1979; 64:18–22.

39. Global strategy for asthma management and prevention. NHLBI/WHO Workshop report. *Global Initiatives for Asthma*. Publication Number 95-3659, January 1995.

40. Sbarbaro JA. Compliance with therapy: How great a problem? J Respir Dis 1986; 6: 44–49.

41. Petheram IS, Jones DA, Collins JV. Assessment and management of acute asthma in the elderly: A comparisons with younger asthmatics. Postgrad Med J 1982; 58: 149–151.

42. Idris AH, McDermott MF, Raucci JC, et al. Emergency department treatment of severe asthma. Chest 1993; 103:665–672.

43. Chapman KR, Verbeek PR, White JG, Rebuck HS. Effect of a short course of prednisone in the prevention of early relapse after the emergency room treatment of acute asthma. N Engl J Med 1991; 324:788–794.

44. Black PN, Woodhouse A, Burmeister S. How frequently should nebulized salbutamol be administered in acute asthma? Am Rev Respir Dis 1993; 147:A57.

45. Fanta CH, Rossing TH, McFadden ER. Glucocorticosteroids in acute asthma: A critical control trail. Am J Med 1983; 74:845–851.

46. Siegel D, Sheppard D, Gelb A. Aminophylline increases the toxicity but not the efficacy of an inhaled beta-adrenergic agonist in the treatment of acute exacerbations of asthma. Am Rev Respir Dis 1985; 132:283–287.

47. Littenberg B. Aminophylline treatment in severe, acute asthma. JAMA 1988; 259: 1678–1683.

48. Powell JR, Vozek S, Hopewell P, et al. Theophylline disposition in acutely ill hospitalized patients. Am Rev Respir Dis 1978; 118:229–239.

49. Sessler CN. Theophylline toxicity: Clinical features of 116 consecutive cases. Am J Med 1990; 88:567–576.

50. Seaton A. Asthma in elderly. In Weiss EB, Segal MS, Stein M, eds. *Bronchial Asthma: Mechanisms and Therapeutics* 2d ed. Boston: Little Brown, 1985:854–856.

51. Rebuch AJ. Nebulized anticholinergic and sympathomimetic treatment of asthma and chronic obstructive airway disease in the emergency room. Am J Med 1987; 82: 59–64.

52. Goodman DE, Israel E, Rosenberg M, et al. The influence of age, diagnosis, and gender on proper use of metered-dose inhalers. Am J Respir Crit Care Med 1994; 150: 1256–1261.

53. Wasterman DE, Benatar SR, Potgieter PD, et al. Identifications of the high-risk asthmatic patient: Experience with 39 patients undergoing ventilation for status asthmaticus. Am J Med 1979; 66:565–572.

54. Rouby JJ, Laurent P, Gosnach M, et al. Risk factors and clinical relevance of nosocomial maxillary sinusitis in the critically ill ICU patient. Am J Respir Crit Care Med 1994; 150:776–783.

55. Haake R, Schlichtig R, Ulstad DR, et al. Barotrauma. Chest 1987; 91:608–615.

56. Rossi A, Gottfried SB, Zocchi L, et al. Measurement of static compliance of the total respiratory system in patients with acute respiratory failure during mechanical ventilation: The effect of intrinsic positive end-expiratory pressure. Am Rev Respir Dis 1985; 131:672–677.

57. Smith TC, Marini JJ. Impact of PEEP on lung mechanics and work of breathing in severe airflow obstruction. J Appl Physiol 1988; 65:1488–1499.

58. Pepe PE, Marini JJ. Occult positive end-expiratory pressure in mechanically ventilated patients with airflow obstruction: The "auto-PEEP" effect. Am Rev Respir Dis 1982; 126:166–170.

59. Feihl F, Perret C. Permissive hypercapnia. Am J Respir Crit Care Med 1994; 150: 1722–1737.

60. Darioli R, Perret C. Mechanical controlled hypoventilation in status asthmaticus. Am Rev Respir Dis 1984; 129:385–387.

61. Hansen-Flaschen J, Cowen J, Raps EC. Neuromuscular blockade in the intensive care unit. Am Rev Respir Dis 1993; 147:234–236.

62. Braman SS, Kaemmerlen JT. Intensive care of status asthmaticus: A 10-year experience. JAMA 1990; 366–371.

63. Pingleton SK. Complications of acute respiratory failure. Am Rev Respir Dis 1988; 137:1463–1493.

9

Patient Education
Creating Partnership Care

GAYLE A. TRAVER

University of Arizona
Tucson, Arizona

Optimal care of patients with a chronic illness requires open communication between the care provider and care recipient. The care of patients with asthma is no exception to this rule. The patient must be an active participant in the setting of treatment goals, determining the approach to therapy, maintaining usual care, and instituting appropriate measures when symptomatology changes. Thus there must not only be open communication but the patient must also be well educated in the management of his or her disease. This chapter discusses the development of reciprocal communication between the care provider and patient, the major educational objectives in an asthma program, and special considerations in the development of educational programs for the elderly.

As discussed in other sections, there is not a "typical" elderly patient with asthma. Some elderly are robust and more active than much younger counterparts, while others are frail elderly; some have had a diagnosis of asthma for many years, while others may be newly diagnosed. In building an environment of open communication, it is important not to make assumptions about the individual because of his or her age. Nor should assumptions be made about the patient's level of understanding of the asthma diagnosis or treatment of asthma or of the patient's quality of life or goals of therapy.

The caregiver must seek information about the patient's knowledge and expectations and be a listener as well as a source of information. It is acknowledged that in today's health care system, it is often difficult for the primary care provider to be the sole person responsible for obtaining the necessary information and providing the patient education required. When certain activities are delegated to others, it is important that there also be open communication between the various persons involved in providing care. For example, a change in the goals (e.g., level of activity) must be known by all providing guidance to the patient, so that conflicting information is not given. Depending on the specific setting, a variety of resources may be used. Nursing personnel, respiratory therapists, social workers, or health educators may be interacting with the patient; interactions may be on a one-to-one basis or they may be in group sessions (educational, support groups). Regardless of the specific setting, the health care system must provide an approach that supports the development of a knowledgeable patient who is actively involved in maintaining his or her optimal level of health, function, and quality of life.

I. Changes with Aging that Affect Educational Programs

Before discussing the specifics of developing the care relationship, some of the changes and/or characteristics associated with aging need to be reviewed. This background helps one to be cognizant of certain problems that may be more evident in the elderly, and it also helps the caregiver to avoid some misconceptions about the elderly. The issues discussed have direct impact on the approaches to patient education.

Living arrangements for the elderly are variable. Although some elderly migrate to the "sun belt" for retirement, the majority remain in their usual community. Data show that even those who move away from their usual area of residence and family make a second move later in life to be near family (1–3); it is often the frail elderly who make the move back to a location near family. It is important to remember, however, that the majority of elderly live independently in the community (2,3). Men, when widowed, tend to remarry, while women are less likely to do so (4). Thus it is frequently the elderly female patient who lives alone; it has been estimated that women live alone for an average of 15 years (2–4). For those with respiratory symptoms, the fear of breathlessness is even more overwhelming when they are alone.

The elderly women who live alone are also much more likely to have a decreased income. This finding is especially true of the present elderly population, where women did not have sufficient social security quarters for full benefits (2,4). Elderly persons with limited income will often have difficulty paying for the prescribed medications; compliance may be a problem of inability to purchase the drugs, not an inability to follow the plan of care.

Depression is commonly associated with the elderly, but overall estimates of its prevalence in this age group vary widely. Major depression is probably less than 3%; the estimates of depressive symptoms range from 13–27%. The greatest risk is for those in the over-75 age group (5). In the chronically ill elderly, the prevalence of depression increases to 25–50% (6). Many believe that depression is associated with chronic and disabling conditions rather than age alone. Whether the significant factor is age or chronic illness, elderly patients with asthma should be considered susceptible to depression. Although data are not available, assuming that depression is more prevalent in those with disabling conditions, one could anticipate that depression would be more common in elderly persons with poorly controlled asthma as opposed to those with well-controlled disease. It is also known that some of the medications used to treat asthma (e.g., corticosteroids) may also contribute to depression. The same can be said for medications used to treat some of the comorbid conditions that may be seen in the elderly with asthma (e.g., antiparkinsonian drugs, antihypertensives) (7). Depression, when present, may affect the perception of symptoms, ability to follow a treatment plan, and quality of life. An association between asthma mortality and depression has been noted (8). When present, depression should be treated. It must also be considered when setting goals with the patient and when determining the extent and capabilities of patients in making management decision.

Changes in neurological and sensory function in the elderly have significant effects on the educational approaches and materials developed for the elderly. Memory changes are common, with the major impact being on short-term memory; short-term memory problems include impaired ability to acquire and retrieve recent information (9,10). The requirement for more time to process information should not be confused with cognitive impairment. Cognitive function is usually well maintained well into the eighties. It is important for the clinician/educator to recognize any change in cognitive abilities—not only is such a change abnormal, but it will have a dramatic impact on the patients ability to carry out the care program (10,11). When presenting new information to elderly patients, time must be allowed for processing; it also appears that visual information is more easily acquired than information presented audibly (12). These potential changes in the ability to acquire and then retrieve information accentuate the need to provide the patient with written instructions and explanations.

Sensory changes also affect the approach to education in the elderly. Due to changes in eyesight (decreased visual acuity and color discrimination) (13–15), printed information should be in large-size type. A white, uncluttered background is superior to one with colors. Print is better perceived when it is black on white. Many elderly also have impaired hearing, which may affect communication (14,15).

II. Patient Education

Although asthma educational programs specifically designed for the elderly have not yet been studied, several programs for adults with asthma have been evaluated. The education programs for patients with asthma are designed to give patients the ability to manage themselves. A study by Wilson and colleagues (16) of 18 to 50-year-olds evaluated both group and individual patient education programs as compared with two control conditions, usual care and provision of written material. The group sessions consisted of four 90-min weekly sessions. The investigators found that those patients enrolled in formal educational programs demonstrated greater symptom control, improved metered-dose inhaler (MDI) technique, and fewer acute-care visits. They also saw a trend for the patients in the group classes to demonstrate more improvement than those instructed individually.

Mayo and colleagues (17) provided patient education to a group of patients who had a history of frequent emergency room visits or hospitalizations for asthma exacerbations. The patients were followed in a special asthma clinic and education was given on a one-to-one basis. There was no time limit on the program. The evaluation of the program demonstrated a significant decrease in emergency room visits.

European studies have utilized an inpatient setting for asthma education and have demonstrated similar results. Even with the inpatient programs, cost-effectiveness of the asthma education could be demonstrated (18–21).

As is evident from the variation of program design among the published studies on asthma education, there is no *one* way that the asthma patient should be educated. There are, however, basic educational areas that should be covered. Therefore, this section is not written as an outline of a specific educational program, but rather to provide guidelines for the various components required in a program of asthma management.

A. Knowledge of the Disease Process

It is important that the meaning of the diagnosis "asthma" be discussed with the patient. Some elderly patients may have had the diagnosis for many years and thus their understanding of the disease may include some of the old misconceptions; for example, they may have been told that asthma is a psychological disease—you bring it on yourself. Some patients who are newly diagnosed may be disbelieving, as they may have heard that only young people get asthma.

Today, asthma education in all age groups stresses the inflammatory aspect of the disease. Having some understanding of the chronic inflammatory nature of asthma helps one to understand the chronicity of the disease and the need to continue medications even when one is not feeling ill or wheezy. During this early educational process, it is important that terminology be clarified. The educator and the patient must have similar definitions for words: Has the patient heard the word *dyspnea* before? what does *bronchi* mean? and so on. Explanations will vary according to the style of the educator and the background of the patient; one should not "talk down" to the patient nor should the educator's vocabulary be at too high a level. Similarly, written material should be at an appropriate level. Although it is usually recommended that patient education materials be written at a seventh- to ninth-grade level, studies have reported that much of the available asthma education material is at higher levels (22).

B. Goal Setting

As the patient gains an understanding of the asthma diagnosis, the caregiver/educator needs also to assess the patient's present functional status, preferences, and expectations. Inherent to this assessment is the caregiver's knowledge of the presence of potentially nonreversible airways obstruction and other coexisting medical problems that could affect functional status. The terms *preferences* and *expectations* are helpful to define an approach to patients who may not be able to attain a "normal" functional status. Preferences define the way we would ideally like to be—if there were no limitations of any kind. Expectations are more realistic and may often be more fluid and dynamic over time. Functional status, preferences, and expectations are all components involved in setting goals for the patient's care. In young persons with asthma, the usual goals include normal lung function and normal activity. Although these goals are also appropriate for some elderly persons with asthma, they are not appropriate for others. It is also important to remember that goals and expectations change over time. Some patients respond so well to therapy that higher expectations become appropriate. In others, expectations may need to be lowered due to the development of new comorbid conditions or the development of more fixed airways obstruction.

C. Prevention

The foremost point under the topic of prevention is smoking cessation. As discussed in earlier chapters, the diagnosis of asthma is not excluded by a present or past smoking history, although patients with asthma are less likely than patients with chronic obstructive lung disease (COPD) to have a smoking history greater than 25 pack-years. The question of allergen avoidance is more difficult to answer in the elderly patient, where it is frequently not possible to identify specific allergens that trigger an asthma exacerbation. If a trigger is identified, avoidance techniques should be discussed. Some of the common approaches may be difficult to accomplish in the elderly. As the major allergens associated with asthma are indoor, the avoidance techniques usually include cleaning and eliminating dust reservoirs (carpets, overstuffed furniture, etc.). Some elderly may not have the energy for aggressive cleaning and may not be able to afford outside help with it. If a specific allergy to house dust mites has not been identified, this aggressive cleaning should not be demanded. Basic housekeeping is needed. If the educator is unsure of the ability of the patient to perform basic household chores, a home visit may significantly contribute to the evaluation. Many home care agencies and some suppliers of durable medical equipment (such as nebulizers or oxygen canisters) can help to provide this information.

Another important area of prevention in the elderly is immunization. The educational program should include the need for a yearly influenza vaccination and a pneumococcal vaccination every 6 years. Because of changes in the immune system of the elderly, reimmunization for pneumococcus is recommended every 6 years in those between 60 and 75 years of age, and every 3–4 years in those over 75 (23).

D. Monitoring

Just as is true with all patients with asthma, elderly patients with asthma must be taught to monitor their symptoms. Symptom monitoring both with and without peak flow measures has been used. Sufficient data are not yet available to say what approach to monitoring should be taught in this age group. Some believe that the effects of aging on normal lung function may adversely affect the validity of peak flow measures (8), while others comment on the difficulty the elderly may have in reading and recording peak flow values. In patients with a significant amount of nonreversible airways obstruction, the peak flow readings may be very low, making small changes difficult to interpret. A large epidemiological study of peak expiratory flow rates in an elderly population (24) demonstrated a fall in peak flow with age to levels of about 270 L/min in males and <200 L/min in females aged 85 and older. In terms of variability, another study of peak flow measures in a group of patients with a mean age of 62 years found that a change of 60 L/min was needed to demonstrate a significant increase or decrease in function (25). This amount of variability may not be seen in patients with marked irreversible obstruction or in the very elderly.

There are also reasons to support the use of peak flow meters in the elderly. Some data indicate that the elderly may be less aware of increasing bronchoconstriction than younger adults (26,27). A study by Noseda et al. (28) looked at the differences in perception between patients with COPD and those with asthma. The mean age of the entire sample was 63 years; the ages for the COPD and asthma groups were not reported. This study found that patients with asthma were better perceivers than patients with COPD and that among the COPD patients some were good perceivers and others were poor perceivers. Other studies of patients with asthma have found significant numbers of young and old to be nonperceivers (29,30). Some of the differences in these findings are probably due to study design, as some investigators looked at bronchodilator response while others studied methacholine response. Regardless, the caregiver/educator must be alert to the possibility that a patient is a poor perceiver. In such a patient, it is assumed that peak flow monitoring would be indicated, as early decreases in function would not be recognized by changes in symptomatology alone.

In those situations where peak flow monitoring is used, the patient must be carefully instructed. Most of the peak flow meters come with written instructions—but one must make sure that the print is large enough to be easily readable. Videotapes and written materials are also available from various pharmaceutical companies, the National Asthma Education and Prevention Program (NAEPP), and other sources (31). Regardless of the approach used to present the information, patients must be observed using a peak flow meter that is of the same type they will be using at home. One must make sure that the patient can not only use the peak flow meter correctly but that he or she can read and record the results.

Use of the peak flow meter should always include symptom monitoring. It is extremely helpful to know if the patient's symptoms vary with changes in peak flow. If symptoms do not increase with falls in peak flow, the patient may be a nonperceiver. In such instances, continued peak flow monitoring is very helpful. Use of the peak flow meter in conjunction with symptom monitoring can also help in educating the patient to interpret symptoms and recognize symptom changes. Often patients are "not sure" if symptoms are "real." The peak flow readings help the patient to build a reference system to judge the severity of symptom changes.

It is important that the caregiver/educator review patients' recordings of peak flow and symptom diaries at every visit or contact. During the educational process, it is also important to determine the patient's use of such diaries. There are some patients who record peak flows and symptoms very faithfully; others do not (32). One study of adults demonstrated a 26% error rate in recording values from home spirometry (33). The educator must be confident that the peak flows and/or symptoms reported are valid; this also means that the patient must be free to state when and why he or she did not record peak flow or symptoms. (In other words, the patient should not be forced to "make up" numbers when none are available.)

If the patient's symptom perceptions are good, measurement of daily peak flow may not be necessary over the long term (although some would disagree). Some patients initially use peak flow to determine their usual level. They may then use simple symptom monitoring (without a diary) when their asthma is under good control. With changes in symptomatology, peak flow monitoring is again instituted in order to obtain objective measures and to confirm perceived changes. In the elderly patient with comorbid cardiac conditions, peak flow readings can be very helpful in differentiating shortness of breath related to asthma from shortness of breath due to other causes. Regardless of the monitoring program ultimately used, the patient must have a valid, reliable system for detecting and confirming changes in physiological status.

Attaining a monitoring system that works for the patient is a process. Several studies in younger subjects and adults have demonstrated that both symptom monitoring and peak flow monitoring are effective (34,35). The goal is to find the monitoring system that works for the individual patient. The caregiver/ educator and patient must also decide at what level the patient will interpret the results of monitoring. This aspect is covered under "The Integrated Plan of Care," below.

E. Medications

It is extremely important that the patient understand the purpose of the medications prescribed as well as how and when those medications are to be taken. A recent study demonstrated that patients with asthma often have "antimedication" attitudes, regardless of their attitudes about having asthma or their level of function (36). Thus the educator must also evaluate and attempt to overcome "antimedication" attitudes. Because many of the elderly with asthma have other comorbid conditions, the caregiver/educator must also be aware of the other medications the patient takes—not only because of potential interactions but to assure that medications for one problem are not confused with medications for another.

In the elderly person with asthma, the presence of other comorbid conditions may also affect the intensity of pharmacological intervention. For example, the decision to use oral steroids over long periods of time may be influenced by the presence or severity of osteoporosis; the use of beta agonists may be influenced by the presence of cardiac dysrhythmias. These interactions as well as the patient's functional status and quality of life influence the ultimate pharmacological plan. Thus, the setting of goals by the caregiver and patient influences the selection of medications and how they will be used. The pros and cons of more medication to control asthma versus the potential impact on lifestyle and quality of life need to be discussed with the patient. When a short burst of corticosteroids or a moderate increase in the chronic level of steroid therapy effects a major improvement in symptomatology and mobility there is usually little question; improvement is seen by the patient and caregiver and the risks are low. On the other hand, when oral corticosteroids produce only a slight additional improvement in lung function but expose the patient to multiple real or potential side effects, the question of continuing therapy must be carefully considered. The management of the patient's asthma should not detract from his or her total quality of life.

Patients must be educated in use of the various medications. They should be able to state the purpose of each medication; the difference between bronchodilators and anti-inflammatories is especially important. Written handouts are very helpful, as they allow the patient to review the content more than once. Simple verbal descriptions may be forgotten or unknowingly modified by the patient over time.

Although the schedule of "when" to take medications may seem to be clear-cut to professionals, it may not be so clear to the patient. For example, patients often believe that they should not take multiple medications at the same time. Other common misconceptions are that there should be 5 min between all inhaler doses, including inhaled steroids, and that oral prednisone should be divided into several doses during the day (because 5-mg tablets are often used, patients assume that multiple pills of the same kind should not all be taken at one time). These misconceptions may affect the plan of care in a variety of ways. For example, patients may take too few puffs of inhaled medicine due to the time involved, and prednisone in divided doses may contribute to side effects.

Because elderly patients are more likely to be on complicated medical regimens, it is frequently difficult for them to remember all of their medications and when to take them. This complexity, coupled with the potential for a change in short-term memory, makes learning the medication plan a major educational goal. There are various ways to help patients remember when to take medications. Some simply remember their medications and take them; some use pill dispensers; some place a written schedule of all of the day's medications on the refrigerator or the bathroom mirror; some require a reminder from a caregiver. Because many patients use multiple inhalers, it is not unusual for them to confuse inhalers. One solution is to label each inhaler with its specific use. Of course, one must also assure that the correct canister is placed in the correct mouthpiece. Written schedules of steroid bursts are usually required by all patients. A calendar with each daily dose is very helpful; the patient can then "cross off" each dose. On every visit, it is helpful to have the patient list all medications taken, including dose and schedule. Avoid listing the medication and allowing the patient to simply reply in the affirmative. This procedure of having the patient recite medications also contributes to detecting changes in memory and cognition that may occur over time.

One of the most important goals of any educational program for patients with asthma is the optimal delivery of aerosolized medications. The elderly are not immune to the problems that face other age groups, but they also have some additional problems as a result of the aging process.

Although it can be simple and effective to use, the metered-dose inhaler (MDI) also presents many problems. Multiple studies have demonstrated that the majority of patients have poor inhaler technique (37–40). Some studies have looked specifically at such problems in the elderly (41,42). Regretfully, it must also be noted that several studies (43,44) have documented that even many health professionals are unable to use an MDI correctly. The picture is further confounded by the fact that experts do not agree on all the specifics of inhaler technique. Finally, the special problems of the elderly are added to the picture. Hand strength decreases as one ages (41); in addition, many elderly have coexisting arthritic problems, which further impair their ability to activate the inhaler.

Several aspects of technique have universal acceptance. These include the following: shake the inhaler before each activation, use only one MDI activation per breath, inhale through the mouth with slow inspiratory flow rates, and follow the maximal inspiration with a breath hold. Aspects where there continue to be disagreement include exhaling to functional residual capacity (FRC) or to residual volume (RV) prior to activation of the MDI, tipping the head back or not, and using an open or closed mouth around the inhaler (38,39,43,45,46).

Although there is no agreement in the literature about inhaler technique, it is important that all of those educating the patient within a given setting are consistent on this subject. All patients must be observed using the inhaler during the instruction process; simply providing written instruction is not sufficient. Placebo inhalers are available from the pharmaceutical companies for use in teaching sessions. One successful demonstration by the patient should not be considered adequate. It is usually recommended that inhaler technique be checked at the visit following initial instruction and then at least every 6 months; for many, more frequent observation and reinstruction may be needed.

Because problems with inhaler technique are more common in the elderly, most clinicians caring for elderly patients recommend the use of a reservoir device to improve lower airway deposition and reduce side effects from large particles deposited in the oropharynx. Perhaps most importantly, the reservoir device is very forgiving of inadequate inhaler technique. (Note that a reservoir or holding chamber device is recommended versus a simple spacer device.) The type of reservoir selected usually varies with the preference of the clinician, but it should also be recognized that some patients will have more success with one type of device over another. For example, some have difficulty selectively mouth breathing and do better with a reservoir bag, which they can see deflate when they inhale; the bag-type devices are also helpful for patients who are confused and who may receive their medications with the assistance of another. Because the design of the various reservoir devices varies, the instructions for use also vary; the caregiver/educator must be aware of these differences.

Some patients find use of the reservoir devices very inconvenient, especially when away from home. During the educational process, it may be found that the inconvenience is adversely affecting the medication program. Some newer alternative approaches for administering inhaled bronchodilators may be helpful. Examples of these techniques include the breath-activated pressurized inhalers, the dry powder inhalers, and the disk inhalers. Some of these devices have been specifically studied in the elderly and found to be helpful (47,48). They also eliminate the need to depress the canister to activate it. Because many elderly patients have decreased hand strength, with or without arthritis, activation of the

MDI, especially at the correct time during the inspiratory maneuver, can be especially difficult. The new devices avert this problem.

Some patients are unable to use an MDI or one of the newer devices and require a compressor unit and small-volume nebulizer for the administration of aerosolized medications. The small-volume nebulizers may also be used for short periods during an acute exacerbation, where one is concerned about the total dose delivered. To improve drug delivery, it is recommended that a reservoir device be placed on the exhalation side. When prescribing a small-volume nebulizer for an elderly patient, one must assure that he or she can assemble and clean the equipment. Most suppliers of durable medical equipment instruct patients in the use of a small-volume nebulizer. The educator must not assume, however, that the patient has been adequately instructed, because one educational session is frequently not adequate; also, many patients purchase second-hand units and never receive formal instruction. If a multiple-dose bottle of medication is prescribed, the clinician must assure that the patient can read the dropper. Most elderly patients do better with unit-dose drugs, so that measuring and mixing are not necessary.

A major concern when educating a patient in the use of the small-volume nebulizer is clarifying when to use the MDI and when to use the nebulizer. Many patients continue to use the MDI of the same type drug even when using a small-volume nebulizer. It often requires multiple discussions to be sure that the patient understands that the nebulizer treatments are replacing an MDI treatment.

Inhaled corticosteroids are always administered via an MDI with a spacer or reservoir device. (One brand of inhaled corticosteroids includes a spacer device as part of the delivery system.) Depending on patient preference and ability to comply, these drugs may be administered on a twice-a-day schedule or more frequently. The twice-a-day schedule has the advantages that one is less likely to forget doses and that administration of the drug is done prior to brushing the teeth, thus assuring that the mouth is rinsed after use. The major disadvantage is that a large number of inhalations must often be taken in order to obtain the desired daily dose. As the higher-dose inhaled steroids become available in the United States, this latter problem will be less significant. Since the important factor in efficacy of inhaled steroids is total daily dose versus the dosing schedule, a schedule that is convenient for the patient is frequently determined during the educational process.

F. Other Measures

Depending on the problems presented by the individual patient, additional content may be included in the asthma teaching program. One example is the use of breathing techniques. Teaching the patient to use a controlled breathing pattern with a slow, prolonged exhalation during an increase in shortness of breath is helpful to many, especially those with a significant component of fixed airways obstruction. Other patients profit from instruction in relaxation techniques (50,51). It is hoped that, with good pharmacological management, episodes of acute shortness of breath due to asthma would be rare. Finally some patients need encouragement to participate in regular exercise—walking, riding a stationary bicycle, and so on.

III. The Integrated Plan of Care

All of the above components of a patient education program become integrated into the total plan of care. For the plan of care to be truly successful, the patient must know how to prevent exacerbations, to monitor his or her disease, to recognize an exacerbation early, and to institute the appropriate measures. Thus patient education is not just *how* to do something but includes *when* to do something. Knowing when and how to treat an asthma exacerbation is not always straightforward. The question is often quite complex in the elderly due to the existence of comorbid problems.

Some interpretation and initiation of action is always required. Will decreases in function be recognized and simply reported to the professional caregiver for direction of action to be taken? Or will the patient independently take action, and to what extent? An increasingly popular approach to facilitate patient self-management of an asthma exacerbation is the use of "zones" of peak flow (31). Once the patient's "personal best" or usual peak flow is determined, levels are set to determine action. The classic zones are shown in Table 1. The patient then has a pharmacological plan to initiate for each zone. If the zone approach is used, the patient must be given written instructions with the actual limits of peak flow he or she is to follow. The written instructions also include what medications and actions to add at each level. Some have printed the zones and symptoms on a "credit card." One side of the card (credit-card sized) lists peak flow zones and associated actions; the other side of the card lists symptom changes and associated actions (49,52). When used as part of an educational and care program, the card was found to help patients make decisions about care measures.

Early in the educational process, it is probable that a large proportion of patients will want to report changes prior to taking action. The caregiver/educator must be available to confirm the patient's interpretations and guide interventions. Studies have demonstrated that telephone follow-up can be helpful in the problem-solving process (53). Others find that the use of group sessions for education offer additional support—there are usually relatively frequent sessions early in the process and the learning process is enhanced when patients hear of similar decision making by other patients. One study found that even for supposedly well-educated patients, there were significant gaps between knowledge about treatment and actual practice (54); in the study, the patients could tell

Table 1 Peak Flow Zones Used for Asthma Self-Management

Green zone	Asthma is in good control
	Peak flow is 80–100% of personal best
Yellow zone	Caution zone, need to get asthma back under control
	Peak flow is 50–79% of personal best
Red zone	Danger zone, need to call doctor or go to hospital immediately
	Peak flow is less than 50% of personal best

investigators what to do, but when presented with a scenario, they frequently did not apply that knowledge. Others have looked at the impact of personality factors on effective self-management (55). In other words, one cannot assume that the educational program will result in effective self-management by the patient. The educational process for elderly patients with asthma must be ongoing. The educator/clinician must be alert to changes in the patient's status (due to asthma or other conditions) and must be available for questions, review, and reinforcement of decisions made. Asthma self-management is truly a joint process—one whose ultimate success is determined by open and available communication between the professional and the patient.

Abbreviations

MDI	metered-dose inhaler
FRC	functional residual capacity
RV	residual volume

References

1. Speare A, Meyer JW. Types of elderly residential mobility and their determinants. J Gerontol 1988; 43:S74–S78.
2. Neugarten BL. Social and psychological characteristics of older people. In: Cassel CK, Riesenberg DE, Sorensen LB, Walsh JR, ed. Geriatric Medicine, 2d ed. New York: Springer-Verlag, 1990:28–37.
3. Serow WJ, Sly DF, Wrigley JM. Population aging in the United States. New York: Greenwood Press, 1990.
4. Carstensen LL. Selectivity theory: Social activity in life-span context. In: Schaie KW, Lawton MP, eds. Annual Review of Gerontology and Geriatrics. New York: Springer, 1991:195–216.
5. Devons C. Suicide in the elderly. Geriatrics 1996; 51:67–72.
6. Pachana NA, Gallagher-Thompson D, Thompson LW. Assessment of depression. In:

Lawton MP, ed. Annual Review of Gerontology and Geriatrics. New York: Springer, 1994:234–256.
7. Reynolds C. Recognition and differentiation of elderly depression in the clinical setting. Geriatrics 1995; 50:S6–S15.
8. National Heart, Lung and Blood Institute. National Asthma Education Program Panel. Considerations for Diagnosing and Managing Asthma in the Elderly. NIH pub. no. 96-3662, February 1996.
9. West RL, Crook TH, Barron KL. Everyday memory performance across the life span: Effects of age in noncognitive individual differences. Psychol Aging 1992; 7:72–82.
10. Morris JC, McManus DQ. The neurology of aging: Normal vs pathologic change. Geriatrics 1991; 46:47–54.
11. Jutagir R. Psychological aspects of aging: When does memory loss signal dementia? Geriatrics 1994; 49:45–53.
12. Ciocom JO, Potter JF. Age-related changes in human memory: Normal and abnormal. Geriatrics 1988; 43:43–48.
13. Carter TL. Age-related vision changes: A primary care guide. Geriatrics 1994; 49: 37–45.
14. Lichtenstein MJ. Hearing and visual impairments. Clin Geriatr Med 1992; 8: 173–182.
15. Kick E. Patient teaching for elders. Nurs Clin North Am 1989; 24:681–686.
16. Wilson SR, Scamagas P, German DF, et al. A controlled trial of two forms of self-management education for adults with asthma. Am J Med 1993; 94:564–576.
17. Mayo PH, Richman J, Harris HW. Results of a program to reduce admissions for adult asthma. Ann Intern Med 1990; 112:864–871.
18. Trautner C, Richter B, Berger M. Cost-effectiveness of a structured treatment and teaching programme on asthma. Eur Respir J 1993; 6:1485–1491.
19. Worth H. Patient education in asthmatic adults. Monaldi Arch Chest Dis 1993; 48: 155–158.
20. Muhlhauser I, Richter B, Kraut D, et al. Evaluation of a structured treatment and teaching programme on asthma. J Intern Med 1991; 230:157–164.
21. van der Schoot TAW, Kaptein AA. Pulmonary rehabilitation in an asthma clinic. Lung 1990; 168(suppl):495–501.
22. Sarma M, Alpers JH, Prideaux DJ, Kroemer DJ. The comprehensibility of Australian educational literature for patients with asthma. Med J Aust 1995; 162:360–363.
23. Musher D. Streptococcus pneumoniae. In: Mandell G, Bennett J, Dolin R, eds. Principles and Practice of Infectious Diseases, 4th ed. New York: Churchill Livingstone, 1995:1811–1826.
24. Cook NR, Evans DA, Scherr PA, et al. Peak expiratory flow rate in an elderly population. Am J Epidemiol 1989; 130:66–78.
25. Dekker FW, Schrier AC, Sterk PJ, Dijkman JH. Validity of peak expiratory flow measurement in assessing reversibility of airflow obstruction. Thorax 1992; 47: 162–166.
26. Connolly MJ, Crowley JJ, Charan NB, et al. Reduced subjective awareness of bronchoconstriction provoked by methacholine in elderly asthmatic and normal subjects as measured on a simple awareness scale. Thorax 1992; 6:410–413.
27. Barnes P. Poorly perceived asthma. Thorax 1992; 47:408–409.

28. Noseda A, Schmerber J, Prigogine T, Yernault J. Perceived effect on shortness of breath of an acute inhalation of saline or terbutaline: Variability and sensitivity of a visual analogue scale in patients with asthma or COPD. Eur Respir J 1992; 5: 1043–1053.

29. Rubinfeld AR, Pain M. Perception of asthma. Lancet 1976; 1:882–884.

30. Kendrick A, Higgs C, Whitfield M, Laszlo G. Accuracy of perception of severity of asthma: Patients treated in general practice. Br Med J 1993; 307:422–424.

31. National Heart, Lung and Blood Institute; National Asthma Education and Prevention Program. Nurses: Partners in Asthma Care. Pub. No. 95-3308, NIH; October 1995.

32. Chmelik F, Doughty A. Objective measurements of compliance in asthma treatment. Ann Allergy 1994; 73:527–532.

33. Chowiencyzk P, Parkin DH, Lawson CP, Cochrane GM. Do asthmatic patients correctly record home spirometry measurements? Br Med J 1994; 309:1618.

34. Charlton I, Charlton G, Broomfield J, Mullee MA. Evaluation of peak flow and symptoms only self management plans for control of asthma in general practice. Br Med J 1990; 130:1355–1359.

35. Malo JL, L'Archeveque J, Trudeau C, et al. Should we monitor peak expiratory flow rates or record symptoms with a simple diary in the management of asthma? J Allergy Clin Immunol 1993; 91:702–709.

36. Osman LM, Russell IT, Friend JA, et al. Attitudes to asthma medication. Thorax 1993; 48:827–830.

37. Shim C, Williams MH. The adequacy of inhalation of aerosol from canister nebulizers. Am J Med 1980; 69:891–894.

38. Kumana CR, So SY, Lauder IJ, et al. An audit of antiasthmatic drug inhalation technique and understanding. J Asthma 1993; 30:263–269.

39. Larsen JS, Hahn M, Ekholm B, Wick KA. Evaluation of conventional press-and-breathe metered-dose inhale technique in 501 patients. J Asthma 1994; 31:193–199.

40. McFadden E. Improper patient techniques with metered dose inhalers: Clinical consequences and solutions to misuse. J Allergy Clin Immunol 1996; 2:278–283.

41. Armitage J, Williams S. Inhaler technique in the elderly. Age Ageing 1988; 17:275–278.

42. Allen S, Prior A. What determines whether an elderly patient can use a metered dose inhaler correctly? Br J Dis Chest 1986; 80:45–49.

43. Guidry GG, Brown WD, Stogner S, George RB. Incorrect use of metered dose inhalers by medical personnel. Chest 1992; 101:31–33.

44. Jones J, Holstege C, Riekse R, et al. Metered-dose inhalers: Do emergency health care providers know what to teach? Ann Emergency Med 1995; 26:308–311.

45. Nimmo C, Chen D, Martinusen S, et al. Assessment of patient acceptance and inhalation technique of a pressurized aerosol inhaler and two breath-actuated devices. Ann Pharmacother 1993; 27:922–926.

46. Labrune S, Chinet T, Huchon G. Inhaled therapy in asthma: Metered-dose inhaler experience. Monaldi Arch Chest Dis 1994; 49:254–257.

47. Diggory P, Bailey R, Vallon A. Effectiveness of inhaled bronchodilator delivery systems for elderly patients. Age Ageing 1991; 20:379–382.

48. Chapman KR, Love L, Brubaker H. A comparison of breath-actuated and conventional metered-dose inhaler inhalation techniques in elderly subjects. Chest 1993; 104:1332–1337.

49. D'Souza W, Crane J, Burgess C, et al. Community-based asthma care: Trial of a "credit card" asthma self-management plan. Eur Respir J 1994; 7:1260–1265.

50. Lehrer PM, Sargunaraj D, Hochron S. Psychological approaches to the treatment of asthma. J Consult Clin Psychol 1992; 6:639–643.

51. Lehrer PM, Hochron SM, Mayne T, et al. Relaxation and music therapies of asthma among patients prestabilized on asthma medication. J Behav Med 1994; 17:1–24.

52. D'Souza W, Burgess C, Ayson M, et al. Trial of a "credit card" asthma self-management plan in a high-risk groups of patients with asthma. J Allergy Clin Immunol 1996; 97:1085–1092.

53. Roberts J, Browne G, Streiner D, et al. Problem-solving counselling or phone-call support for outpatients with chronic illness: Effective for whom? Can J Nurs Res 1995; 27:111–137.

54. Kolbe J, Vamos M, James F, et al. Assessment of practical knowledge of self-management of acute asthma. Chest 1996; 109:86–90.

55. Richards JM, Dolce JJ, Windsor RA, et al. Patient characteristics relevant to effective self-management: Scales for assessing attitudes of adults toward asthma. J Asthma 1989; 26:99–108.

10

Coexisting Conditions that Complicate Asthma Management in the Elderly

HENRY GONG, JR.

University of Southern California School of Medicine
Los Angeles, California

I. Introduction

The advancing average age of the general population is relatable to an elderly population that is growing in size and living longer (1). Since the 1970s, the population above age 65 has grown twice as quickly as the rest of the population in the United States. By the year 2030, one in five persons in the United States (approximately 35 million people) is expected to be older than 65 years. Mortality rates even at advanced ages are falling (2). As survival increases, more elderly individuals will develop chronic medical conditions. These trends in the elderly population clearly challenge the diagnostic and management skills of health professionals.

Diseases of the airways are important causes of morbidity and mortality in elderly persons as well as in the general population. Asthma has become a prominent topic because of its public health significance and related impacts on medical diagnosis (or misdiagnosis), decision making, interventions, and outcomes (3–5). Older adults with asthma constitute a distinct clinical group because of difficulties in diagnosis and medical management. This review addresses one major clinical aspect of asthma in the elderly, i.e., the coexisting medical conditions that can complicate asthma management. Older asthmatics frequently have multiple comorbidities and associated drug therapies, placing them at risk for adverse drug interactions (6,7). This review summarizes the medical conditions of elderly asthmatics and the potential clinical interactions between asthma and coexisting disorders and/or their treatments in this age group, while pointing out the limitations of knowledge in these areas. Issues related to the pathophysiology of asthma in the elderly, clinical evaluation, differential diagnosis, and the educational, monitoring, environmental, and pharmacological components of asthma management are discussed elsewhere (3–5).

II. Overview

A. Medical Conditions in the Elderly

The management of diseases and disabilities in elderly patients can be complicated and challenging. Many clinicians have heretofore emphasized a single disorder in diagnosis and management. However, this singular approach ignores the "whole patient" who has several concurrent medical conditions and is treated, not infrequently, with various medications (polypharmacy) by different physicians. The emergence of an increasing pool of elderly patients, managed care, and the discipline of gerontology has significantly altered this approach and escalated the importance of recognizing and understanding comorbid conditions and potential disease-drug interactions. The general approach to managing elderly patients should be based on certain gerontologic principles (8,9) (Table 1). The anticipation of disease or complications can result in better preventive and therapeutic interventions and healthier outcomes.

The pattern of death among the elderly is generally similar to that of the population as a whole, although there are some differences in the rankings of the leading causes. Leading causes of death among those 65 years of age and older are heart disease, malignant neoplasms, and cerebrovascular disease (10) (Table 2).

In general, the occurrence of acute conditions decreases with advancing age, while that of chronic conditions increases. Most major illnesses in the elderly result from preexisting conditions that contribute to a greater risk of developing further disease progression or complications. Older persons have an average of five concurrent medical conditions (9). The most prevalent chronic conditions among the aged are arthritis, hypertension, and heart disease (11) (Table 3). Trends in chronic illnesses are dynamic; shifts in disease prevalence follow changes in diagnosis, technology, and therapies. Modification of risk factors and treatment have mitigated some diseases, so that onset may be delayed or modified and survival is prolonged. For example, the federally funded National Long Term Care Surveys compared the 1982 and 1989 prevalences of 16 medical conditions in Medicare-eligible community residents aged 65 and older and identified as chronically disabled on screening interviews (12). The survey identified chronic

Table 1　Important Clinical Principles in Managing Diseases in Elderly Patients

1. Multiple diseases commonly coexist.
2. The spectrum of illness is relatively unique.
3. Illness may present in unusual ways.
4. The aging process per se is too often blamed for health problems.
5. Health problems are frequently underreported.
6. The symptom(s) or disease may not require pharmacological therapy. Use of over-the-counter medication should be reviewed with the patient.
7. The risks of treatment, drug interactions, and the patient's ability to comply with the treatment regimen must be reviewed.
8. Most medications should be started at a low dose and the dose increased or adjusted slowly.
9. Therapy must be closely monitored for efficacy and side effects.
10. Goals for health care should become more functional than curative in chronic diseases.

Source: Refs. 8 and 9.

Table 2　Death Rates for 10 Leading Causes of Death Among Older People, by Age Group, 1984

Cause of death (per 100,000)	<65 years	65–74 years	75–84 years	85+ years
All causes	*5,103*	*2,848*	*6,398*	*15,223*
Diseases of the heart	2,186	1,103	2,749	7,251
Malignant neoplasms	1,042	835	1,272	1,604
Cerebrovascular diseases	476	177	626	1,884
Chronic obstructive pulmonary diseases	199	141	270	331
Pneumonia and influenza	182	54	216	883
Diabetes	95	59	126	217
Accidents	87	50	107	257
Atherosclerosis	83	17	88	488
Nephritis, nephrotic syndrome, nephrosis	58	27	76	201
Septicemia	41	20	52	142
All other causes	654	365	816	1,965

Source: Ref. 11.

Table 3 Leading Chronic Conditions per 1000 Persons and Percent with Activity Limitations Due to Chronic Disease by Age Group, United States, 1985

	All ages	Under 18 years	18–44 years	45–64 years	65+ years
Chronic condition (per 1000)					
Arthritis	28.6	2.2	52.1	268.5	472.8
Hypertension	125.1	2.3	64.1	258.9	414.5
Hearing impairment	90.7	19.2	49.8	159.0	294.4
Heart condition	82.6	21.2	40.1	129.0	304.5
Orthopedic impairment	112.6	33.2	25.3	160.6	170.8
Sinusitis	139.0	59.6	164.4	184.8	154.5
Cataracts	25.0	2.1	1.8	24.4	164.0
Diabetes	26.2	1.9	9.1	51.9	103.8
Visual impairment	36.4	10.8	32.8	43.7	96.5
Tinnitus	26.1	0.7	15.0	49.8	91.7
Activity limitation (%)					
None	86.0	94.9	91.6	76.6	60.4
Limitation, not in a major activity	4.5	1.5	2.8	5.9	15.5
Limitation in a major activity	9.5	3.7	5.7	17.5	24.1

Source: Ref. 11.

disability episodes and associated morbidity (Table 4). Between 1982 and 1989, prevalences significantly decreased for arthritis, arteriosclerosis, dementia, hypertension, stroke, circulatory disease, and emphysema in this elderly noninstitutionalized cohort. On the other hand, Parkinson's disease, other heart disease (e.g., congestive heart failure), pneumonia, bronchitis, and hip fractures increased. Asthma prevalence remained stable. As expected, disabilities that accompany both acute and chronic conditions increase and accumulate with advancing age.

Patients 65 years of age and older are the largest consumers of pharmaceuticals in the United States and use 40% of all prescription and over-the-counter medications (9). The types and number of coexisting medical conditions make the elderly patient especially prone to polypharmacy: the average older person takes 4.5 medications and fills 13 prescriptions every year (13). The risk of drug interactions increases with the age of the patient and number of medications (14). Because of age-related physiological changes in homeostatic mechanisms and supervening diseases, elderly persons tend to be less tolerant of many drugs, some of which may also adversely interact with diseases. For example, 10–30% of geriatric hospital admissions are due to drug toxicity (15,16) and 1 of every 1000 older patients admitted to a hospital dies of an adverse drug reaction (17). It is estimated that the rate of adverse effects is 4% for persons receiving 5 or fewer

Table 4 Morbidity Prevalance in U.S. Noninstitutional Elderly Population, National Long-Term-Care Surveys, 1982 and 1989

Condition	1982 observed ($n = 6088$)	1989 observed ($n = 4463$)	Difference between 1989 observed proportion and 1982 standardized (%)
1. Arthritis	68.8%	63.1%	−8.0[a]
2. Parkinson's	0.8	1.3	0.5[a]
3. Diabetes	11.0	12.4	1.0
4. Cancer	6.2	5.7	−0.8
5. Arteriosclerosis	20.7	14.9	−6.5[a]
6. Dementia	2.8	1.7	−1.2[a]
7. Heart attack	3.7	3.2	−0.7
8. Other heart	19.5	22.9	2.7[a]
9. Hypertension	44.5	39.5	−6.5[a]
10. Stroke	3.4	2.6	−0.9[a]
11. Circulation	40.7	32.1	−10.0[a]
12. Pneumonia	2.9	4.8	1.8[a]
13. Bronchitis	9.5	12.1	2.2[a]
14. Emphysema	8.6	6.4	−2.4[a]
15. Asthma	6.5	6.3	−0.4
16. Broken hip/ fractures	0.5	0.9	0.4[a]
Average number of conditions	2.50	2.29	−11.2[a]

[a]$p < 0.05$, t-test.
Source: Ref. 12.

drugs, 10% for those receiving 6–10 drugs, and 28% for those receiving 11–15 drugs (18). Unfortunately, little information about the efficacy and safety of many new drugs in elderly persons is typically available. Most clinical drug trials exclude the old and infirm; the actual incidence and severity of drug toxicity are unknown until after approval by the U.S. Food and Drug Administration and widespread use (9). Thus, adverse drug reactions occur commonly in elderly patients but are often preventable.

B. Asthma in the Elderly

Estimates of the prevalence of asthma in the elderly differ greatly from country to country and even within the same country because of different diagnostic criteria, types of surveyed groups, and health care systems (19,20). The prevalence of asthma in the elderly has ranged between 3 and 7% in most population studies (21–24). In the United States, the prevalence of asthma in 1989 was 5.2% among people 65 years of age and older (22). An American population study estimated that current asthma was present in 3.8% of men and 7.1% of women aged 65 years and older (23). Thus, asthma is not uncommon, especially as the elderly segment of the population increases.

Elderly asthmatics can be categorized into two groups: those with long-standing or recurrent asthma since childhood or early adulthood and those with clinical asthma that develops de novo during advanced age. The former pattern is considered more common. Up to 85% of asthmatics experience their first symptoms before age 40 years (25). During a 20-year follow-up in the Normative Aging Study (in which men with chronic medical conditions, including asthma, were excluded at screening), only 53 (mean age 61 years) of 1298 subjects (4.1%) reported ever having physician-diagnosed asthma and 16 subjects (1.2%) reported active asthma (26). However, asthma in the elderly is complicated by (1) the high frequency of coexisting irreversible airflow obstruction, i.e., chronic obstructive pulmonary disease (COPD) (6,7,27–29), and (2) indifference or misdiagnosis, which delays the recognition and proper treatment of asthma (30,31). A study of elderly asthmatics in a pulmonary clinic revealed that 48% developed asthma at greater than 65 years of age (28). Furthermore, approximately half of elderly asthmatics in a large population study reported the onset of clinical asthma after the age of 40 years, although asthmatic-type symptoms were usually present for many years before the diagnosis, and recall bias may have been a factor (27,32).

The health consequences of asthma in the elderly are substantial. Between 1975 and 1980, all ambulatory visits for asthma in the United States increased from 2.71 to 2.85 visits per 100 population, largely related to persons 15–44 years of age and those 65 years of age and older (33). Between 1969 and 1990, asthmatics 65 years of age and older had the highest annual hospitalization rates for asthma of any age group, although the trend has leveled off to about 3.2 per 1000 population since 1985. Asthmatics tend to continuously take at least two antiasthma medications, excluding courses of antibiotics and corticosteroids (6). Functional status greatly influences everyday life in elderly people, particularly when they have chronic disease(s). Elderly asthmatics who are being treated for symptoms report greater dependency in activities of daily living, poor health, and impaired mobility than nonasthmatic controls (34). Following adjustments for medical and nonmedical factors, patients treated for asthma still have a greater risk of disability in daily life and poorer subjective health than controls. Dyspnea is the main factor for disability in elderly subjects treated for asthma (34,35), although wheezing remains a predominant symptom in most studies (19).

Although mortality rates from asthma increase with age and across time in almost all age groups, most deaths occur in patients more than 50 years of age (36). The 1991 death rates for the age groups of 55–59 and 60–64 years were 2.8 and 4.2 per 100,000 general population in the United States, respectively, compared to less than 2 per 100,000 for all other age groups. Aging may partly account for the upward trend in asthma mortality, although age-adjusted death rates still indicate overall increases in mortality since the late 1970s. Advanced age is a definite risk factor for mortality in asthmatic patients following discharge from the intensive care unit (after requiring first-time mechanical ventilation for acute asthma); approximately 60% of posthospitalization deaths occur within the year following discharge and are usually due to a new asthma attack (37). The causes for the high risk of fatal or near fatal asthma in this age group include, in addition to aging, less awareness or reporting of moderate airflow obstruction than is the case with younger patients (7,38,39), delays in self-referral (7), inadequate anti-inflammatory airways therapy (3–5), and other risk factors for severe asthma (5,40–43), such as comorbid medical conditions (6,7) and adverse drug interactions.

III. Limitations of this Review

Ideally, a review on comorbid medical conditions in elderly asthmatics should draw on a large volume of peer-reviewed published data. Unfortunately, such a substantial database is not as yet available. Most publications about asthma in the elderly during recent decades have focused on the concept of asthma per se in this age group and the difficulty of differential diagnosis. Whereas data are available on age-related differences in pharmacokinetics, pharmacodynamics, and interactions of drugs (but not necessarily in elderly asthmatics), relatively few reports have examined disease-drug interactions in the elderly with asthma. To date, an analysis of comorbidity in elderly asthmatics must be based upon a limited number of sources, such as investigations of small series of patients, care reports, and inferential statements in various reviews. Vital statistics are plentiful and another useful source of information. The diseases most frequently associated with aging, as determined from vital statistics, are more likely to be comorbid disorders in elderly asthmatic patients. However, the data do not adequately link asthma with comorbid conditions or drug therapies. Furthermore, less common conditions, not necessarily related to aging, must also be considered. Indeed, elderly patients with asthma may develop concurrent medical problems or disorders that may be associated more frequently with younger adults or that unexpectedly result from treatment of the comorbid disorder. Thus, this review must synthesize a mixture of published reports and reviews, extrapolate information from other age groups, and exercise certain clinical assumptions and judgments. This review attempts to indicate areas of knowledge and uncertainty, with the expectation that future studies will shed more light on specific comorbid conditions in this asthmatic age group.

IV. Comorbid Conditions in Elderly Asthmatics

Table 5 summarizes medical conditions in the elderly that may exist concurrently and can potentially influence or complicate asthma or its management. This list is

Table 5 Medical Conditions that May Interact with Asthma in the Elderly Due to the Coexisting Condition and/or Concurrent Treatments

---

Chronic obstructive pulmonary disease (COPD)
Smoking
Bronchogenic carcinoma
Cardiovascular diseases
Pulmonary embolism
Arthritis
Neurological and psychiatric conditions
Sleep apnea
Upper respiratory infections and rhinitis
Lower respiratory infections
Gastroesophageal reflux and aspiration
Diabetes mellitus
Hypothyroidism
Hyperthyroidism
Adrenocortical insufficiency

---

not all-inclusive and is deliberately simplistic in order to direct attention to likely or possible patterns of interactions. Changing patient status, clinical judgment, and individual circumstances may result in different scenarios or actions. An attempt is made to categorize the interactions between diseases and between drugs used to treat either condition. The following discussion examines major clinical interactions between asthma and comorbid conditions, some of which must also be considered in the differential diagnosis of new or worsening asthma-like symptoms in the elderly. Not all possible interactions necessarily occur frequently, and not all interactions are firmly documented or, if documented, fully understood. Many interactions may be of concern for younger as well as elderly asthmatics.

General principles regarding drug interactions are reviewed elsewhere (44–47). Drugs used intermittently or chronically to treat nonasthmatic diseases can adversely affect the asthmatic patient by exacerbating the asthma either through pharmacological or idiosyncratic mechanisms (e.g., beta blocker–and aspirin-induced bronchospasm) or undesirable interactions with asthma drugs (e.g., pharmacokinetic alterations in theophylline metabolism) (45). Most clinically significant drug interactions are produced by altering the bioavailability or clearance of a drug by another. Induction of metabolic enzymes (e.g., hepatic cytochrome P-450 mixed-function oxidative enzymes) is a principal means of increasing drug clearance. Drugs that are primarily eliminated by enzyme metabolism or active secretion are very susceptible to drug interactions, particularly when concurrent drugs are metabolized by the same pathway, resulting in higher plasma levels of the drug that "loses" the competition.

A. Chronic Obstructive Pulmonary Disease

Disease Interactions

Approximately 14 million persons in the United States have chronic obstructive pulmonary disease (COPD)—about 12.5 million with chronic bronchitis and about 1.7 million with emphysema. Chronic airflow obstruction in population-based studies in the United States range from 4–6% of adult white males and from 1–3% of adult white females (48). Death rates are similar for men and women before the age of 55 years, but they rise dramatically for men thereafter. At age 70 years, the death rate for men is more than double that for women, and at 85 and older, the male rate is more than 3.5 times that for females (49). The presumptive diagnosis of chronic bronchitis and/or emphysema in the symptomatic elderly patient, especially in males with a smoking history, is frequently made whenever irreversible airflow obstruction is documented. The question whether chronic irreversible airways obstruction in elderly asthmatics is related to long-standing asthma (possibly mimicking COPD) and/or to coexisting COPD illustrates the difficulties in defining asthma in the elderly in research studies as well as in the physician's office (19,27,28). Correct diagnosis is important because severe chronic asthma responds better to therapy (50) and has a better prognosis than smoking-related COPD, independent of smoking history (51). Asthmatics over 34 years of age with COPD have worse survival than expected (52).

Drug Interactions

The types and dosing regimens of medications used for COPD (53,54) are similar to those used for asthma, except that ipratropium bromide is emphasized more for COPD treatment, whereas anti-inflammatory medications (corticosteroids, cromolyn, and nedocromil) are primary treatment for asthma, regardless of age. However, since the diagnostic separation of asthma and COPD is frequently impossible to make in the elderly ex-smoker or smoker, therapeutic distinctions in most cases may not be clinically critical, since the elderly asthmatic patient with irreversible airways obstruction can effectively receive similar medications, including corticosteroids and ipratropium (19).

B. Smoking

Disease Interactions

Tobacco smokers are predisposed to develop COPD, lung cancer, and cardiovascular disorders as well as unstable asthma and sudden death. Education about smoking hazards and smoking cessation efforts have made considerable headway in reducing the smoking habits of the population. However, some individuals with asthma and COPD continue to smoke and have persistent problems with stopping this habit, in part due to nicotine addiction and for psychological reasons (42,55). Cigarette smoking, probably mediated by nicotine and/or adrenergic stimulation, also reduces lower esophageal sphincter pressure (56), which, in turn, facilitates possible gastroesophageal reflux (GER) and asthmatic symptoms via a vagally induced reflex. Some smokers maintain adequate asthma control (usually with multiple medications, including oral corticosteroids), whereas other asthmatics (the majority) cannot tolerate low levels of environmental tobacco smoke (57). The underlying mechanisms for these differences are not known. A prospective controlled study (58) of the effects of inhaled budesonide in smoking and non-smoking middle-aged asthmatics clearly demonstrated that the smoking group was resistant to corticosteroid treatment—based on results of lung function, histamine challenge, and blood markers of inflammation—unlike the responsive nonsmoking asthmatics. The use of β-agonists remained unchanged in the smoking group but was reduced substantially among the nonsmokers. The mechanism for this functional steroid resistance in smoking asthmatics is likely related to complex immunological interactions among oxidants, elastase-mediated injury, activated neutrophils and eosinophils, and their mediators, which perpetuate airway inflammation. A major conclusion is that smoking is harmful in asthmatics due in part to smoking-induced accelerated decline in lung function, the development of COPD (51,52,59), and resistance to anti-inflammatory drug therapy. This smoking effect is in addition to the possible progressive decline in lung function associated with asthma of long duration (6,59).

Drug Interactions

Theophylline continues to be widely prescribed for asthma (6,7). Paradoxically, older asthmatic patients tend to be more compliant with taking oral theophylline than inhaled antiasthma medications (60), despite theophylline-related side effects (6,7) and risk of toxicity (47). Theophylline is the major respiratory drug that has clinically significant pharmacokinetic interactions with smoking (61). Smoking of tobacco (or marijuana), even passively (62), increases the elimination of theophylline and requires upward adjustment of the theophylline dose to maintain a therapeutic level (47). On the other hand, theophylline elimination decreases following smoking cessation, requiring a downward dose adjustment to prevent theophylline toxicity.

C. Bronchogenic Cancer

Disease Interactions

The risk for bronchogenic carcinoma increases independently with age (notably, after age 69 years) and is a common malignancy in the elderly, particularly in former or current smokers. Lung cancer is more common across all age groups when airflow obstruction is present compared with persons with normal airflow (63). A strong relationship between airflow obstruction and lung cancer was also observed in the multicenter Lung Health Study (64,65). Interestingly, an inverse relationship between allergy-related diseases (including asthma) and lung cancer has been suggested (66–68). Although populations with allergy-related disorders appear to be at decreased risk for lung cancer, many elderly patients with asthma and/or COPD continue to smoke or are ex-smokers, rendering them at continued risk for tobacco-related lung cancers. Bronchogenic carcinoma may worsen asthma by producing localized or diffuse bronchitis or obstructive pneumonia, or, if centrally located, by increasing airways resistance and work of breathing. A high index of suspicion is necessary to recognize this diagnostic possibility in the elderly asthmatic, who may have unexplained worsening of bronchospasm that is unresponsive to intensified therapy or new symptoms or findings, such as hemoptysis, wet cough, unilateral or localized wheezing, or obstructive pneumonia on chest radiographs (30). Localized wheezing may be audible when a bronchogenic or metastatic carcinoma or tracheal tumor narrows a large airway. These symptoms may initially be attributed to asthma or COPD.

Drug Interactions

Radiation-induced bronchitis or fibrosis may make control of asthma more difficult. Infused vinca alkaloids (vinblastine, vindesine) may precipitate acute dyspnea and severe bronchospasm, most frequently when combined with mitomycin C (69). The relationship to underlying asthma is unclear.

D. Cardiovascular Diseases

Disease Interactions

Cardiovascular diseases are more prevalent in elderly than in middle-aged individuals (Table 3): coronary artery disease (CAD) affects 15% of men and 9% of women by age 70 years; congestive heart failure (CHF) affects over 2 million people, with 400,000 new cases and 900,000 hospitalizations every year; senile calcific aortic stenosis affects 48% of patients over age 70 years undergoing aortic valve replacement; premature ventricular complexes and bundle branch block increase in frequency with age; and atrial fibrillation affects 4% of people older than 60 years (70). Heart disease and cerebrovascular disease are the first and third major causes of death in the elderly (Table 2), and hypertension is one of their major risk factors. Hypertension is one of the most common comorbid conditions in elderly asthmatics (6,7). Despite the prevalence of cardiovascular diseases in elderly people, the relationship between cardiovascular disease, and its risk factors, to asthma has received limited epidemiological investigation. The Cardiovascular Health Study (CHS) found a 6% prevalence of asthma in 5201 subjects over age 65 years (24). Cross-sectional multivariate analyses of data from 309 elderly asthmatics (mean age, 72 years) indicated that asthma was significantly associated with higher levels of high-density lipoprotein cholesterol (HDL-C) and plasma fibrinogen, but not with cardiovascular diseases (CHF, coronary, cerebrovascular, and peripheral vascular diseases) (24). Nonsmoking men with asthma were more likely to have prevalent CAD and smoking men and women with asthma were more likely to report CHF and to have left ventricular hypertrophy by electrocardiographic (ECG) criteria. Longitudinal population studies are needed to confirm the CHS findings and to clarify the relationships between geriatric asthma and cardiovascular disease.

Clinically, concomitant heart disease can significantly complicate the management of asthma in the elderly patient:

1. Signs and symptoms of asthma may be confused with those of myocardial dysfunction and vice versa ("cardiac asthma").
2. Congestive heart failure and pulmonary edema can cause and exacerbate wheezing, dyspnea, and hypoxemia (30), which may temporarily improve with inhaled bronchodilators. Patients with left ventricular failure have increased airway reactivity, which is unaffected by diuretic therapy (71,72).
3. Hypoxemia, tachycardia, and hypertension associated with worsening or severe asthma may lead to myocardial ischemia or CHF.

Drug Interactions

Cardiovascular Drugs

Cardiopulmonary drug interactions are well documented in the medical literature (73–80), owing to the high frequency of cardiorespiratory illnesses and related multidrug usage in clinical practice. A number of commonly used cardiovascular medications can worsen asthma. Nonselective $beta_1$ (β_1) antagonists (e.g., propranolol, nadolol, and timolol) are frequently used for treatment of angina pectoris, post–acute myocardial infarction (MI), and hypertension. However, these agents can trigger sudden and severe bronchospasm in asthmatic patients (5,75,79). Propranolol also increases theophylline levels (Table 6) and nonspecific airways hyperreactivity in asthmatics. The so-called cardioselective β_1-antagonists (e.g., atenolol, metoprolol), beta blockers with intrinsic sympathomimetic (β_2) effects (e.g., pindolol), and the mixed α/β-antagonist labetalol may be better tolerated in the majority of bronchospastic patients, usually beginning with low doses (5,75,79). The ultra-short-acting intravenous beta blocker esmolol is usually well tolerated in asthmatics with unstable angina. Beta blockers with combined β-antagonist activity may be used for post-MI therapy in asthmatics (5,79).

Calcium-channel blockers, angiotensin-converting enzyme inhibitors (ACEIs),

Table 6 Drug Interactions Likely to Cause at Least a 20% Change in the Rate of Elimination of Theophylline

Drugs that decrease theophylline elimination	Drugs that increase theophylline elimination
Alcohol (0.9 g/kg)	Aminoglutethimide
Allopurinol (≥ 600 mg per day)	Carbamazepine
Cimetidine	Isoproternol (intravenous)
Ciprofloxacin	Moricizine
Clarithromycin	Phenytoin
Disulfiram	Rifampin
Enoxacin	Sulfinpyrazone
Erythromycin	
Estrogen	
Fluvoxamine	
Interferon	
Methotrexate	
Mexiletine	
Pentoxifylline	
Propafenone	
Propranolol	
Tacrine	
Thiabendazole	
Ticlopidine	
Troleandomycin	
Verapamil	
Zileuton	

When given in their usual doses, drugs that decrease the elimination of theophylline will increase steady-state serum concentrations, whereas drugs that increase elimination will decrease steady-state serum concentrations.
Source: Ref. 47.

and diuretics are desirable cardiovascular agents for asthmatics. Calcium-channel blockers and ACEIs are widely used and do not trigger bronchoconstriction. Calcium-channel blockers are useful in treating hypertension and CAD, since this drug class modestly prevents specifically (allergen-) and nonspecifically induced bronchospasm. However, verapamil and, to a lesser extent, diltiazem also inhibit theophylline metabolism (47). In patients with hypertension or left ventricular dysfunction/CHF, ACEI therapy may occasionally produce cough (5–15% incidence), but asthmatics are no more predisposed to this side effect than nonasthmatics (78,79).

Aspirin is widely used in cardiac patients to reduce the risk of myocardial infarction and stroke, but it may provoke severe bronchospasm, especially in patients with the triad of bronchial asthma, rhinosinusitis, and nasal polyps with aspirin sensitivity (76,81). Aspirin-sensitive asthmatic patients should avoid ingestion of aspirin and other nonsteroidal anti-inflammatory drugs (NSAIDs), but they may still achieve cardiovascular protection from the antiplatelet drug ticlopidine (82). However, ticlopidine significantly increases theophylline elimination (from 8.8 to 12.2 hr) with a comparable reduction in total plasma clearance in healthy volunteers (83).

Some antiarrhythmic agents can precipitate bronchoconstriction by different mechanisms: edrophonium (cholinergic stimulation); adenosine (release of mast cell mediators); sotalol (direct blockade of β_2-adrenoreceptors) (80). These medications are relatively contraindicated in asthmatics and must be used with caution. Mexiletine, used in managing ventricular arrhythmias, does not produce bronchoconstriction but significantly inhibits theophylline clearance.

Intravenous (but not oral) dipyridamole is used in thallium cardiac stress testing but precipitates acute bronchospasm in 0.15% of patients, presumably by inducing the release of mast cell mediators (84). The bronchoconstrictor adenosine frequently produces adverse cardiopulmonary side effects during pharmacological stress testing and requires more interventions with aminophylline than dipyridamole (85).

Antiasthma Drugs

Medications commonly used to treat asthma may adversely affect cardiovascular function. Bronchodilators—such as theophylline, beta$_2$ (β_2) agonists, epinephrine, ephedrine, and their combinations—can aggravate or induce adverse changes in gas exchange and hemodynamics that result in arrhythmias, angina pectoris, or hypertension by virtue of their pharmacological (adrenergic) actions. Intravenous aminophylline may be very risky in some patients with increased susceptibility to tachycardia and arrhythmia (5). The use of relatively β_2-selective agents reduces but does not eliminate cardiovascular side effects (86). Inhaled bronchodilators delivered by metered-dose inhaler (MDI) cause fewer systemic effects than nebulized or oral preparations, although the total delivered dose is likely the critical factor (5). Inhaled ipratropium bromide is a safe bronchodilator in this setting, since it is virtually devoid of hemodynamic effects (87–90). Oral corticosteroid therapy may induce sodium retention, hypertension, CHF, and hyperlipidemia. Inhaled corticosteroids lack these side effects and are effective and safe in the cardiac setting (91–93).

E. Pulmonary Embolism

Disease Interactions

Deep venous thrombosis in the lower extremities is a common complication in the elderly because of predisposing risk factors such as sedentary lifestyle, physical limitations, CHF, malignancy, and prolonged recuperation (immobilization) following surgery (30). Fracture of a hip or extremity secondary to osteoporosis or a fall is particularly commonplace in the elderly. Although pulmonary embolism is a rare cause of audible wheezing, localized release of bronchoconstrictive mediators during an embolic episode can precipitate generalized bronchospasm and acute asthma in a patient with underlying reactive airways.

Drug Interactions

There are no known adverse drug interactions between anticoagulants and asthma or antiasthma therapy. For example, theophylline metabolism is not altered by heparin or warfarin. Heparin has been found to demonstrate anti-inflammatory and antiallergic properties, such as the inhibition of histamine release, degranulation of stimulated mast cells, and attenuation of antigen- and exercise-induced bronchoconstriction in humans (94–96). The protective effect of heparin in induced bronchoconstriction is achieved by the inhaled route of administration and does not affect the partial thromboplastin time.

F. Arthritis

Disease Interactions

Arthritis is the leading chronic condition in the elderly (Table 3) and is commonly present in elderly asthmatics (6,7). Asthma may be difficult to manage in arthritic patients with significant physical restrictions in their upper extremities. The coordination necessary in using MDIs is generally less critical with the use of spacers in most elderly asthmatics with arthritis, although a subgroup of impaired patients may require hand-held nebulizers or oral medications. Inadequate hand strength may result in patients actuating the MDI either too late or not at all (97,98).

Drug Interactions

Aspirin and other NSAIDs are frequently used to treat arthritis but may cause severe and sudden asthma exacerbation in susceptible individuals (81). All NSAIDs with cyclooxygenase-inhibitory properties cross-react with aspirin. Although 10–20% of patients with asthma have idiosyncratic (non–IgE mediated) reactions to aspirin or NSAIDs, there appears to be a spectrum of responses. The widespread therapeutic use of NSAIDs in the elderly requires careful, individualized physician advisement when asthma is present (99). A history of worsening asthma or nasal or ocular symptoms after NSAID ingestion is usually adequate to identify sensitive patients.

Corticosteroids are effective anti-inflammatory therapy for many non-pulmonary conditions (e.g., arthritis) as well as for asthma. Fortunately, most elderly asthmatics use low doses of oral corticosteroids for control of comorbid rheumatological conditions. The elderly patient is very susceptible to adverse side effects from corticosteroid therapy (100–102). Systemic complications of oral corticosteroids—such as osteoporosis (including fractures of ribs and vertebrae), cataracts, hypothalamic-pituitary-adrenal axis suppression, diabetes mellitus, and hypertension—are related to the duration and dose of steroid therapy. These side effects (with clinical significance) have not been associated with inhaled corticosteroids at standard doses (91–93).

G. Neurological and Psychiatric Conditions

Disease Interactions

Central Nervous System

Physical and cognitive limitations are frequently present in elderly patients with Alzheimer's disease, vascular dementia, depression, psychoses, and other neuropsychiatric conditions. The prevalence of parkinsonism (bradykinesia, gait disturbance, rigidity, and tremor) increases with age and is very common among people over 65 years of age (103). These debilitating conditions may interfere with optimal drug administration, dosing regimens, and compliance in asthmatic patients. Ineffective hand-breath coordination and impaired cognitive status can significantly worsen MDI technique (98,104,105). Manual dexterity, hand strength, and coordination are important components for MDI actuation and are likely to be impaired in patients with cerebrovascular accidents, neuromuscular weakness, or tremors related to parkinsonism. The faulty MDI technique results in an inadequate amount of medication delivered to the lower airways, limited bronchodilation, and wasted medication (with concomitant costs) (106). Severely impaired patients may be incapable of using the MDI (even with a spacer device) or dry-powder breath-actuated inhalers (primarily because they cannot load the capsules). They will require a hand-held nebulizer (107) or breath-activated MDI (105), assuming that they have sufficient inspiratory airflow. Alternatively, oral bronchodilator preparations or using a two-handed technique or a grip aid for the MDI can be considered.

Psychological stress and psychiatric disorders are important predisposing factors for life-threatening asthma (40,41). Depression, personality disorders, schizophrenia, alcohol abuse, recent family loss or disruption, and recent unemployment clearly complicate asthma management and predict increased risks of morbidity and death from asthma (42,43). Denial of disease(s), inappropriate anxiety, noncompliance with medications and appointments, inordinate amounts of time and care required by concomitant disorders, abuse of medical resources, and a fear of some medications (corticosteroids) by both the patient and physician, even after a life-threatening asthma exacerbation, are other notable risk factors. Psychoactive, antipsychotic, and antidepressant drugs must always be administered with caution and monitoring in older persons (9). Asthmatics who use major tranquilizers or other psychoactive drugs appear to be at an increased risk of death or near death from asthma and hospital readmission (108,109). Patients who discontinue their antipsychotic drugs are at higher risk for serious complications of asthma.

Visual impairment increases with age (Table 3). Macular degeneration, cataracts, glaucoma, diabetic retinopathy, and other causes of visual impairment are frequently present in elderly patients and are major causes of blindness in the elderly, many of whom are unaware of their impaired vision (110). These conditions can compromise asthma management by limiting the patient's ability to select the correct MDI or oral medication (especially during an asthma attack), accurately read instructions or numbers on the peak flowmeter, and measure liquid medications.

Spinal Cord Injury

Patients with spinal cord injury (SCI) represent an underevaluated respiratory group. The mean age of injury and duration of long-term survival are increasing in the population with SCI. In the multicenter National Spinal Cord Injury Database (111), individuals over the age of 60 years represented 8.5% of the database's cases in 1991, compared with 4.5% for the 1973–1977 period. Aging-associated spinal osteoarthritis is a particular risk for cervical-level SCI in elderly persons (112). Survivors of the acute event are vulnerable to subsequent atelectasis, sputum retention, pneumonia, and pulmonary emboli as well as ventilator assistance. Although the prevalence of preexisting COPD is low (3%) in the National SCI Database (111), asthma is not listed in this source or in other references (113,114). Whether this absence is related to diagnostic issues, lack of suspicion, or actual rarity is unclear. Asthma, more than likely, is underdiagnosed in SCI patients, particularly in those with cervical tetraplegia who are likely to be asymptomatic (due to absent or altered perceptions) or who complain of atypical symptoms. In one survey of patients with complete SCI (C6–S5 lesions) (115), 18% complained of chronic cough, 18% of chronic sputum production, 24% of persistent wheeze, and 50% of any wheeze. Approximately 40–50% of otherwise healthy tetraplegic patients have a significant bronchodilator response following inhalation of metaproterenol (116) or ipratropium bromide (117) despite an underlying restrictive ventilatory defect. Eight otherwise healthy SCI subjects (C4–C7 injuries) demonstrated significant airways reactivity to methacholine inhalation (PC20-FEV$_1$ less than 5 mg/ml), which was completely blocked by pretreatment with ipratropium (118). Similarly, another study (119) compared methacholine responsiveness in otherwise healthy tetraplegic nonsmokers with and without chronic therapy with baclofen, a commonly used muscle relaxant. The mean PC20-FEV$_1$ in the control group was 1.42 mg/ml, as compared with 15.0 mg/ml in the baclofen group ($p = 0.001$), suggesting that gamma-aminobutyric acid (GABA) and the GABA agonist baclofen inhibit cholinergic, neurally mediated bronchoconstriction. The above data indicate that the typical restrictive ventilatory impairment in cervical tetraplegia "masks" an obstructive component as a result of interrupted sympathetic innervation of the airways (originating in the upper six thoracic ganglia) and an intact parasympathetic nerve supply (efferent cholinergic nerves pass from the vagal nuclei of the brainstem via the vagus nerve to synapse in ganglia within the airway wall). Such unopposed cholinergic tone can be expected to enhance bronchial responsiveness. Thus, cervical SCI represents a unique situation of purely neurally mediated bronchial hyperreactivity (with PC20s well within the typical asthmatic range) (119). Whether these findings may explain why some patients with cervical SCI complain of respiratory symptoms (e.g., dyspnea) out of proportion to their impaired lung function or without clinically obvious respiratory complications remains to be investigated. Clinicians in this situation might consider an evaluation of airways responsiveness and/or a trial of an inhaled anticholinergic bronchodilator.

Drug Interactions

Physicians must be aware of the asthmogenic drug interactions of certain antidepressants, e.g., acute asthma from tartrazine-containing antidepressants and vasopressor effects resulting from the combination of monoamine oxidase inhibitors (MAOIs) and tyramine and possibly epinephrine. Extreme caution should be used if any antidepressant is given to an allergic patient with myocardial ischemia who is also receiving epinephrine injections. Theophylline increases the renal clearance of lithium, which may necessitate an adjustment of the dose of the latter to control acute mania in bipolar disorders (47).

Topically applied ophthalmic solutions for glaucoma therapy, such as nonselective β_1-antagonists (e.g., timolol, betaxolol, carteolol, levobunolol, metipranolol), anticholinesterases, and parasympathomimetic drugs (e.g., pilocarpine, carbachol), may severely exacerbate asthma because of systemic absorption (99,120,121). Eyedrops containing an NSAID (e.g., indomethacin, flurbiprofen, suprofen, ketorolac, and diclofenac) for treating conjunctivitis can provoke an asthma attack following absorption (99). Acute angle-closure glaucoma has rarely been reported to result from nebulized ipratropium (122,123), although this complication may relate more to faulty technique than to the inhaled drug.

Beta blockers (propranolol, timolol), NSAIDs (e.g., naproxen), or calcium-channel blockers are used as prophylaxis for frequent or severe migraine headaches (124). As indicated previously, beta blockers and NSAIDs are contraindicated in asthmatics, whereas calcium-channel blockers are preferred.

The anticonvulsants phenytoin, carbamazepine, and phenobarbital are potent inducers of hepatic cytochrome P-450 mixed-function oxidase activity. These drugs significantly reduce steady-state theophylline concentrations by increasing its systemic clearance. For example, phenytoin increases theophylline clearance by 30–65%. Asthmatic patients will need a higher than usual theophylline dose to maintain a therapeutic level during combination therapy. Serum theophylline concentration should be checked several days after these anticonvulsants are added to the regimen to make appropriate adjustment of the theophylline dosage.

Seizures in the elderly require careful diagnosis and management, especially in the presence of asthma (125–128). Theophylline toxicity may be associated with seizures, particularly in patients with underlying central nervous system lesions. Seizures may be confused with nonischemic tonic attacks, which are related to hypoxia during severe asthma attacks (127) and can lead to respiratory arrest and anoxic encephalopathy. Both types of neural events respond poorly to anticonvulsants alone and require appropriate monitoring of serum theophylline concentrations if the drug is continued. Theophylline should probably be avoided in patients with underlying neurologic disease, since this drug may precipitate seizures at even subtherapeutic plasma concentrations in these patients (128).

Subcutaneous terbutaline can acutely decrease systemic vascular resistance and result in severe hypotension in tetraplegic patients with recent cervical injury and autonomic dysfunction (129). Thus, subcutaneous β-adrenergic agents should be administered with great caution in this setting.

The use of oral corticosteroids is associated with psychoses in 2.4% and acute psychological changes in 3% of cases (91). Fewer than ten patients have been reported to develop psychiatric symptoms during inhaled glucocorticoid therapy (usually with budesonide) (91–93). Symptoms improved with stopping the inhaled steroid.

H. Sleep Apnea

Disease Interactions

The frequency of sleep disorders (e.g., snoring, obstructive sleep apnea) increases with aging, especially in men and postmenopausal women (130). The coexistence of asthma and obstructive sleep apnea is rare, although reports about combined sleep apnea and COPD (including "asthma" in some cases) have appeared (131–133). Sleep apnea should be considered in asthmatic patients with heavy snoring or obstructing nasal polyps or those who have erythrocytosis (5). Heavy snoring may precede the onset of unstable asthma. The coexistence of the two disorders defines a special high-risk group in that sleep-related hypoxemia and cardiovascular consequences may be more marked than that observed in patients with sleep apnea alone, in addition to interference with the control of asthma during the day and night. Nocturnal or sleep-related asthma is very common in uncontrolled asthma and is most severe and potentially fatal during the early morning hours (134). Asthmatic patients with sleep apnea may have severe nocturnal asthma attacks, including respiratory arrests, which do not respond to maximal bronchodilator and steroid therapy (135). Sleep apnea in asthmatic patients is regarded as a major risk factor for fatal asthma (43), partly related to daytime sleepiness, cognitive impairments, personality changes associated with sleep apnea, and resulting noncompliance (136). Therapy with nasal continuous positive airway pressure (CPAP) can improve nocturnal obstructive episodes, asthma symptoms, and lung function (135,137). Treatment of chronic nasal obstruction, surgical resection of anatomically obstructing pharyngeal tissue, and, occasionally, tracheostomy may be required.

Drug Interactions

There are no known adverse drug interactions with asthma or its therapy. Theophylline may be considered as a respiratory stimulant in patients with central sleep apnea.

I. Upper Respiratory Infections and Rhinitis

Disease Interactions

Acute respiratory infections are responsible for significant morbidity and mortality in the elderly population. They are ranked as the fifth leading cause of death in persons aged 65 and older and are diagnosed in at least 6% of hospitalized persons aged 65 and older (138,139). The incidence of acute respiratory illness in community-based populations of noninstitutionalized elderly is relatively low (i.e., 2.5 to 3.5 episodes of illness per 100 person-months of observation), which is consistent with the notion that viral respiratory rates decrease with increasing age (140). However, these infection rates are generally derived from healthy older people living independently in the community and may underestimate the incidence of acute respiratory infections in frail elderly, who are most likely to develop serious sequelae. For example, seniors concentrated in day-care programs, nursing homes, and hospitals may be more susceptible and likely to be exposed to more contagious infections than counterparts living at home. One prospective day-care study (141) found an overall rate of 10.8 acute respiratory infections per 100 person-months, primarily with infections by respiratory syncytial virus, influenza A, and coronavirus. Chronic cardiac conditions (69%) and nonspecified chronic pulmonary disease (13%) were present in the 165 subjects (average age, 79 years). Wheezing was present in 4% at baseline and 19% in those who were ill, mostly associated with influenza A and bacterial infections. Although the mechanisms of transmission are numerous, exposure to infected individuals, particularly children, appears to be a definite risk factor (140,141).

   The relationship between respiratory tract infections and asthma in adult patients is established for viral or nonbacterial upper respiratory infections (URIs) and bacterial sinusitis (142–146). Although not all viruses exacerbate asthma in all patients, URIs with rhinovirus, influenza, and parainfluenza clearly induce or provoke acute airway inflammation and bronchial hyperreactivity, which lead to temporary (in most cases), symptomatic bronchospasm in healthy nonasthmatics and worsening asthma in adult asthmatics (145). Elderly asthmatics appear to be as susceptible as younger asthmatics. Viral URIs can profoundly affect asthmatics by producing airways obstruction (particularly in the small airways) and increasing airways hyperreactivity to both nonspecific stimuli and allergens (143,147). Viral URIs can increase the propensity to develop late asthmatic reactions after allergen exposure; this response can persist for weeks after infection (147). Antibody-documented infection with *Chlamydia pneumoniae* has been found to be associated with wheezing, asthmatic bronchitis, and asthma in some elderly adults (148). Whether acute reinfection or repeated or prolonged exposure to this organism has a causal or coincidental factor in adult-onset asthma remains to be determined.

Sinusitis occurs frequently in the elderly (Table 3) and is a common comorbid problem in elderly asthmatics (6,7). The association between asthma exacerbations and sinusitis is clinically apparent—e.g., persistent asthma may improve once the sinusitis is properly treated (5). However, firm evidence that sinusitis causes or worsens asthma remains controversial (144). The theories for an association range from bacterial seeding of the lungs with secondary bronchitis to a parasympathetic nasobronchial reflex resulting in bronchospasm (142,144,149). Bacterial sinusitis frequently occurs in nonatopic adults who may have coexisting nasal polyps.

Rhinorrhea or rhinitis from any cause is a common comorbid condition in elderly asthmatics (6,7) and can aggravate asthma regardless of the patient's age. Rhinorrhea is the most common physical finding in viral respiratory infections in a day-care setting (141). Most patients with nasal polyps are over 40 years of age and have a chronic history of perennial rhinitis (149). Exacerbation of allergic rhinitis in an atopic asthmatic commonly affects the lower airways.

Drug Interactions

Appropriate antibiotic and symptomatic (drainage) therapy of active sinusitis can effectively reduce asthmatic symptoms and bronchodilator requirements. Rhinorrhea or allergic rhinitis can be effectively treated with nasally administered ipratropium bromide or corticosteroids, cromolyn, or oral antihistamines, respectively, without adverse interactions with asthma. In fact, asthmatic symptoms and airway hyperresponsiveness may improve with use of nasal steroids in patients with allergic rhinitis (150). Newer-generation, nonsedating antihistamines, such as terfenadine, loratadine, and cetirizine, may be used safely and effectively in most asthmatics (5,151–154). There is a strong clinical impression that improving upper respiratory symptoms with nonsedating histamine (H_1)-receptor antagonists in patients with concomitant allergic rhinitis and asthma may facilitate the control of asthma. This action may be related to their modest bronchodilatory properties (cetirizine) and partial inhibition of allergic and nonallergic asthmatic reactions (5). Antihistamines must still be considered as useful adjuncts and not as primary therapy in the allergic asthmatic (5,151,152). Initial concern about an anticholinergic drying effect on airway mucus (as in the older antihistamines) has not been clinically evident in the nonsedating antihistamines, which are devoid of anticholinergic properties. The nonsedating antihistamines do not produce adverse drug interactions with antiasthma therapy. However, terfenadine and astemizole can produce ECG prolongation of the QTc interval, torsades de pointes, cardiac arrest, and other ventricular arrhythmias, either after overdosing (e.g., with hepatic dysfunction) or in combination with ketoconazole or certain macrolide antibiotics.

J. Lower Respiratory Infections

Disease Interactions

Bacterial and nonbacterial pneumonias are very common and important diseases in the elderly, in whom the initial diagnosis is frequently missed because of atypical symptoms and signs (155). Some types of bacterial pneumonia, such as *Legionella* pneumonia, are more frequent in persons of age 50 years and older, particularly in those who smoke, have chronic airflow obstruction, or are taking corticosteroids (156,157). Community-acquired pneumonia caused by the TWAR strain of *Chlamydia* affects primarily young adults but can also cause severe pneumonia (requiring hospitalization) in many older adults and persons with chronic cardiopulmonary or renal disease (158). Infection with drug-resistant tuberculosis or atypical mycobacteria has not emerged as a significant problem in chronic asthmatics, unlike that in patients infected with the human immunodeficiency virus (HIV). Respiratory tract colonization or infections by bacteria or nonbacterial agents may increase airway inflammation and reactivity. However, the consensus is that most bacterial infections provoke asthma in only a few asthmatics, regardless of age (143,145,146).

Allergic bronchopulmonary aspergillosis (ABPA) may complicate the management of asthma in the geriatric patient (159). It is not unusual for mild to moderate asthma that has been responsive to bronchodilators alone to evolve into corticosteroid-dependent asthma following the development of ABPA. Wheezing may be related to either uncontrolled bronchospasm and/or mucoid impaction of proximal bronchi. Asthma may also be worsened by the development of severe fibrotic lung disease (ABPA stage V or chronic hypersensitivity pneumonitis), producing combined irreversible obstructive and restrictive ventilatory defects.

Drug Interactions

Antimicrobial therapy of bronchitis or pneumonia in asthmatics generally does not interact adversely with the control of asthma except possibly when theophylline is administered. Ciprofloxacin and other fluoroquinolones (enoxacin, norfloxacin), clarithromycin, and erythromycin decrease serum concentrations of theophylline, whereas rifampin increases steady-state serum levels of theophylline (47). Measurement of the serum theophylline concentration several days after initiation of the antibiotic is indicated to adjust the theophylline dosage and avoid toxicity or subtherapeutic levels. Rifampin significantly increases the hepatic metabolism of corticosteroids and can worsen control of steroid-dependent asthma (160). The oral corticosteroid dose can be increased (or replaced with inhaled corticosteroids) to maintain optimal control and tapered when rifampin therapy is discontinued.

Influenza and pneumococcal vaccinations are recommended in all persons age 65 years and older (including asthmatics) (5), although there remains some doubt about the efficacy of the latter in preventing pneumococcal pneumonia in the elderly (110). Asthma medications generally do not interfere with or are influenced by routine vaccinations (5).

Most adequately monitored elderly patients with steroid-dependent asthma are not at increased risk for bacterial or fungal pneumonia or reactivated tuberculosis (100,101). Inhaled corticosteroids do not increase the risk of respiratory infection (91–93). Prophylaxis with isoniazid is not indicated in older tuberculin-positive patients taking inhaled corticosteroids because of the increased risks of isoniazid-induced hepatotoxicity (5).

K. Gastroesophageal Reflux and Aspiration

Disease Interactions

Gastroesophageal reflux (GER) occurs commonly in patients with asthma. Depending on the diagnostic criteria, 45–65% of adults with asthma have significant GER (161). Asthmatics tend to have a higher incidence of both hiatal hernia and GER than nonasthmatics (162). This relationship appears to increase with age (162). Patients with both disorders have difficult to manage or "refractory" asthma if the GER is not recognized and treated. Reflux should be suspected in elderly patients who have asthma that becomes unusually resistant to routine therapy and is associated with heartburn, nocturnal respiratory symptoms, or cough (163).

The interaction between asthma and GER remains controversial, but evidence supports the long-standing beliefs that GER, with or without hiatal hernia, can either cause or worsen asthma and, conversely, that asthma and/or its therapy can cause or contribute to GER (5,164–168). The most frequently considered mechanisms are pulmonary aspiration of refluxed gastric contents and neurally (vagally) mediated reflex bronchoconstriction secondary to acidic irritation (esophagitis) of distal esophageal nerve endings. The latter mechanism is probably the predominant cause of reflux-induced bronchospasm (5). Some patients with unexplained cough but no reflux symptoms (e.g., heartburn) have occult GER resulting in reflex bronchoconstriction (163). Studies with 24-hr esophageal pH monitoring may clearly demonstrate acute decreases in esophageal pH that precede or occur simultaneously with wheezing or cough. On the other hand, asthma itself may aggravate or even cause GER by (1) flattening the diaphragm and relaxing the phrenoesophageal ligament and (2) increasing the pressure gradient between the intra-abdominal and intrathoracic cavities during acute asthma. Significantly obese asthmatics on chronic oral corticosteroid therapy may be especially at risk for unstable asthma and GER because of thoracoabdominal alterations and decreases in respiratory muscle strength, total lung capacity, and vital capacity (169). These patients should benefit from weight reduction and reliance on inhaled corticosteroids.

Aspiration is a common problem in elderly individuals because of waning gag reflex or diminished mental status from sedatives, alcohol, and neuropsychiatric disorders, including seizures. Asthma can be exacerbated by aspiration of a foreign body or stomach contents due to airways irritation. Subsequent bronchoscopic evaluation and removal of inhaled substances may also exacerbate asthmatic symptoms.

Drug Interactions

Antireflux therapy (meal regulation, weight loss, elevation of head of bed, avoidance of tobacco and alcohol, antacids, histamine (H_2)-receptor antagonists, metoclopramide, cisapride, omeprazole, and surgery) may be effective in reducing asthma symptoms (5). Although these therapies have not uniformly improved the asthma or bronchial hyperresponsiveness (167), prolonged, aggressive antireflux therapy and high doses of acid-suppressive therapy may be necessary for improving the asthmatic component (170).

Some asthmatic patients may have difficulty in controlling coexisting peptic ulcer disease, gastritis, or esophagitis because of ongoing therapy with theophylline (which increases gastric acid secretion) and possibly corticosteroids. Inhaled corticosteroids should replace systemic corticosteroids whenever possible in these asthmatic patients (5). Cimetidine strongly inhibits microsomal enzymes and produces high serum theophylline levels, which can further worsen control of the peptic ulcer as well as cause theophylline toxicity.

Asthma therapy with theophylline or oral beta agonists may exacerbate GER by decreasing the lower esophageal sphincter (LES) pressure. Although this finding may not be clinically relevant in many patients, a vicious cycle can potentially be established between asthma, bronchodilator therapy, and GER (164), and some patients may benefit from discontinuation of this therapy. Inhaled albuterol appears to have no effect on LES pressure or esophageal motility (171). Corticosteroids are not contraindicated in asthmatic patients with GER, whereas cholinergic stimulants such as bethanecol should be avoided (5).

L. Diabetes Mellitus

Disease Interactions

Although asthma and diabetes mellitus are both common chronic diseases in the population, their concurrence is less than expected (172–174). This infrequent combination is likely to be related to genetic discordance of the two diseases (78). The coexistence of asthma and diabetes occurs mainly in people after age 40 years (6,7,173).

Information about the physiological and clinical interactions of diabetes mellitus and asthma is scant and largely speculative (175,176). The adrenergic system in young adult nondiabetic asthmatics may alter insulin release and reduce hypoglycemic effects, resulting in "protection" against diabetes (175). An important consideration in diabetic asthmatics is diabetic autonomic neuropathy, which reduces resting vagally mediated bronchomotor tone (177). This, in turn, may limit the capability for increased nonspecific bronchial reactivity and acute bronchospasm and possibly result in improved asthmatic control. Clinically, when diabetes develops or both diseases coexist, the severity of the asthma generally improves (173). Such a neurally mediated protective effect has been physiologically supported by bronchoprovocation studies in small numbers of young adults with asthma and diabetes (178,179), but the clinical relevance to the general diabetic-asthmatic population and specifically the elderly remains uncertain. Nevertheless, the combination of the two diseases is not wholly protective, in that diabetics with autonomic neuropathy are susceptible to an increased risk of respiratory failure as a consequence of diminished ventilatory responses to hypoxia (180), hemodynamic or ventilatory sensitivity to beta-adrenergic agonists (129), and exposure to cholinergic agents, sedatives, and anesthetics (181) as well as acute respiratory and nonrespiratory infections.

Drug Interactions

The balance between asthmatic and diabetic control is generally possible in most patients with mild-moderate asthma and diabetes mellitus, especially when as-needed inhaled bronchodilators, inhaled corticosteroids, diet, oral antidiabetic agents, and occasional insulin treatment are appropriately used. However, difficult treatment issues can occur in patients with both severe asthma and diabetes mellitus. Oral or parenteral corticosteroid therapy for severe asthma or other conditions may significantly complicate glucose control and insulin therapy. The asthma should be stabilized and controlled first and then any insulin dosage adjusted to prevent significant hyperglycemia or hypoglycemia (182). On the other hand, effective treatment of hyperglycemia with exogenous insulin may result in exacerbation of asthma or emergence of latent asthma in some patients (172,173,182). Insulin dosage can be altered (alternated) without too much difficulty in patients receiving alternate-day prednisone (182). Emphasis on inhaled corticosteroids (or cromolyn or nedocromil sodium) for anti-inflammatory therapy is recommended to minimize diabetogenic effects, although efficient delivery systems (e.g., spacers) and some newer, more potent topical corticosteroids may elicit more dose-related systemic effects (92,183). The metabolic effects of β_2-agonist therapy, regardless of route of administration, include hypokalemia and hyperglycemia, although there is generally less effect via the inhaled route with standard doses (86). Ipratropium bromide and theophylline are alternative bronchodilators without adverse metabolic consequences. Thus, therapy of the asthmatic patient with diabetes requires monitoring of blood levels of glucose, potassium, and other electrolytes.

M. Thyroid Disease

Disease Interactions

Hypothyroidism

Thyroid dysfunction increases with aging, particularly in women older than 50 years of age. Hypothyroidism is more common in elderly than younger patients, with a prevalence of overt and mild disease in 2–3% of men and 6–10% of women (110). Subclinical hypothyroidism is a relatively common biochemical disorder that occurs in asymptomatic individuals, affecting 9–16% of women older than 60 years of age (184). Approximately 20–50% of these individuals appear to develop overt hypothyroidism within 4–8 years (184). The combination of thyroid disease and asthma has been reportedly infrequently in the medical literature. One retrospective study found only 12 patients (12.5%) with coexisting asthma and hypothyroidism out of 96 patients with hypothyroidism (185). Most asthmatic patients affected by thyroid disease develop respiratory symptoms after age 60 years. However, younger adults with both conditions have also been reported (186–189).

Hypothyroidism is clinically associated with stable or improved asthma. However, rapid drug restoration to the euthyroid state may be associated with worsening airways obstruction (185,187,189) as well as myocardial ischemia. Thus, slow and cautious therapy of hypothyroidism is necessary in elderly patients with asthma.

Hyperthyroidism

The prevalence of unsuspected thyrotoxicosis ranges from 2–20 cases per 1000 persons; the annual incidence of thyrotoxicosis ranges from 1–5 cases per 10,000 persons (110). Hyperthyroidism in patients over age 60 years accounts for 10–15% of all cases of thyrotoxicosis (190). Few studies have been conducted on the prevalence of subclinical hyperthyroidism, although it occurs less frequently (1–12%) than subclinical hypothyroidism (184). A retrospective study found only 5 patients (2.4%) with coexisting asthma or asthmatic bronchitis and hyperthyroidism in 209 patients with hyperthyroidism (185). The onset of hyperthyroidism worsens asthma and its control in most patients, regardless of age (185,186,188). Asthma, the side effects of adrenergic antiasthma medications, and hyperthyroidism may be clinically confusing, since they share common symptoms—such as anxiety, tachycardia, palpitations, dyspnea, hyperventilation, diaphoresis, weight loss, and tremor (186). The biochemical basis for the action of thyroxine in asthma is unknown, although an accelerated effect on corticosteroid metabolism is possible (187,188). The interplay of the autonomic nervous system in hyperthyroidism favors bronchodilation (191). An early case report (188) indicated that asthmatic symptoms and increased bronchial reactivity to histamine inhalation decreased to a nonasthmatic level in a young asthmatic following treatment of moderately severe hypothyroidism (Graves' disease). Although this case report suggests that increased nonspecific bronchial reactivity might be a physiological mechanism for asthma severity in hyperthyroidism, subsequent controlled studies have indicated otherwise. Studies of triiodothyronine-induced thyrotoxicosis in normal volunteers (192) and bronchoprovocation with carbachol in hyperthyroid patients (191) showed no effect on lung function and airways reactivity and even reduced airways reactivity. Thus, hyperthyroidism may worsen asthma by a mechanism other than increasing airways reactivity, e.g., adding respiratory stress to hyperthyroid-induced restrictive ventilatory defect (193,194) by increasing minute ventilation and respiratory muscle weakness (193–195), or by accelerating the metabolism and excretion of antiasthma drugs, including theophylline and corticosteroids (187,192). A physiological evaluation of asthmatics would be useful to investigate these mechanisms. It is probably not cost-effective to routinely obtain thyroid function tests in all asthmatic patients or in difficult-to-control asthmatics unless clinical evidence of hyperthyroidism is present (192).

Drug Interactions

As noted above, thyroid dysfunction alters drug pharmacokinetics–i.e., hyperthyroidism generally increases while hypothyroidism decreases drug elimination. In most cases, hyperthyroidism results in enhanced drug elimination by induction of hepatic cytochrome P-450 microsomal isoenzymes or enhanced renal excretion

(196). Thus, the metabolism of theophylline and corticosteroids is significantly decreased in hypothyroidism and increased in hyperthyroidism (196–198). Theophylline toxicity in hypothyroid patients is a distinct predisposition unless therapy is titrated and monitored with theophylline levels (199). Correction of the thyroid dysfunction results in a normalization of theophylline pharmacokinetics.

The correction of the hyperthyroid state in patients with intractable asthma results in clinically improved asthma and decreased nonspecific airways reactivity (186,188). However, treatment of asthma in the hyperthyroid patient is complicated by the hyperadrenergic state. Standard doses of epinephrine or intravenous aminophylline can produce severe hyperexcitability and even worsening of bronchospasm in hyperthyroid patients with asthma (186,187). This response may be a clue that occult hyperthyroidism is present in such patients (186). Adrenergic antiasthma drugs should be used cautiously or not at all in asthmatic patients with hyperthyroidism, and corticosteroid dosing may need to be increased during the hyperthyroid state (5). Inhaled steroids and ipratropium bromide may be effectively used in these circumstances. Nonselective beta blockers improve respiratory muscle strength in thyrotoxicosis (195) but are contraindicated in asthmatic patients.

Exogenous iodine, such as potassium iodide or iodinated glycerol, is not infrequently used in respiratory treatment as a mucolytic expectorant (5). Iodine-based oral medications may result in hyperthyroidism, hypothyroidism, or euthyroid goiter in elderly patients (185,200,201). Hypothyroidism is the most common metabolic complication of iodine intake (185). Hyperthyroidism is more likely to occur in older male patients and patients with preexisting thyroidal disorders (e.g., goiter and Graves' disease), although persons without known thyroid disease are not exempt (200,201). Worsening of asthma and greater difficulty in its control can occur with the induced hyperthyroid state. Iodine withdrawal and, if clinically necessary, addition of antithyroid drugs and corticosteroids are useful therapies.

N. Adrenocortical Insufficiency

Disease Interactions

Adrenal disorders are not common in the older population, although it is possible that they are underdiagnosed (202). Acute adrenal insufficiency is rare but may occur in the elderly as a result of anticoagulation-related hemorrhage into the adrenal glands, withdrawal of exogenous corticosteroids, sepsis, postoperative states, myocardial infarction, and adrenal metastases. Chronic adrenal insufficiency may be due to granulomatous infections such as tuberculosis or histoplasmosis, autoimmune disease (Addison's disease), malignancy, or idiopathic causes. Patients with coexisting Addison's disease and asthma have been rarely reported (203), but adrenocortical insufficiency may unmask new-onset asthma and cause unusually severe attacks. Little evidence exists that asthma is associated with pituitary or adrenal insufficiency (5).

Drug Interactions

There are no known adverse drug interactions. Appropriate corticosteroid replacement readily corrects the adrenal insufficiency and dramatically improves the asthmatic condition. Asthmatic patients who are treated preoperatively with corticosteroids can undergo surgical procedures with a low incidence of complications, including adrenocortical insufficiency (204). Overall, in the absence of previous or concomitant oral glucocorticoid therapy, doses less than 1500 μg/day of inhaled corticosteroids produce no clinically significant effect on pituitary-adrenal function (92). Indeed, a low rate of inhaled glucocorticoid-related side-effects has proved to be the case, and there are no reported cases of symptomatic adrenal insufficiency attributed to inhaled corticosteroids alone (93).

V. Summary

Recognition of coexisting medical conditions and their interactions with asthma and its therapy is critical in the proper management of asthmatic patients of any age and, in particular, in the elderly. Unlike younger asthmatics, elderly asthmatics are more likely to have comorbid medical conditions. Concurrent conditions may influence the diagnosis and management of asthma in clinically important ways. The diagnosis of either condition may be complicated by nonspecific, similar, or misleading symptoms and laboratory results. The coexisting condition and/or its treatment may worsen the control of asthma or, conversely, asthma and/or its therapy may complicate management of the other disease. Elderly patients are likely to be prescribed multiple respiratory and nonrespiratory drugs. For example, aspirin, NSAIDs, and beta-blocking medications are among the most commonly prescribed medications in elderly patients. Pharmacokinetic and pharmacodynamic effects of concurrent medications may aggravate asthma, complicate the effective control of asthma, and require modification of usual treatment. Thus, all elderly asthmatics should be evaluated for concomitant disorders and monitored for adverse drug-related side effects or interactions, especially when unstable asthma is not fully explicable despite standard therapy.

Abbreviations

ABPA	allergic bronchopulmonary aspergillosis
ACEI	angiotensin-converting enzyme inhibitor

CAD   coronary artery disease
CHF   congestive heart failure
CHS   cardiovascular Health Study
COPD   chronic obstructive pulmonary disease
CPAP   continuous positive airway pressure
GABA   gamma-aminobutyric acid
GER   gastroesophageal reflux
MAOI   monoamine oxidase inhibitor
MDI   metered-dose inhaler
MI   myocardial infarction
NSAID   nonsteroidal anti-inflammatory drug
$PC20\text{-}FEV_1$ provocative concentration of inhaled methacholine that induces a
                 20% decrease in forced expired volume in 1 sec (FEV_1)
SCI   spinal cord injury
URI   upper respiratory infection

Acknowledgment

The author thanks the Working Group on the Management of Asthma in the Elderly and the staff of the National Asthma Education and Prevention Program (NAEPP), Division of Lung Diseases, NHLBI, NIH, for providing ideas and criticisms during the development of the *NAEPP Working Group Report: Considerations for Diagnosing and Managing Asthma in the Elderly*, which formed the foundation for this chapter.

References

1. Kane RL, Ouslander JG, Abrass IB. The elderly patient: Demography and epidemiology. In: Kane RL, Ouslander JG, Abrass IB, eds. Essentials of Clinical Geriatrics, 3d ed. New York: McGraw-Hill, 1994:19–43.
2. Cassel CK, Brody JA. Demography, epidemiology, and aging. In: Cassel CK, Riesenberg DE, Sorensen LB, Walsh J, eds. Geriatric Medicine, 2d ed. New York: Springer-Verlag, 1990:16–27.
3. National Heart, Lung, and Blood Institute. Guidelines for the Diagnosis and Management of Asthma. Bethesda, MD: U.S. Department of Health and Human Services, National Institute of Health, pub. no. 91-3042, 1991.
4. National Heart, Lung, and Blood Institute. Considerations for Diagnosing and Managing Asthma in the Elderly. Bethesda, MD: U.S. Department of Health and Human Services, National Institute of Health, pub. no. 96-3662, 1996.
5. Spector SL, Nicklas RA, eds. Practice parameters for the diagnosis and treatment of asthma. J Allergy Clin Immunol 1995; 96(part 2):821–824.

6. Bailey WC, Richards JM Jr, Manzella BA, et al. Characteristics and correlates of asthma in a university clinic population. Chest 1990; 98:821–828.

7. Bailey WC, Richards JM Jr, Brooks CM, et al. Features of asthma in older adults. J Asthma 1992; 29:21–28.

8. Irvine PW. Patterns of disease: The challenge of multiple illnesses. In: Cassel CK, Riesenberg DE, Sorensen, Walsh JR, eds. Geriatric Medicine, 2d ed. New York: Springer-Verlag, 1990:96–103.

9. Hobson M. Medications in older patients. West J Med 1992; 157:539–543.

10. National Center for Health Statistics. Advance report of final mortality statistics, 1984. Monthly Vital Statistics Report 35. No. 6, suppl 2, September 1986.

11. U.S. Department of Health and Human Services. Current Estimates from the National Health Interview Survey, United States, 1985. Series 10, no. 160, September 1986.

12. Manton KG, Stallard E, Corder L. Changes in morbidity and chronic disability in the U.S. elderly population: Evidence from the 1982, 1984, and 1989 National Long Term Care Surveys. J Gerontol 1995; 50B:S194–S204.

13. Beers MH, Ouslander JG. Risk factors in geriatric drug prescribing: A practical guide to avoiding problems. Drugs 1989; 37:105–112.

14. Lamy PP. The elderly and drug interactions. J Am Geriatr Soc 1986; 34:586–592.

15. Williamson J, Chopin JM. Adverse reactions to prescribed drugs in the elderly: A multicenter investigation. Age Ageing 1980; 9:73–80.

16. Popplewell PY, Henschle PJ. Acute admissions to a geriatric assessment unit. Med J Aust 1982; 1:343–344.

17. Porter J, Jick H. Drug-related deaths among medical inpatients. JAMA 1977; 237:879–881.

18. May FE, Steward RB. Drug interactions and multiple drug administration. Clin Pharmacol Ther 1977; 22:322–328.

19. Traver GA, Cline MG, Burrows B. Asthma in the elderly. J Asthma 1993; 30:81–91.

20. Bardana EJ Jr. Is asthma really different in the elderly patient? J Asthma 1993; 30:77–79.

21. Ford R. Aetiology of asthma: A review of 11,551 cases (1958 to 1968). Med J Aust 1969; 1:628–631.

22. National Heart, Lung, and Blood Institute Data Fact Sheet. Asthma Statistics. May 1992.

23. Burrows B, Barbee RA, Cline MG, et al. Characteristics of asthma among elderly adults in a sample of the general population. Chest 1991; 100:935–942.

24. Enright PL, Ward BJ, Tracy RP, Lasser EC. Cardiovascular Health Study Research Group: Asthma and its association with cardiovascular disease in the elderly. J Asthma 1996; 33:45–53.

25. Broder I, Barlow PP, Horton RJM. The epidemiology of asthma and hay fever in a total community, Tecumseh, Michigan: I. Description of study and general findings. 1962; 33:315–323.

26. O'Connor GT, Sparrow D, Segal M, Weiss ST. Risk factors for ventilatory impairment among middle-aged and elderly men: The Normative Aging Study. Chest 1993; 103:376–382.

27. Dodge RR, Burrows B. The prevalence and incidence of asthma and asthma-like symptoms in a general population sample. Am Rev Respir Dis 1980; 122:567–575.

28. Braman SS, Kaemmerlen JT, Davis SM. Asthma in the elderly: A comparison between patients with recently acquired and long-standing disease. Am Rev Respir Dis 1991; 143:336–340.

29. Postma DS, Lebowitz MD. Persistence and new onset of asthma and chronic bronchitis evaluated longitudinally in a community population sample of adults. Arch Intern Med 1995; 155:1393–1399.

30. Braman SS, Davis SM. Wheezing in the elderly: Asthma and other causes. Geriatr Clin North Am 1986; 2:269–283.

31. Banerjee DK, Lee GS, Malik SK, Daly S. Underdiagnosis of asthma in the elderly. Br J Dis Chest 1987; 81:23–29.

32. Burrows B, Lebowitz MD, Barbee RA, Cline MS. Findings before diagnoses of asthma among the elderly in a longitudinal study of a general population sample. J Allergy Clin Immunol 1991; 88:870–877.

33. Weiss KB, Gergen PJ, Wagener DK. Breathing better or wheezing worse? The changing epidemiology of asthma morbidity and mortality. Annu Rev Publ Health 1991; 14:491–513.

34. Najjari C, Tessier JF, Barberger-Gateau P, et al. Functional status of elderly people treated for asthma-related symptoms: A population based case-control study. Eur Respir J 1994; 7:1077–1083.

35. Lee HY, Stretton TB. Asthma in the elderly. Br Med J 1972; 4:93–95.

36. Sly RM. Changing asthma mortality. Ann Allergy 1994; 73:259–268.

37. Marquette CH, Saulnier F, LeRoy O, et al. Long-term prognosis of near-fatal asthma: A 6-year follow-up study of 145 asthmatic patients who underwent mechanical ventilation for a near-fatal attack of asthma. Am Rev Respir Dis 1992; 146:76–81.

38. Connolly MJ, Crowley JJ, Charan NB, et al. Reduced subjective awareness of bronchoconstriction provoked by methacholine in elderly asthmatic and normal subjects as measured on a simple awareness scale. Thorax 1992; 47:410–413.

39. Kikuchi Y, Okabe S, Tamura G, et al. Chemosensitivity and perception of dyspnea in patients with a history of near-fatal asthma. N Engl J Med 1994; 330:1329–1334.

40. Rea HH, Scragg R, Jackson R, et al. A case-controlled study of deaths from asthma. Thorax 1986; 41:833–839.

41. Boulet L-P, Deschesnes F, Turcotte H, Gignac F. Near fatal asthma: Clinical and physiologic features, perception of bronchoconstriction, and psychologic profile. J Allergy Clin Immunol 1991; 88:838–846.

42. Patterson R, Greenberger PA, Patterson DR. Potentially fatal asthma: The problem of noncompliance. Ann Allergy 1991; 67:138–142.

43. Greenberger PA: Potentially fatal asthma. Chest 1992; 101(suppl):401S–402S.

44. Montamat SC, Cusak BJ, Vestal RE. Management of drug therapy in the elderly. N Engl J Med 1989; 321:303–309.

45. Kelly HW. Pharmacologic problems in the allergic patient with multiple medical problems. Immunol Allergy Clin North Am 1991; 11:17–29.

46. Tietze KJ, Hussar DA. Avoiding drug interactions in respiratory medicine. J Respir Dis 1992; 13:1669–1685.

47. Weinberger M, Hendeles L. Theophylline in asthma. N Engl J Med 1996; 334: 1380–1388.

48. Higgins MW, Thom TG. Incidence, prevalence, and mortality: Intra- and inter-county differences. In: Hensley MJ, Saunders NA, eds. Clinical Epidemiology of Chronic Obstructive Pulmonary Disease. New York: Marcel Dekker, 1990:23–43.

49. Feinlieb M, Rosenberg HM, Collins JG, et al. Trends in COPD morbidity and mortality in the United States. Am Rev Respir Dis 1989; 140(suppl):S9–S18.

50. Burrows B, Bloom JW, Traver GA, Cline MG. The course and prognosis of different forms of chronic airways obstruction in a sample from the general population. N Engl J Med 1987; 317:1309–1314.

51. Burrows B. Predictors of loss of lung function and mortality in obstructive lung diseases. Eur Respir Rev 1991; 1:340.

52. Silverstein MD, Reed CE, O'Connell EJ, et al. Long-term survival of a cohort of community residents with asthma. N Engl J Med 1994; 331:1537–1541.

53. Ferguson GT, Cherniack RM. Management of chronic obstructive pulmonary disease. N Engl J Med 1993; 328:1017–1022.

54. American Thoracic Society. Standards for the diagnosis and care of patients with chronic obstructive pulmonary disease. Am J Respir Crit Care Med 1995; 152 (suppl):S77–S120.

55. Hillerdahl G, Rylander R. Asthma and cessation of smoking. Clin Allergy 1984; 14:45–47.

56. Richter J, Castell D. Gastroesophageal reflux. Ann Intern Med 1982; 97:93–102.

57. Jindal SK, Gupta D, Singh A. Indices of morbidity and control of asthma in adult patients exposed to environmental tobacco smoke. Chest 1994; 106:746–749.

58. Pedersen B, Dahl R, Karlström R, et al. Eosinophil and neutrophil activity in asthma in a one-year trial with inhaled budesonide: The impact of smoking. Am J Respir Crit Care Med 1996; 153:1519–1529.

59. Lange P, Ulrik CS, Vestbo J, for the Copenhagen City Heart Study Group. Mortality in adults with self-reported asthma. Lancet 1996; 347:1285–1289.

60. Kelloway JS, Wyatt RA, Adlis SA. Comparison of patients' compliance with prescribed oral and inhaled asthma medications. Arch Intern Med 1994; 154:1349–1352.

61. Schein JR. Cigarette smoking and clinically significant drug interactions. Ann Pharmacother 1995; 29:1139–1148.

62. Matsunga SK, Plezia PM, Karol MD, et al. Effects of passive smoking on theophylline clearance. Clin Pharmacol Ther 1989; 46:399–407.

63. Tockman MS, Anthonisen NR, Wright EC, Donithan MG, the Intermittent Positive Pressure Breathing Trial, the Johns Hopkins Lung Project for the Early Detection of Lung Cancer. Airways obstruction and the risk for lung cancer. Ann Intern Med 1987; 106:512–518.

64. Anthonisen NR, Connett JE, Kiley JP, et al. Effects of smoking intervention and the use of an inhaled anticholinergic bronchodilator on the rate of decline of FEV_1: The Lung Health Study. JAMA 1994; 272:1497–1505.

65. Petty TL. Lung cancer and chronic obstructive pulmonary disease. Med Clin North Am 1996; 80:645–655.

66. Ford RM. Primary lung cancer and asthma. Ann Allergy 1978; 40:240–242.

67. Vena JE, Bona JR, Byers TE, et al. Allergy-related diseases and cancer: An inverse association. Am J Epidemiol 1985; 122:66–74.

68. McDuffie HH, Cockcroft DW, Talebi Z, et al. Lower prevalence of positive atopic skin tests in lung cancer patients. Chest 1988; 93:241–246.

69. Twohig KJ, Matthay RA. Pulmonary effects of cytotoxic agents other than bleomycin. Clin Chest Med 1990; 11:31–54.

70. Duncan AL, Vittone J, Fleming KC, Smith HC. Cardiovascular disease in elderly patients. Mayo Clin Proc 1996; 71:184–196.

71. Cabanes LTR, Weber SN, Matran R, et al. Bronchial hyperresponsiveness to methacholine in patients with impaired left ventricular function. N Engl J Med 1989; 320:1317–1322.

72. Pison C, Malo J, Rouleau J, et al. Bronchial hyperresponsiveness to inhaled methacholine in subjects with chronic left heart failure at a time of exacerbation and after increasing diuretic therapy. Chest 1989; 96:230–235.

73. Ziment I. Management of hypertension in the asthmatic patient. Chest 1983; 83(suppl):392–395.

74. George RB. Management of hypertension in patients with obstructive airway disease. Chest 1985; 88(suppl):190S–193S.

75. Gradman AH, Kohl-Lachs SL. Managing hypertension in patients with obstructive airway disease. J Respir Dis 1990; 11:68–80.

76. Nicklas RA. Treatment of the elderly asthmatic patient with heart disease. Immunol Allergy Clin North Am 1991; 11:183–199.

77. Heine DL, Gradman AH. The challenge of managing angina in patients with COPD. J Respir Dis 1992; 13:766–781.

78. Chapman KR, Rebuck AS. Therapeutic approaches in the cardiac-hypertensive-diabetic patient. In: Weiss ED, Stein M, eds. Bronchial Asthma. Mechanisms and Therapeutics, 3d ed. Boston: Little, Brown, 1993:1038–1044.

79. Zitnik RJ. Drug-induced lung disease: Cardiovascular agents. J Respir Dis 1996; 17:293–298.

80. Zitnik RJ. Drug-induced lung disease: Antiarrhythmic agents. J Respir Dis 1996; 17:254–270.

81. Zeitz HJ. Bronchial asthma, nasal polyps, and aspirin sensitivity: Samter's syndrome. Clin Chest Med 1988; 9:567–576.

82. Balsano F, Rizzon P, Violi F, et al. Antiplatelet treatment with ticlopidine in unstable angina: A controlled multicenter trial. Circulation 1990; 82:17–26.

83. Anonymous. Antiplatelet agents: Ticlopidine HCl. In: Olin BR, ed. Drug Facts and Comparisons. St. Louis: Wolters Kluwer, 1996:85c–85g.

84. Ranhosky A, Kempthorne-Rawson J. The safety of intravenous dipyridamole thallium myocardial perfusion imaging. Circulation 1990; 81:1205–1209.

85. Johnston DL, Daley JR, Hodge DO, et al. Hemodynamic responses and adverse effects associated with adenosine and dipyridamole pharmacologic stress testing: A comparison in 2,000 patients. Mayo Clin Proc 1995; 70:331–336.

86. Nelson HS. β-adrenergic bronchodilators. N Engl J Med 1995; 333:499–506.

87. Gross NJ. Ipratropium bromide. N Engl J Med 1988; 319:486–494.

88. Gross NJ, Bankwala Z. Effects of an anticholinergic bronchodilator in arterial blood gases of hypoxemic patients with chronic obstructive pulmonary disease: Comparison with a beta-adrenergic agent. Am Rev Respir Dis 1987; 136:1091–1094.

89. Ashutosh K, Dev G, Steele D. Nonbronchodilator effects of pirbuterol and ipratropium in chronic obstructive pulmonary disease. Chest 1995; 107:173–178.

90. Siefkin AD. Optimal pharmacologic treatment of the critically ill patient with obstructive airways disease. Am J Med 1996; 100(suppl 1A):54S–61S.

91. Barnes PJ, Pedersen S. Efficacy and safety of inhaled corticosteroids in asthma: Report of a workshop held in Eze, France, October 10, 1992. Am Rev Respir Dis 1993; 148(suppl):S1–S26.

92. Barnes PJ. Inhaled glucocorticoids for asthma. N Engl J Med 1995; 332:868–875.

93. Robinson DS, Geddes DM. Inhaled corticosteroids: Benefits and risks. J Asthma 1996; 33:5–16.

94. Martineau P, Vaughan LM. Heparin inhalation for asthma. Ann Pharmacother 1995; 29:71–73.

95. Ahmed T, Garrigo J, Danta I. Preventing bronchoconstriction in exercise-induced asthma with inhaled heparin. N Engl J Med 1993; 329:90–95.

96. Garrigo J, Danta I, Ahmed T. Time course of the protective effect of inhaled heparin on exercise-induced asthma. Am J Respir Crit Care Med 1996; 153:1702–1707.

97. Armitage JM, Williams SJ. Inhaler technique in the elderly. Age Ageing 1988; 17:275–278.

98. Gray SL, Williams DM, Pulliam CC, et al. Characteristics predicting incorrect metered-dose inhaler technique in older subjects. Arch Intern Med 1996; 156:984–988.

99. Anderson CJ, Bardana EJ. Asthma in the elderly: Interactions to be wary of. J Respir Dis 1995; 16:965–976.

100. Lieberman P, Patterson R, Kunske R. Complications of long-term steroid therapy for asthma. J Allergy Clin Immunol 1972; 49:329–336.

101. Kwong FK, Sue MA, Klaustermeyer WB. Corticosteroid complications in respiratory disease. Ann Allergy 1987; 58:326–330.

102. Hollister JR, Bowyer SL. Adverse side effects of corticosteroids. Semin Respir Med 1987; 8:400–405.

103. Bennett DA, Beckett LA, Murray AM, et al. Prevalence of Parkinsonian signs and associated mortality in a community population of older people. N Engl J Med 1996; 334:71–76.

104. Allen SC, Prior A. What determines whether an elderly patient can use a metered dose inhaler correctly? Br J Dis Chest 1986; 80:45–49.

105. Diggory P, Bailey R, Vallon A. Effectiveness of inhaled bronchodilator delivery systems for elderly patients. Age Ageing 1991; 20:379–382.

106. McFadden ER Jr. Improper patient techniques with metered dose inhalers: Clinical consequences and solutions to misuse. J Allergy Clin Immunol 1995; 96:278–283.

107. Hoffman NB, Laucka PV. Dexamethasone aerosol use in an asthmatic nursing-home patient with Parkinson's disease and dementia. Drug Intell Clin Pharm (DICP) Ann Pharmacother 1990; 24:707–708.

108. Crane J, Pierce N, Burgess C, et al. Markers of risk of asthma death or readmission in the 12 months following a hospital admission for asthma. Int J Epidemiol 1992; 21:737–744.

109. Joseph KS, Blais L, Ernst P, Suissa S. Increased morbidity and mortality related to asthma among asthmatic patients who use major tranquilizers. Br Med J 1996; 312:79–83.

110. Scheitel SM, Fleming KC, Chutka DS, Evans JM. Geriatric health maintenance. Mayo Clin Proc 1996; 71:289–302.

111. Go BK, DeVivo MJ, Richards JS. The epidemiology of spinal cord injury. In: Stover SL, DeLisa JA, Whiteneck GG, eds. Spinal Cord Injury. Clinical Outcomes from the Model Systems. Gaithersburg, MD: Aspen Publishers, 1995:21–51.

112. Menter RR, Hudson LM. Effects of age at injury and the aging process. In: Stover SL, DeLisa JA, Whiteneck GG, eds. Spinal Cord Injury. Clinical Outcomes from the Model Systems. Gaithersburg, MD: Aspen Publishers, 1995:272–288.

113. DeVivo MJ, Black KJ, Stover SL. Causes of death during the first 12 years after spinal cord injury. Arch Phys Med Rehabil 1993; 74:248–254.

114. Ditunno JF Jr, Formal CS. Chronic spinal cord injury. N Engl J Med 1994; 330:550–556.

115. Ashba J, Garshick E, Tun CG, et al. Spirometry—Acceptability and reproducibility in spinal cord injured patients. J Am Paraplegia Soc 1993; 16:197–203.

116. Spungen AM, Dicpinigaitis PV, Almenoff PL, Bauman WA. Pulmonary obstruction in individuals with cervical spinal cord lesions unmasked by bronchodilator administration. Paraplegia 1993; 31:404–407.

117. Almenoff PL, Alexander LR, Spungen AM, et al. Bronchodilatory effects of ipratropium bromide in patients with tetraplegia. Paraplegia 1995; 33:274–277.

118. Dicpinigaitis PV, Spungen AM, Bauman WA, et al. Bronchial hyperresponsiveness after cervical spinal cord injury. Chest 1994; 105:1073–1076.

119. Dicpinigaitis PV, Spungen AM, Bauman WA, et al. Inhibition of bronchial hyperresponsiveness by GABA-agonist baclofen. Chest 1994; 106:758–761.

120. Everitt DE, Avorn J. Systemic effects of medications used to treat glaucoma. Ann Intern Med 1990; 112:120–125.

121. Prakash UBS, Rosenow EC III. Pulmonary complications from ophthalmic preparations. Mayo Clin Proc 1990; 65:521–529.

122. Shah P, Dhurjon L, Metcalfe T, Gibson JM. Acute angle closure glaucoma associated with nebulised ipratropium bromide and salbutamol. Br Med J 1992; 304:40–41.

123. Hall SK. Acute angle-closure glaucoma as a complication of combined β-agonist and ipratropium bromide therapy in the emergency department. Ann Emerg Med 1994; 23:884–887.

124. Anonymous. Drugs for migraine. Med Lett 1995; 37:17–20.

125. Zwillich CW, Sutton FD Jr, Neff TA, et al. Theophylline-induced seizures in adults: Correlation with serum concentrations. Ann Intern Med 1975; 82:784–787.

126. Yarnell PR, Chu N-S. Focal seizures and aminophylline. Neurology 1975; 25:819–822.

127. Keene DL, Melmed CA, Andermann F, Baxter DW. Anoxic tonic seizures due to asthma: A serious complication in adults. Can J Neurol Sci 1981; 8:177–179.

128. Covelli HD, Knodel AR, Heppner BT. Predisposing factors to apparent theophylline-induced seizures. Ann Allergy 1985; 54:411–415.

129. Pingleton SK, Schwartz O, Szymanski D, Epstein M. Hypotension associated with terbutaline therapy in acute quadriplegia. Am Rev Respir Dis 1982; 126:723–725.

130. White DP. Disorders of breathing during sleep: Introduction, epidemiology, and incidence. Semin Respir Med 1988; 9:529–533.

131. Guilleminault C, Cummiskey J, Motta J. Chronic obstructive airflow disease and sleep studies. Am Rev Respir Dis 1980; 122:397–406.

132. Alford NJ, Fletcher EC, Nickeson D. Acute oxygen therapy in patients with sleep apnea and COPD. Chest 1986; 89:30–38.

133. Sampol G, Saagles MT, Roca A, et al. Nasal continuous positive airway pressure with supplemental oxygen in coexistent sleep apnoea–hypopnoea syndrome and severe chronic obstructive pulmonary disease. Eur Respir J 1996; 9:111–116.

134. Martin RJ. Nocturnal asthma. Clin Chest Med 1992; 13:533–550.

135. Chan CS, Woolcock AJ, Sullivan CE. Nocturnal asthma: role of snoring and obstructive sleep apnea. Am Rev Respir Dis 1988; 137:1502–1504.

136. Roth TR, Roehrs TA, Conway WA. Behavioral morbidity of apnea. Semin Respir Med 1988; 9:554–559.

137. Guilleminault C, Quera-Salva MA, Powell N, et al. Nocturnal asthma: Snoring, small pharynx and nasal CPAP. Eur Respir J 1988; 1:902–907.

138. National Center for Health Statistics. Monthly Vital Statistics Report. August 13, 1991; 39:N13.

139. National Center for Health Statistics. Detailed diagnoses and procedures. National Hospital Discharge Survey. Series 13, no. 108, 1991.

140. Hodder SL, Ford AB, FitzGibbon PA, et al. Acute respiratory illness in older community residents. J Am Geriatr Soc 1995; 43:24–29.

141. Falsey AR, McCann RM, Hall WJ, et al. Acute respiratory tract infection in daycare centers for older persons. J Am Geriatr Soc 1995; 43:30–36.

142. Cook JL. Infection in asthma. Semin Respir Med 1987; 8:259–270.

143. Frick WE, Busse WW. Respiratory infections: Their role in airway responsiveness and pathogenesis of asthma. Clin Chest Med 1988; 9:539–549.

144. Friday GA Jr, Fireman P. Sinusitis and asthma: Clinical and pathogenetic relationships. Clin Chest Med 1988; 9:557–565.

145. Busse WW. The relationship between viral infections and onset of allergic diseases and asthma. Clin Exp Allergy 1989; 19:1–9.

146. Cazzola M, Matera MG, Rossi F. Bronchial hyperresponsiveness and bacterial respiratory infections. Clin Ther 1991; 13:157–171.

147. Lemanske RF, Dick EC, Swenson CA, et al. Rhinovirus upper respiratory infection increases airway hyperreactivity and late asthmatic reactions. J Clin Invest 1989; 83:1–10.

148. Hahn DL, Dodge RW, Golubjatnikov R. Association of Chlamydia pneumoniae (TWAR) infections with wheezing, asthmatic bronchitis, and adult onset asthma. JAMA 1991; 266:225–230.

149. Slavin RG. Relationship of nasal disease and sinusitis to bronchial asthma. Ann Allergy 1982; 49:76–80.

150. Watson WTA, Becker AB, Simons FER. Treatment of allergic rhinitis with intranasal corticosteroids in patients with mild asthma: Effect on lower airway responsiveness. J Allergy Clin Immunol 1993; 91:97–101.

151. Rafferty P. Antihistamines in the treatment of clinical asthma. J Allergy Clin Immunol 1990; 88:647–650.

152. Bousquet J, Godard Ph, Michel FB. Antihistamines in the treatment of asthma. Eur Respir J 1992; 5:1137–1142.

153. Wood-Baker R, Holgate ST. Histamine antagonists. In: Weiss EB, Stein M, eds. Bronchial Asthma. Mechanisms and Therapeutics, 3d ed. Boston: Little, Brown, 1993:884–888.

154. Grant JA, Nicodemus CF, Findlay SR, et al. Cetirizine in patients with seasonal rhinitis and concomitant asthma: Prospective, randomized, placebo-controlled trial. J Allergy Clin Immunol 1995; 95:923–932.

155. Bentley DW. Bacterial pneumonia in the elderly. Hosp Pract [Off] 1988; 23(12): 99–116.

156. England AC, Fraser DW, Plikaytis BD, et al. Sporadic legionellosis in the United States: The first thousand cases. Ann Intern Med 1981; 94:164–170.

157. Marston BJ, Lipman HB, Breiman RF. Surveillance for legionnaire's disease. Arch Intern Med 1994; 154:2417–2422.

158. Marrie TJ, Grayston T, Wang S-P, Kuo C-C. Pneumonia associated with the TWAR strain of Chlamydia. Ann Intern Med 1987; 106:507–511.

159. Greenberger PA, Patterson R. Allergic bronchopulmonary aspergillosis: Model of bronchopulmonary disease with defined serologic, radiologic, pathologic and clinical findings from asthma to fatal destructive lung disease. Chest 1987; 91(suppl): 165S–171S.

160. Powell-Jackson PR, Gray BJ, Heaton RW, et al. Adverse effect of rifampin administration on steroid-dependent asthma. Am Rev Respir Dis 1983; 128:307–310.

161. Gonzalez ER, Castell DO. Respiratory complications of gastroesophageal reflux. Am Fam Physician 1988; 37:169–172.

162. Mays EE. Intrinsic asthma in adults: Association with gastroesophageal reflux. JAMA 1976; 236:2626–2628.

163. Irwin RS, Zawacki JK, Curley FJ, et al. Chronic cough as the sole presenting manifestation of gastroesophageal reflux. Am Rev Respir Dis 1989; 140:1294–1300.

164. Barish CF, Wu WC, Castell DO. Respiratory complications of gastroesophageal reflux. Arch Intern Med 1985; 145:1882–1888.

165. Wald JA, Fernandez E. Gastroesophageal reflux and asthma: Pathogenesis, diagnosis, and therapy. Semin Respir Med 1987; 8:324–331.

166. Gurevitch MJ, Valenzuela JE. Lung and gastroesophageal disorders. Semin Respir Med 1988; 9:254–261.

167. Nelson HS. Is gastroesophageal reflux worsening your patient's asthma? J Respir Dis 1990; 11:827–844.

168. Simpson WG. Gastroesophageal reflux disease and asthma: Diagnosis and management. Arch Intern Med 1995; 155:798–803.

169. Melzer E, Souhrada JF. Decrease of respiratory muscle strength and static lung volumes in obese asthmatics. Am Rev Respir Dis 1980; 121:17–20.

170. Harding SM, Richter JE, Guzzo MR, et al. Asthma and gastroesophageal reflux: Acid suppressive therapy improves asthma outcome. Am J Med 1996; 100:395–405.

171. Schindlbeck NE, Heinrich C, Huber RM, Muller-Lissner SA. Effects of albuterol (salbutamol) on esophageal motility and gastroesophageal reflux in healthy volunteers. JAMA 1988; 260:3156–3158.

172. Abrahamson EM. Asthma, diabetes mellitus, and hyperinsulinemia. J Clin Endocrinol 1941; 1:402–406.

173. Helander E. Asthma and diabetes. Acta Med Scand 1958; 162:165–174.
174. Hermansson B, Holngren G, Samuelson G. Juvenile diabetes mellitus and atopy. Hum Hered 1971; 21:504–508.
175. Szczeklik A, Pieton R, Sieradzski J. Alterations in both insulin release and its hypoglycemic effects in atopic bronchial asthma. J Allergy Clin Immunol 1980; 66:424–427.
176. Lasser E. Asthma and diabetes mellitus: A biochemical basis for antithetical features. Med Hypoth 1987; 23:95–106.
177. Douglas NJ, Campbell IW, Ewing DJ, et al. Reduced airway vagal tone in diabetic subjects with autonomic neuropathy. Clin Sci 1981; 61:581–584.
178. Heaton RW, Guy RJC, Gray BJ, et al. Diminished bronchial reactivity to cold air in diabetic patients with autonomic neuropathy. Br Med J 1984; 289:149–151.
179. Villa MP, Cacciari E, Bernardi F, et al. Bronchial reactivity in diabetic patients: Relationship to duration of diabetes and degree of glycemic control. Am J Dis Child 1988; 142:726–729.
180. Eagleton LE, Soler NG. Hypoventilation in response to hypoxemia in diabetics (abstr). Chest 1981; 80:367.
181. Page MM, Watkins PJ. Cardiorespiratory arrest and diabetic autonomic neuropathy. Lancet 1978; 1:14–16.
182. Tinkelman D, King S. Severe asthma and volatile diabetes mellitus in the same patient: A treatment dilemma. J Allergy Clin Immunol 1979; 64:223–226.
183. Lipworth BJ. New perspectives on inhaled drug delivery and systemic bioactivity. Thorax 1995; 50:105–110.
184. Surks MI, Ocampo E. Subclinical thyroid disease. Am J Med 1996; 100:217–223.
185. Korsager S, Kristensen HPO. Iodine-induced hypothyroidism and its effect on the severity of asthma. Acta Med Scand 1979; 205:115–117.
186. Settipane GA, Schoenfeld E, Hamolsky MW. Asthma and hyperthyroidism. J Allergy Clin Immunol 1972; 49:348–355.
187. Bush RK, Ehrlich EN, Reed CE. Thyroid disease and asthma. J Allergy Clin Immunol 1977; 59:398–401.
188. Cockcroft DW, Silverberg JDH, Dosman JA. Decrease in non-specific bronchial reactivity in an asthmatic following treatment of hyperthyroidism. Ann Allergy 1978; 41:160–163.
189. Rowe MS, MacKechnie HLN. Hypothyroidism with coexistent asthma: Problems in management. South Med J 1984; 77:401–402.
190. David PJ, David FB. Hyperthyroidism in patients over the age of 60 years: Clinical features in 85 patients. Medicine 1974; 53:161–181.
191. Israel RH, Poe RH, Cave WT Jr, et al. Hyperthyroidism protects against carbachol-induced bronchospasm. Chest 1987; 91:242–245.
192. Irwin RS, Pratter MR, Stivers DSH, Braverman LE. Airway reactivity and lung function in triiodothyronine-induced thyrotoxicosis. J Appl Physiol 1985; 58:1485–1488.
193. Stein M, Kimbel P, Johnson RL Jr. Pulmonary function in hyperthyroidism. J Clin Invest 1961; 40:348–363.
194. Mier A, Brophy C, Wass JAH, et al. Reversible respiratory muscle weakness in hyperthyroidism. Am Rev Respir Dis 1989; 139:529–533.

195.	Wang YT, Poh SC. Lung function and respiratory muscle strength after propranolol in thyrotoxicosis. Aust NZ J Med 1986; 16:495–500.

196.	Vozeh S, Otten M, Staub J-J, Follath F. Influence of thyroid function on theophylline kinetics. Clin Pharmacol Ther 1984; 36:634–640.

197.	Bauman JH, Teichman S, Wible DA. Increased theophylline clearance in a patient with hyperthyroidism. Ann Allergy 1984; 52:94–96.

198.	Pokrajac M, Simic D, Varagic VM. Pharmacokinetics of theophylline in hyperthyroid and hypothyroid patients with chronic obstructive pulmonary disease. Eur J Clin Pharmacol 1987; 33:483–486.

199.	Aderka D, Shavit G, Garfinkel D, et al. Life-threatening theophylline intoxication in a hypothyroid patient. Respiration 1983; 44:77–80.

200.	Huseby JS, Bennett SW, Hagensee ME. Hyperthyroidism induced by iodinated glycerol. Am Rev Respir Dis 1991; 144:1403.

201.	Becker CS, Gordon JM. Iodinated glycerol and thyroid dysfunction: Four cases and a review of the literature. Chest 1993; 103:188–192.

202.	Ackermann RJ. Adrenal disorders: Know when to act and what tests to give. Geriatrics 1994; 49:32–37.

203.	Green M, Lim KH. Bronchial asthma with Addison's disease. Lancet 1971; 1:1159–1162.

204.	Kabalin CS, Yarnold PR, Grammar LC. Low complication rate of corticosteroid-treated asthmatics undergoing surgical procedures. Arch Intern Med 1995; 155:1379–1384.

AUTHOR INDEX

Italic numbers give the page on which the complete reference is listed.

A

Abboud, R., 78, *90*, 151, *174*

Abrahamson, E.M., 243, 244, *256*

Abrass, I.B., 99, *116*, 137, *167*, 219, *248*

Abuan, T.H., 80, 82, *91*, 138, 151, *167*

Abu-Ghazaleh, R., 36, *48*, *49*

Ackerman, S.J., 44, *51*

Ackermann, R.J., 246, *258*

Adame, D., 80, *91*

Adelroth, E., 56, 61, 63, *65*

Adelson, J., 146, *173*

Aderka, D., 246, *258*

Adler, S., 107, 111, *119*

Adlis, S.A., 228, 230, *251*

Adolphson, C., 42, *50*

Ahmed, T., 96, 99, 113, *115*, *117*, 233, *253*

Ahrens, R.C., 150, *174*

Aikawa, T., 56, 61, *64*

Aikman, S.L., 139, *168*

Alexander, L.R., 235, *254*

Alford, N.J., 237, *255*

Alhashimi, M.M., 156, *177*

Ali, N.J., 160, *179*

Allegra, L., 14, 16, *30*, 108, *119*

Allen, M.S., 105, *118*

Allen, S.C., 8, *29*, 141, 151, *170*, *174*, 211, *217*, 234, *253*

Almenoff, P.L., 235, *254*

Almind, M., 22, 23, *31*

Almy, T.P., 122, 127, *132*

Alpers, J.H., 207, *216*

Alt, H.L., 124, *132*

Altose, M.D., 80, *91*, 101, *117*, 123, *132*

Amico, C.A., 185, *200*

Andermann, F., 237, *254*

Anderson, A.E., Jr., 60, *66*

Anderson, C.J., 233, 236, *253*

Anderson, G.P., 139, *167*

Anderson, H.R., 10, *29*

Anderson, J.A., 56, 57, 61, *64*, 139, *167*

Anderson, J.R., 61, *66*

Andersson, K.E., 160, *179*

Andrade, W.P., 161, *181*

Anliker, M., 155, *176*

Annesi, I., 16, 17, *30*, *31*

Antal, E.J., 146, *172*

Anthonisen, N.R., 15, *30*, 71, 84, *89, 92*, 105, *118*, 229, *251*

Antic, R., 105, *118*

Antonini, M.T., 5, *27*, 61, *66*

Armanini, D., 153, *175*

Armitage, J.M., 141, *170*, 211, 212, *217*, 233, *253*

Armstrong, X., 2, *26*

Arnold, A., *90*

Arrighi, H.M., 13, *29*

Arsura, E.L., 142, *171*

Ascione, F.J., 127, 130, *133*

Ashba, J., 235, *254*

Ashutosh, K., 232, *253*

Asmundsson, T., 58, *66*

Au, W.Y., 146, *172*

Aubert, J.D., 45, *51*

Aubier, M., 144, *171*

Auerbach, H., 7, *28*

Austen, K.F., 56, 61, *64*

Avorn, J., 236, *254*

Ayres, J.G., 106, 111, *118*

Ayson, M., 214, *218*

Azzawi, M., 38, *49*

B

Bach, D., 56, 61, *64*

Backer, V., 44, *51*

Baier, H., 103, *118*

Bailey, R., 212, *217*, 234, *253*

Bailey, W.C., 101, *117*, 123, 124, 125, 129, 130, *132*, *133*, 220, 224, 225, 228, 229, 233, 239, 243, *249*

Bakke, P.S., 80, *91*

Baldwin, C.J., 143, *171*

Balsano, F., 232, *252*

Banerjee, D.K., 8, *28*, 93, 95, 101, 102, 108, *115*, 224, *250*

Bankwala, Z., 232, *252*

Baram, D., 161, *180*

Barbee, R.A., 2, 5, 16, 17, 18, *26, 30, 31*, 34, *47*, 61, *66*, 97, 98, 102, 108, 111, 112, *116*, 123, 126, 127, 129, 130, *132, 133*, 185, 186, 190, *200*, 223, 224, *249, 250*

Barberger-Gateau, P., 94, *115*, 123, *132*, 224, *250*

Bardana, E.J., Jr., 102, 108, 111, *118, 119*, 223, 233, 236, *249, 253*

Barden, J.M., 162, *181*

Barett, L.A., 56, *64*

Barish, C.F., 242, 243, *256*

Barker, A.F., 111, *119*, 186, *200*

Barker, J., 103, *118*

Barlow, P.P., 224, *249*

Barnes, N.C., 162, *181*

Barnes, P., 208, *216*

Barnes, P.J., 101, 114, *117, 120*, 136, 137, 139, 140, 144, 151, 152, 153, 157, 158, 159, 160, 161, *166, 168, 171, 174, 175, 178, 179, 180*, 184, *199*, 232, 234, 237, 241, 244, 247, *253*

Barreuther, A.D., 141, *170*

Barrio, J.L., 103, *118*

Barron, K.L., 205, *216*

Baskerville, J.C., 160, *179*

Basner, R.C., 16, *30*

Baste, V., 80, *91*

Bateman, E.D., 161, *181*

Bates, D.V., 69, *89*

Bates, M.E., 36, *48*

Bauer, L.A., 146, *173*

Bauer, W., 36, *48-49*

Baughman, R.P., 105, *118*

Bauman, J.H., 246, *258*

Bauman, W.A., 235, 236, *254*

Baumgarth, N., 41, *50*

Baxter, D.W., 237, *254*

Bayley, A., 105, *118*
Beaglehole, R., 11, 12, *29*
Beasley, R., 3, *26*, 56, 57, *65*, 140, *169*, 184, *199*
Beck, G.J., 22, 23, *31*
Becker, A.B., 7, *28*, 239, *255*
Becker, C.S., 246, *258*
Beckett, L.A., 234, *253*
Beecher, H.K., 106, *118*, 185, *200*
Beers, M.H., 222, *249*
Bekir, S., 144, *172*
Bel, E.H., 161, *180*
Benatar, S.R., 196, *202*
Benater, S.R., 113, *120*
Bengtsson, B., 142, *170*
Benner, S.E., 60, *66*
Bennett, D.A., 234, *253*
Bennett, S.W., 246, *258*
Bentley, D.W., 240, *256*
Berger, M., 206, *216*
Berger, R., 83, *92*
Berkowitz, J.S., 155, *177*
Berkowitz, R., 150, *174*
Bernardi, F., 243, *257*
Bernstein, D.I., 34, *47*
Bernstein, I.L., 34, *47*, 160, 161, *180*
Berry, G., 5, *27*
Berscheid, B.A., 5, *27*
Bertin, L., 141, *169-170*
Bertorelli, G., 3, *26*
Bertrand, C., 41, *50*
Bewtra, A., 5, *27*, 99, *116*
Bighley, L., 144, *172*
Birch, S., 99, 108, *117*, *119*
Birmingham, J., 155, *176*
Birt, J.A., 158, *178*
Bittar, G., 146, *173*
Bjornsson, E., 126, *133*
Black, K.J., 235, *254*
Black, L.F., 77, *90*
Black, P.N., 194, *201*
Blais, L., 235, *253*

Blaser, K., 36, *48*
Blazer, D.G., 122, 124, *132*, *178*
Bleecker, E.R., 162, *181*
Blom, H., 77, *90*
Bloom, J.W., 21, 22, *31*, 141, 152, *170*, *175*, 227, *251*
Blouin, R.A., 99, *116*, 138, 146, *167*, *173*
Blumenstein, B.A., 161, *181*
Bochner, B.S., 36, *48*
Bode, E., 40, *50*
Bode, F., 105, *118*
Boer, C., 36, *48*
Boer, L., 36, 40, *48*, *50*
Bohannon, A.D., 154, *176*
Bohrod, M.G., 57, *65*
Boivin, J.F., 140, *169*
Boman, G., 126, *133*
Bona, J.R., 229, *252*
Bonnaud, F., 5, *27*, 61, *66*
Bonner, J.C., 45, *51*
Booth, H., 60, *66*
Boschetto, P., 153, *175*
Bosco, L.A., 7, *28*
Bosken, C.H., 44, 45, *51*, 57, 58, *65*, *66*
Bosquet, J., 57, *65*
Boulet, L.P., 113, *120*, 150, 161, *174*, *180*, 225, 234, *250*
Bourey, R.E., 155, *177*
Boushey, H.A., 140, *169*, 184, *199*, *200*
Bousquet, J., 3, 12, *26*, *29*, 35, 36, *47*, 57, 62, *65*, 184, *199*, 239, 240, *255*
Bowyer, S.L., 234, *253*
Boye, N.P., 146, *172*
Bradley, B.L., 38, *49*
Braman, S.S., 5, 17, 18, 19, *27*, 34, *47*, 61, *66*, 93, 94, 96, 97, 98, 102, 103, 104, 106, 108, 112, *115*, *117*, *119*, 126, *133*, 150

[Braman] 157, 163, *174*, 185, 186, 192, 196, 198, *200*, *202*, 224, 227, 229, 233, *250*

Brambilla, C., 141, *169-170*

Brand, P.L.P., 5, *27*, 80, 84, *91*, 139, 153, *168*

Braun, P., 36, *48*

Braun, R.K., 36, *48-49*

Braverman, L.E., 245, *257*

Bredesen, J.E., 146, *172*

Breiman, R.F., 240, *256*

Brenner, M., 150, *174*

Brewster, C.E.P., 56, *65*

Brey, F.J., 153, *175*

Brisman, J., 4, *26*

Britto, S.A., 139, *168*

Britton, J.R., 5, *27*, 161, *180*

Broder, I., 8, *28*, 224, *249*

Brody, A.R., 45, *51*

Brody, J.A., 162, *182*, 219, *248*

Broll, J., 155, *176*

Brooks, C.M., 101, *117*, 123, 124, *132*, 220, 224, 225, 228, 229, 233, 239, 243, *249*

Broomfield, J., 210, *217*

Brophy, C., 245, *257*

Brown, D.C., 142, *171*

Brown, J.B., 126, *133*

Brown, L., 41, *50*

Brown, M.J., 142, *171*

Brown, P.J., 23, *31*, 61, *67*, 96, *116*

Brown, W.D., 211, 212, *217*

Browne, G., 214, *218*

Brubaker, H., 212, *217*

Bruijnzeel, P.L., 161, *180*

Bruns, F.J., 107, 111, *119*

Brussino, L., 109, 110, *119*

Bryant, D.H., 151, *174*

Bucca, C., 109, 110, *119*

Buist, A.S., 13, 16, *30*, 98, *116*, 165, *182*

Bukowskyj, M., 144, 148, *171*

Bulpitt, C.J., 23, *31*

Burch, R., 44, *51*

Burdo, H., 13, *29*

Burgess, C., 214, *218*, 235, *253*

Burk, J., 161, *180*

Burki, N.K., 150, *174*

Burmeister, S., 194, *201*

Burney, P.G., 5, 7, *27*, *28*

Burr, M., 8, 17, 18, 19, *29*, 93, 97, 98, *115*

Burrows, B., 2, 5, 6, 8, 14, 15, 16, 17, 18, 20, 21, 22, *26*, *27*, *30*, *31*, 34, *47*, 61, *66*, 85, 86, *92*, 97, 98, 102, 108, 111, 112, *116*, 123, 127, 129, *132*, *133*, 185, 186, 190, *200*, 223, 224, 227, 228, *249*, *250*, *251*

Buseck, P.R., 61, *66*

Bush, R.K., 139, *167*, 244, 245, 246, *257*

Buske Kirschbaum, A., 44, *51*

Busse, W.W., 40, *50*, 157, 161, *178*, *181*, 238, 239, 240, *255*

Butchers, P.R., 137, *166*

Byard, P.J., 99, *116*

Byers, T.E., 229, *252*

C

Cabanes, L.R., 103, 104, *118*, 230, *252*

Cacciari, E., 243, *257*

Cagle, P., 58, *66*

Caldwell, J.R., 153, 156, *175*, *177*

Calhoun, W.J., 36, *48*

Callerame, M.L., 57, *65*

Campbell, I.W., 243, *257*

Cane, R.D., 77, *90*

Capewell, S., 160, *179*

Capron, A., 161, *180*

Cardell, B.S., 53, 56, 57, 59, 60, 61, *64*

Carliner, N.H., 107, *119*

Caron, M.G., 139, *168*
Carrizo, S.J., 161, *180*
Carroll, N., 57, *65*
Carrozzi, L., 80, *91*
Carstairs, J.R., 136, *166*
Carstensen, L.L., 204, *215*
Carter, T.L., 205, *216*
Cartier, A., 127, *133*, 142, 161, *170, 180*
Casaburi, R., 80, 87, *91, 92*
Casanova, J.E., 107, 111, *119*
Casscells, W., 45, *51*
Cassel, C.K., 162, *182*, 219, *248*
Cassels-Brown, A., 162, *182*
Castell, D., 228, 241, 242, 243, *251, 256*
Cave, W.T., Jr., 245, *257*
Cazzola, M., 238, 240, *255*
Cerveri, I., 77, 78, *90*
Chadha, T.S., 108, *119*
Chan, C.S., 237, 238, *255*
Chandler, M.H., 150, *174*
Chanez, P., 3, *26*, 35, 36, 45, 46, *47, 51*, 57, 62, *65*, 144, *172*, 184, *199*
Chang, C.H., 112, *119*
Chang, J.T., 15, *30*, 94, *115*
Chapman, K.R., 127, *133*, 140, 141, 142, 151, *169, 170, 174*, 194, *201*, 212, *217*, 230, 231, 243, *252*
Charan, N.B., 101, 103, *117*, 137, 162, *167, 181*, 185, 187, *200*, 208, *216*, 225, *250*
Charles, T., 8, 17, 18, 19, *29*
Charles, T.J., 93, 97, 98, *115*
Charlton, G., 210, *217*
Charlton, I., 210, *217*
Chastang, C., 141, *169-170*
Chatterjee, S.S., 186, *200*
Chau, G., 162, *181-182*
Chediak, A.D., 96, 113, *115*
Chen, D., 212, *217*
Cherniack, N.S., 101, *117*, 123, *132*
Cherniack, R.M., 82, *91*, 149, *173*, 227, *251*

Chervinsky, P., 139, 140, 157, *167, 178*
Chetta, A., 3, *26*, 62, *67*
Cheung, D., 139, *168*
Chilvers, E.R., 36, 37, *49*
Chinet, T., 212, *217*
Chinn, S., 5, 7, *27, 28*
Chmelik, F., 209, *217*
Chopin, J.M., 222, *249*
Chowiencyzk, P., 209, *217*
Christie, R.V., 69, *89*
Christopher, K., 108, *119*, 164, *182*
Chu, N.-S., 237, *254*
Chung, K.F., 103, *118*, 161, *181*
Church, M.K., 37, *49*, 137, *166*
Churg, A., 58, *66*
Chutka, D.S., 235, 241, 244, 245, *254*
Ciocom, J.O., 205, *216*
Citron, M.L., 156, *177*
Clancey, S.M., 156, *177*
Clark, D.F., 71, *89*
Clark, N.M., 122, 127, 130, *132*
Clark, R.A., 79, *91*, 139, *168*
Clark, T.J., 141, *170*
Clifton, G.D., 150, *174*
Cline, M., 15, 16, 17, 18, 21, 22, *30, 31*, 34, *47*, 61, *66*, 85, 86, *92*, 97, 98, 102, 108, 111, 112, *116*, 123, 127, 129, *132, 133*, 185, 186, 190, *200*, 223, 224, 227, *249, 250, 251*
Cloosterman, S.G., 140, *169*
Cluroe, A., 56, 59, 61, *65*
Cochran, J.E., 161, *181*
Cochrane, G.M., 209, *217*
Cockcroft, D.W., 5, *27*, 85, 87, *92*, 126, *133*, 139, 161, *168, 180*, 229, 244, 245, 246, *252, 257*
Coe, C.I., 151, *174*
Coffey, M.J., 161, *181*
Coffman, R.L., 37, *49*
Cohen, C.A., 190, 193, *201*

Cohn, J., 162, *181*
Collins, J.G., 227, *251*
Collins, J.V., 100, 101, 113, *117, 178,* 192, *201*
Collins, S., 139, *168*
Condemi, J.J., 57, *65*
Connett, J.E., 80, 86, *91, 92,* 229, *251*
Connolly, M.F., 185, 187, *200*
Connolly, M.J., 99, 101, 103, *117,* 137, 141, 162, *167, 170, 181,* 208, *216,* 225, *250*
Conolly, M.E., 139, *167-168*
Constantine, H.P., 143, *171*
Conway, W.A., 238, *255*
Cook, D., 99, 101, *116,* 185, *200*
Cook, J.L., 238, 239, *255*
Cook, N.R., 208, *216*
Cooke, N.J., 100, *117*
Cooney, T.P., 60, *66*
Cooper, D.M., 56, 61, *65*
Cooper, S., 161, *180*
Corbin, J.D., 136, *166*
Corder, L., 220, 223, *249*
Corrao, W.M., 108, *119*
Corrigan, C.J., 37, 38, *49, 50*
Cosio, M.G., 142, *170*
Cote, J., 150, *174*
Cotes, J.E., 70, 72, *89*
Cotlier, E., 155, *176*
Coultas, D.B., 98, *116*
Covelli, H.D., 237, *254*
Cowen, J., 198, *202*
Coyle, A.J., 41, 44, *50, 51*
Crain, E.F., 98, *116,* 123, *132*
Crane, J., 140, *169,* 214, *218,* 235, *253*
Crapo, R.O., 78, 79, *90*
Crepea, S.B., 54, 56, *64*
Creticos, P., 161, *180*
Crilly, R.G., 154, 160, *176*
Crompton, G.K., 100, *117*
Crook, T.H., 205, *216*
Cross, D., 190, 193, *201*

Crotty, T.B., 59, *66*
Crowley, J.J., 99, *117,* 162, *181,* 185, 187, *200,* 208, *216,* 225, *250*
Cruickshank, J.M., 186, *200*
Cugell, D.W., 15, *30,* 94, *115*
Cullen, K., 22, 23, *31,* 96, *115,* 123, *132*
Cummiskey, J., 237, *255*
Curley, F.J., 241, 242, *256*
Curtis, R.A., 146, *173*
Cusack, B.J., 144, 146, *172, 173,* 226, *250*
Cuthbert, O.D., 7, *28*
Cutz, E., 56, 61, *65*

D

Dahl, R., 228, *251*
Dales, R.E., 79, *91*
Daley, J.R., 232, *252*
D'Alonzo, G.E., 140, *169*
Daly, S., 93, 95, 101, 102, 108, *115,* 224, *250*
Daniels, K.S., 127, *133*
Danielson, D.A., 156, 164, *177*
Danneskiold-Samsoe, B., 156, *177*
Danson, J., 71, *89*
Danta, I., 233, *253*
D'Aquino, L.C., 87, *92*
Dardevet, D., 156, *177*
Darioli, R., 198, *202*
Darnell, J.C., 158, *178*
Davey, E.N., 60, *66*
David, D.S., 155, *177*
David, F.B., 245, *257*
David, P.J., 245, *257*
Davies, A.O., 139, *168*
Davies, D., 151, *174*
Davies, R.J., 3, *26*
Davies, S.L., 129, 130, *133*
Davila, D.G., 108, *119*
Davis, P.B., 99, *116*
Davis, P.J., 153, *175*

Davis, S.M., 5, 17, 18, 19, *27*, 34,
 47, 61, *66*, 96, 97, 98, 102, 103,
 104, 106, 112, *115*, *117*, 150,
 157, 163, *174*, 185, 186, 192,
 196, *200*, 224, 227, 229, 233, *250*
deBoar, G., 13, *29*
De Carli, M., 40, *50*
Declamer, P.B.S., 186, *200*
Decramer, M., 156, *177*
DeGraff, A.C., 15, *30*, 80, *91*
de Jong, J.W., 140, *169*
Dekker, F.W., 208, *216*
Del Donno, M., 3, *26*, 62, *67*
Del Prete, G.F., 40, *50*
Dent, G., 144, *172*
Dent, L.A., 36, *49*
Derby, L.E., 147, 148, *173*
Dermarkarian, R., 162, *181*
Derrick, E.H., 8, 17, 19, *28*
Deschesnes, F., 113, *120*, 225, 234, *250*
DeSoyza, N., 146, *172*
Despas, P.J., 62, *67*
Desreumaux, P., 37, *49*
Deutsch, R.I., 139, *167-168*
Dev, G., 232, *253*
De Vivo, M.J., 235, *254*
Devons, C., 205, *215*
Dhillon, D.P., 79, 83, *91*
Dhurjon, L., 236, *254*
Diament, M.L., 191, *201*
Dick, E.C., 239, *255*
Dickens, G.R., 143, *171*
Dicpinigaitis, P.V., 235, 236, *254*
Diggory, P., 162, *181-182*, 212, *217*,
 234, *253*
Dijkman, J.H., 208, *216*
Di Lollo, S., 62, *67*
Dinh Xuan, A.T., 88, *92*
Dirksen, A., 44, *51*
Di Stefano, A., 57, *65*
Ditunno, J.F., Jr., 235, *254*
Dixon, C.M., 152, *175*

Djukanovic, R., 3, *26*, 55, 56, *64*, *65*
Dodge, R., 5, 8, 15, *27*, *30*
Dodge, R.R., 224, 227, *250*
Dodge, R.W., 239, *255*
Dohsaka, K., 84, *92*
Doi, S., 38, *50*
Dolce, J.J., 214, *218*
Doll, R., 11, *29*
Dolovich, M.B., 140, 157, *169*
Dominguez, M., 144, 149, 150, *172*
Dompeling, E., 44, *51*, 84, *92*, 96,
 99, *116*, 140, *169*
Doner, H.C., 139, *167*
Donithan, M.G., 229, *251*
Dosman, J.A., 244, 245, 246, *257*
Doughty, A., 209, *217*
Douglas, J.G., 160, *179*
Douglas, N.J., 243, *257*
Dow, I., 141, *170*
Dow, L., 16, *31*
Dowse, G.K., 5, 7, *28*
Doyle, C.A., 22, 23, *31*
Drage, C.W., 101, *117*
Drazen, J.M., 140, *169*
Driesner, N.K., 80, 82, *91*, 138, 151, *167*
D'Souza, W., 214, *218*
Dubucquoi, S., 37, *49*
DuHamel, T., 146, *173*
Duncan, A.L., 229, *252*
Dunn, M., 112, *119*
Dunn, W.F., 108, *119*
Dunnette, S., 36, 42, *48*
Dunnill, M.S., 3, *26*, 53, 56, 57, 60,
 61, *64*, 184, *199*
Durham, S.R., 37, 38, *49*
Dutt, A.K., 146, *172*
Dyer, P.D., 161, *181*
Dykman, T.R., 155, *176*

E

Eagleton, L.E., 243, 257

Easley, C.B., 162, *181*
Ebden, P., 159, *179*
Eckert, R.C., 108, *119*
Edwards, B.J., 154, *176*
Ehrlich, E.N., 244, 245, 246, *257*
Eichacker, P.Q., 104, *118*
Eidelman, D.H., 142, *170*
Einberger, M.M., 150, *174*
Ejea, M.V., 161, *180*
Ekholm, B., 211, 212, *217*
Elias, M., 127, *133*, 142, *170*
Eliasson, O., 15, *30*, 80, *91*
Elliot, J., 57, *65*
Ellis, E.F., 153, *175*
Ellul-Micallef, R., 139, *168*
Empey, D.W., 184, *199*
Enarson, D.A., 5, *28*
Engels, F., 136, *166*
England, A.C., 240, *256*
Enright, P.L., 9, *29*, 71, 73, 74, 76,
    77, 85, 86, 87, *89*, *90*, *92*, 123,
    124, 126, *132*, *133*, 230, *249*
Ensom, R.J., 146, *173*
Eppel, M.L., 146, *173*
Epstein, M., 237, 243, *254*
Erard, F., 41, 42, *50*
Erjefalt, I., 137, *166*
Ernst, P., 140, 157, *169*, *178*, 235, *253*
Erzurum, S.C., 161, *181*
Eschenbacher, W.L., 161, *181*
Evald, T., 22, 23, *31*
Evans, D.A., 208, *216*
Evans, J.M., 144, *172*, 235, 241,
    244, 245, *254*
Evans, P.M., 144, *172*
Evans, R., 10, 11, 13, *29*
Everitt, D.E., 236, *254*
Ewing, D.J., 243, *257*

F

Fabbri, L., 40, *50*, 153, *175*

Fagard, R., 156, *177*
Fairshter, R.D., 191, *201*
Faling, J., 24, *31*
Falk, J., 156, *177*
Falsey, A.R., 238, 239, *255*
Fancourt, G.J., 159, *179*
Fanta, C.H., 104, *118*, 146, *173*, 190,
    194, *201*
Fedullo, P.F., 108, *119*
Feihl, F., 198, *202*
Feinlieb, M., 227, *251*
Feldman, R.D., 99, *116*, 137, *167*
Fenech, F.F., 139, *168*
Fentem, P.H., 151, *174*
Fenwike, J., 11, 12, *29*
Ferguson, G.T., 227, *251*
Ferguson, H., 3, *26*
Fernandez, E., 242, *256*
Field, W.E.H., 60, *66*
Findlay, S.R., 162, *181*, 239, *256*
Findley, L.J., 191, *201*
Finotto, S., 40, *50*
Finucane, K.E., 23, *31*, 61, *67*, 96, *116*
Fireman, P., 238, 239, *255*
Fischer, A.R., 162, *181*
Fischer, J.H., 146, *173*
Fischl, M.A., 190, *201*
Fishman, A.P., 103, *118*
FitzGerald, J.M., 121, 123, *132*, 187,
    200
Fitzgerald, M.X., 123, *132*
FitzGibbon, P.A., 238, *255*
Fiz, J.A., 156, *177*
Fjellbirkeland, L., 150, *174*
Flack, J.M., 142, *171*
Flanigan, T., 156, *177*
Flannery, E.M., 5, 6, *27*, 142, *171*
Flatt, A., 140, *169*
Fleetham, J.A., 60, *66*
Fleming, K.C., 229, 235, 241, 244,
    245, *252*, *254*
Fletcher, C.M., 14, *30*

Fletcher, E.C., 237, *255*
Flodquist-Priestly, G., 141, *170*
Fogh-Andersen, N., 77, *90*
Folgering, H., 138, 151, *167*, 185, 195, *200*
Folkerts, G., 41, *50*
Follath, F., 246, *258*
Forbes, G.B., 156, *177*
Ford, A.B., 238, *255*
Ford, R.M., 3, 7, 8, 17, *26*, 223, 229, *249*, *251*
Foresi, A., 3, *26*, 62, *67*
Formal, C.S., 235, *254*
Fossieck, B.E., Jr., 156, *177*
Fraley, D.S., 107, 111, *119*
Francois, J., 155, *177*
Frankel, A.H., 189, *200*
Fraser, D.W., 240, *256*
Fraunfelder, F.T., 160, *179*, 186, *200*
Frederiksen, J., 22, 23, *31*
Frette, C., 16, 17, *30*, *31*
Frew, A.J., 57, *65*
Frey, B.M., 153, *175*
Frey, F.J., 156, *177*
Frick, W.E., 238, 239, 240, *255*
Friday, G.A., Jr., 238, 239, *255*
Friedman, H.S., 146, *173*
Friend, J.A., 210, *217*
Frieske, D., 124, 127, *132*
Frith, P., 5, *27*
Fryer, A.D., 44, *50*
Fujisawa, T., 36, *48*, *49*
Fuller, R.W., 152, *175*
Funder, J.W., 155, *176*
Furst, D.E., 156, *177*
Furukawa, C.T., 146, 156, 160, *173*, *179*

G

Gabbrielli, S., 62, *67*
Gagnon, G., 87, *92*
Gallagher-Thompson, D., 205, *215*

Gandevia, B., 150, *174*
Garcia, R., 161, *180*
Gardner, E.R., *178*
Gardner, L.B., 190, *201*
Garfinkel, D., 246, *258*
Garrigo, J., 233, *253*
Garshick, E., 235, *254*
Gautrin, D., 87, *92*
Geddes, D.M., 158, 159, 160, 161, *178*, *179*, *181*, 232, 234, 237, 241, 247, *253*
Geha, R.S., 161, *180*
Gelb, A., 142, 149, *170*, 191, 195, *201*
Gelfand, E., 161, *181*
Gemou-Engesaeth, V., 38, *50*
George, R.B., 211, 212, *217*, 230, *252*
Georges, D., 141, 157, *169-70*, *178*
Gerber, M.A., 57, *65*
Gergen, P.J., 10, 11, *29*, 98, 114, *116*, *120*, 123, *132*, 224, *250*
Gerhard, H., 105, *118*
German, D.F., 206, *216*
Gerritsen, J., 20, *31*
Gerritsen, M.E., 43, *50*
Gershon, S., 156, *178*
Gerstman, B.B., 7, *28*
Ghezzo, H., 58, *66*
Gibson, G., 142, *171*
Gibson, G.J., 101, *117*
Gibson, J.M., 236, *254*
Giembycz, M.A., 36, 37, *49*, 144, *172*
Gignac, F., 113, *120*, 225, 234, *250*
Glass, M., 162, *181*
Glavin, F., 56, *64*
Gleich, G.J., 35, 36, 42, 43, 44, *48*, *50*
Gluck, O.S., 155, *176*
Glynn, A.A., 55, *64*
Go, B.K., 235, *254*
Godard, P., 12, *29*, 239, 240, *255*
Godfrey, R.W., 56, 61, 63, *65*
Godfrey, S., 7, *28*
Goldberg, A., 87, *92*, 161, *180*

Golden, J.A., 184, *199*
Goldin, J.G., 161, *181*
Golubjatnikov, R., 239, *255*
Gomez, E., 3, *26*
Gomm, S.A., 151, *174*
Gong, H., Jr., 98, *116*
Gonzalez, E.R., 241, *256*
Goodman, D.E., 195, *202*
Gordon, J.M., 246, *258*
Gosnach, M., 197, *202*
Gothen, I.H., 77, *90*
Gotsch, A., 122, 127, 130, *132*
Gottfried, S.B., 197, *202*
Gould, G.A., 78, 85, *90*
Grad, R., 98, *116*
Gradman, A.H., 230, *252*
Grammar, L.C., 247, *258*
Grant, I.W.B., 100, *117*
Grant, J.A., 239, *256*
Grassi, V., 77, *90*
Graves, E.J., 114, *120*
Gray, B.J., 241, 243, *256, 257*
Gray, S.L., 233, 234, *253*
Grayston, T., 240, *256*
Green, M., 246, *258*
Greenberger, P.A., 225, 228, 234,
    238, 240, *250, 256*
Greenblatt, D.W., 99, *117*
Greening, A.P., 156, 160, 164, *179*
Greiff, L., 137, *166*
Greville, H.W., 23, *31*, 61, *67*, 96, *116*
Grillo, H.C., 105, 112, *118*
Grimby, G., 156, *177*
Gross, N.J., 57, *65*, 84, *92*, 150, 151,
    152, *174*, 232, *252*
Groth, S., 137, *166*
Grove, A., 139, *168*
Grundel, R.H., 43, *50*
Guarnieri, T., 146, *173*
Guidry, G.G., 211, 212, *217*
Guilleminault, C., 237, 238, *255*
Gulsvik, A., 7, *28*, 80, *91*, 150, *174*

Gundel, R.H., 36, 43, *48, 50*
Gupta, D., 228, *251*
Gurevitch, M.J., 187, *200*, 242, *256*
Guy, R.J.C., 243, *257*
Guyatt, G.H., 84, *92*
Guzelian, P.S., 145, *172*
Guzzo, M.R., 106, 112, *118, 119*,
    242, *256*

H

Haahtela, T., 3, 7, *26, 28*, 57, 61, 63,
    65, 152, 157, *175, 178*
Haake, R., 197, *202*
Haffner, C.A., 142, *171*
Hagensee, M.E., 246, *258*
Hahn, B., 155, *176*
Hahn, D.L., 239, *255*
Hahn, M., 211, 212, *217*
Hahn, T.J., 155, *176*
Haile, J.M., 112, *119*
Hall, I.P., 136, *166*
Hall, R.C., *178*
Hall, S.K., 236, *254*
Hall, W.J., 238, 239, *255*
Halloran, E., 156, *177*
Halonen, M., 2, 5, *26, 27*, 151, *174*
Hamelin, B.A., 99, *116*, 138, *167*
Hamid, Q., 38, *50*
Hamolsky, M.W., 244, 245, 246,
    257
Hansen, J.E., 87, *92*
Hansen-Flaschen, J., 198, *202*
Harbaugh, C.V., 142, *170*
Harbers, H., 138, 151, *167*, 185, 195,
    200
Harding, S.M., 106, 112, *118, 119*,
    157, *178*, 242, *256*
Hards, J., 45, *51*
Hargreave, F., 5, *27*, 187, *200*
Harman, E., 144, *172*
Harman, J.W., 54, 56, *64*

Harper, G.D., 161, *180*
Harris, H.W., 114, *120*, 206, *216*
Harris, M.I., 155, *177*
Harris, M.J., 156, *178*
Harrison, R.A., 77, *90*
Harrison, R.N., 186, *200*
Hartnell, A., 36, *48*
Harvey, J.E., 143, *171*
Hasday, J.D., 162, *181*
Hatton, F., 12, *29*
Hayashi, S., 45, *51*
Hayes, J.P., 123, *132*
Haynes, R.C., Jr., 155, 156, 159, *176*
Heaf, P., 11, *29*
Heaton, R.W., 241, 243, *256, 257*
Hedner, J., 139, *168*
Heine, D.L., 230, *252*
Heino, M., 3, *26*, 57, 61, 63, *65*
Heinrich, C., *256*
Helander, E., 243, 244, *257*
Hemstreet, M.P., 126, *133*
Hendeles, L., 143, 144, 145, 150,
    171, 172, 226, 228, 231, 236,
    241, *251*
Henderson, W.R., Jr., 161, *181*
Hendrick, D.J., 101, 103, *117*
Henochowicz, S.I., 140, 156, 160,
    169, 179
Henricks, P.A., 136, *166*
Henschle, P.J., 222, *249*
Heppner, B.T., 237, *254*
Herbison, G.P., 140, 142, *169, 171*
Hermans, J., 161, *180*
Hermansen, F., 137, *166*
Hermansson, B., 243, *257*
Hernandez, J.A., 60, *66*
Herrala, J., 160, *179*
Hetta, J., 126, *133*
Hey, E., 7, *28*
Heyworth, P., 162, *181-82*
Higgins, M., 8, 9, *28, 29*, 73, 74, 76,
    90, 123, 124, *132*, 227, *251*

Higgs, C., 208, *217*
Hillerdahl, G., 228, *251*
Hingston, D.M., 5, *28*
Hirano, T., 137, *166*
Hiroi, J., 137, *166*
Hobson, M., 220, 221, 222, 223,
    234, *249*
Hochron, S.M., 124, *132*, 214, *218*
Hodder, S.L., 238, *255*
Hodge, D.O., 232, *252*
Hodgson, T.A., 11, *29*, 114, *120*
Hodsman, A.B., 155, 160, *176, 179*
Hoffman, B.B., 138, *167*
Hoffman, N.B., 234, *253*
Hofland, I.D., 140, *169*
Hogg, J.C., 57, 58, 61, 62, *65, 66*
Holgate, S.T., 3, *26*, 37, *49*, 56, *65*,
    141, *170*, 184, *199*, 239, *256*
Hollister, J.R., 234, *253*
Holloway, L., 56, 59, 61, *65*
Holmes, W.I., 60, *66*
Holngren, G., 243, *257*
Holstege, C., 211, *217*
Holtzman, M.J., 184, *200*
Hong, C.K., 80, *91*
Hope, J.A., 93, 103, *115*
Hopewell, P., 146, *173*, 195, *201*
Hopp, R.J., 99, *116*
Horne, A., 122, 124, *132*
Horton, R.J.M., 224, *249*
Hossain, S., 56, 61, *65*
Howard, M.C., 37, *49*
Howarth, P.H., 56, *65*
Howell, R.E., 144, *172*
Huang, D., 144, *172*
Hubbard, W.C., 36, *48*
Huber, H.L., 53, 54, 57, 60, *63*
Huber, R.M., *256*
Huchon, G., 212, *217*
Hudson, I., 20, *31*
Hudson, L.M., 235, *254*
Hui, K.P., 162, *181*

Hunt, C., 145, *172*
Hunt, L.W., 13, *29*
Huntley, W., 150, *174*
Huseby, J.S., 246, *258*
Hussar, D.A., 226, *250*
Hyatt, R.E., 77, 87, *90*, *92*

I

Idris, A.H., 193, 196, *201*
Ikram, H., 142, *171*
Ind, P.W., 152, 156, 160, 164, *175*, *179*
Ingram, C.G., 139, *168*
Insel, P.A., 162, *182*
Irvine, P.W., 220, 221, *249*
Irwin, R.S., 5, *28*, 108, 111, *119*,
    241, 242, 245, *256*, *257*
Isawa, T., 137, *166*
Isenberg, S., 124, *132*
Israel, E., 140, 162, *169*, *181*, 195, *202*
Israel, R.H., 245, *257*
Iwamoto, I., 36, *49*

J

Jabara, H.H., 161, *180*
Jackson, D., 41, *50*
Jackson, R., 225, 234, *250*
Jacobs, L., 184, *199*
Jacobson, M., 38, *49*
Jacoby, D.B., 44, *50*
Jaffar, Z., 144, *172*
Jamal, K., 60, *66*
James, A.L., 57, *65*
James, F., 214, *218*
Janin, A., 37, *49*
Janson, C., 126, *133*
Janssen, M., 41, *50*
Jarjor, N., 161, *181*
Järvholm, B., 4, *26*
Jarvinen, M., 157, *178*
Jarvis, E.H., 101, 103, *117*

Jauregui, R., 105, *118*
Jeffery, P.K., 3, *26*, 38, 44, *49*, *51*,
    55, 56, 61, 63, *64*, *65*
Jenkins, C.R., 88, *92*, 157, *178*
Jenkins, L., 124, *132*
Jennings, B.H., 160, *179*
Jewesson, P.J., 146, *173*
Jiang, H., 136, *166*
Jick, H., 222, *249*
Jick, S.S., 147, 148, *173*
Jindal, S.K., 228, *251*
Joad, J.P., 150, *174*
Johansson, S.A., 160, *179*
Johnson, L.R., 16, *30*, 86, *92*
Johnson, R.L., Jr., 243, 245, *257*
Johnston, D.L., 232, *252*
Jones, D.A., 100, 101, 113, *117*, 192, *201*
Jones, G., 154, 160, *176*
Jones, J., 211, *217*
Jones, N.L., 14, *30*
Jonsson, B., 114, *120*
Jorres, R., 139, *167*
Joseph, J.C., 154, 155, *176*
Joseph, K.S., 235, *253*
Joseph, M., 161, *180*
Josephson, G.W., 142, *171*
Jungeblut, A., 124, *132*
Juniper, E., 5, *27*
Jusko, W.J., *172*
Jutagir, R., 205, *216*

K

Kabalin, C.S., 247, *258*
Kaegi, M.K., 36, *48*
Kaemmerlen, J.T., 5, 17, 18, 19, *27*,
    34, *47*, 61, *66*, 96, 97, 98, 102,
    103, *115*, 150, 157, 163, *174*,
    185, 186, 192, 196, 198, *200*,
    202, 224, 227, *250*
Kahaner, K., 156, *178*
Kaila, T., 162, *182*

Kallenbach, J.M., 189, *200*
Kaltenborn, W., 2, *26*
Kamada, A.K., 145, *172*
Kane, R.L., 219, *248*
Kaneko, M., 36, *48*
Kang, B., 5, *27*
Kaptein, A.A., 206, *216*
Karbowiak, I., 153, *175*
Karlström, R., 228, *251*
Karnes, H.T., 145, *172*
Karol, M.D., 228, *251*
Karpick, R.J., 58, *66*
Kassel, O., 37, *49*
Katz, I., 161, *181*
Kaufman, J., 107, 111, *119*
Kaufmann, F., 17, *31*
Kaufmann, M., 156, *178*
Kava, T., 157, *178*
Kawakami, Y., 84, *92*
Kay, A.B., 36, 38, *48, 49, 50*
Kay, J.C., 104, *118*
Keck, E., 155, *176*
Keene, D.L., 237, *254*
Keistinen, T., 10, *29*
Kelloway, J.S., 228, 230, *251*
Kelly, C., 101, 103, *117*
Kelly, H.W., 226, *250*
Kelly, J.G., 146, *173*
Kelly, P., 155, *176*
Kelly, W.J.W., 20, *31*
Kelman, H.R., 122, *132*
Kelsen, S.G., 77, *90*
Kelso, A., 41, *50*
Kemp, J.P., 158, *178*
Kempthorne-Rawson, J., 232, *252*
Kendall, M.J., 99, *116*, 142, *171*
Kendrick, A., 208, *217*
Kennedy, G.J., 122, *132*
Kennedy, H.L., 142, *171*
Kennedy, T.C., 71, *89*
Kephart, G.M., 59, *66*
Kershner, R.M., 162, *182*

Kerstjens, H.A.M., 5, *27*, 80, 84, *91, 92*, 139, 153, *168*
Kesten, S., 84, *92*, 127, *133*, 140, 142, *169, 170*
Kewley, G.D., 156, 160, *179*
Kick, E., 205, *216*
Kidney, J., 144, 149, 150, *172*
Kikuchi, Y., 101, *117*, 185, *200*, 225, *250*
Kilburn, K.H., 58, *66*
Kiley, J.P., 229, *251*
Kim, J.B., 114, *120*
Kim, W.D., 58, *66*
Kimbel, P., 243, 245, *257*
Kincaid, D., 124, 127, *132*
King, S., 244, *257*
Kinnear, B.F., 37, *49*
Kinney, E.L., 142, *170*
Kircher, T., 13, *29*
Kirsch, I., 124, *132*
Kirschbaum, C., 44, *51*
Kirwan, J.P., 155, *177*
Kishi, F., 84, *92*
Kita, H., 35, 36, *48*
Kivelä, S.L., 10, *29*
Klainer, A.S., 105, *118*
Klaustermeyer, W.B., 153, *175*, 234, 241, *253*
Klein, J.J., 149, *173*
Kleinerman, J., 60, 61, *66*, 74, *90*
Kloner, R., 156, *177*
Knodel, A.R., 237, *254*
Knottnerus, I., 160, *179*
Knox, A.J., 61, 62, *67*
Knudson, R.J., 71, 73, 74, *89, 90*, 143, *171*
Kochwa, S., 57, *65*
Koehnke, R., 153, *175*
Koenig, H.G., *178*
Koessler, K.K., 53, 54, 57, 60, *63*
Kohler, C.L., 129, 130, *133*
Kohl-Lachs, S.L., 230, *252*

Kohrt, W.M., 155, *177*
Kok, P.T., 161, *180*
Kolbe, J., 214, *218*
Kolotkin, B., 5, *27*
Kolstad, A., 124, *132*
Kornstad, S., 146, *172*
Korobaeff, M., 17, *31*
Korsager, S., 244, 245, 246, *257*
Kotlikoff, M.I., 136, *166*
Koup, J.R., *172*
Kradjan, W.A., 80, 82, *91*, 138, 151, *167*
Krall, J.F., 137, *167*
Kramer, P.A., 146, *172*
Kraut, D., 206, *216*
Kray, K.T., 140, *169*
Krieger, B.P., 103, 106, *118*
Kristensen, H.P.O., 244, 245, 246, *257*
Kroegel, C., 36, 37, *48*, *49*, 144, *172*
Kroemer, D.J., 207, *216*
Kronenberg, R.S., 101, *117*
Kronmal, R.A., 9, *29*, 71, 73, 74, 76, 77, 85, *89*, *90*, 123, 124, *132*
Krowka, M.J., 87, *92*
Kryger, M., 105, *118*
Kuller, L.H., *90*
Kumana, C.R., 211, 212, *217*
Kume, H., 136, *166*
Kunske, R., 234, 241, *253*
Kuo, C.-C., 240, *256*
Kuwano, K., 44, 45, *51*, 57, 58, *65*
Kwong, F.K., 153, *175*, 234, 241, *253*

L

Labrune, S., 212, *217*
Lacoste, J.Y., 3, *26*, 35, 36, *47*, 57, 62, *65*, 184, *199*
Lacquet, L.M., 156, *177*
Lacronique, J., 157, *178*

Ladenius, A.R., 36, *49*
LaForce, C., 139, 140, *167*
Laitinen, A., 3, *26*, 57, 61, 63, *65*, 152, *175*
Laitinen, L.A., 3, *26*, 57, 61, 63, *65*, 152, *175*, 184, *199*
Lal, S., 93, *115*
Lam, A., 143, *171*
Lamb, D., 57, *65*
Lammert, J.K., 161, *181*
Lamy, P.P., 222, *249*
Landau, L.I., 20, *31*
Lang, D.M., 98, *116*
Lange, P., 137, *166*, 228, *251*
Langlois, J.C., 147, 148, *173*
Lanier, L.L., 37, *49*
Lapa, 36, *48*
Lapinsky, S.E., 189, *200*
L'Archeveque, J., 210, *217*
Larsen, J.S., 211, 212, *217*
Larson, T.V., 98, *116*
Larsson, S., 139, *168*
Lasser, E., 230, 243, *249*, *257*
Laszlo, G., 208, *217*
Laucka, P.V., 234, *253*
Lauder, I.J., 211, 212, *217*
Laurent, P., 197, *202*
Lavan, J., 146, *173*
Lawson, C.P., 209, *217*
Lawson, D.H., 156, 164, *177*
Lawton, M.P., 205, *215*
Leahy, B.C., 151, *174*
Lebowitz, M.D., 2, 5, 16, *26*, *30*, 34, *47*, 85, 87, *92*, 98, 102, *116*, 126, 129, *133*, 185, 186, 190, *200*, 224, *250*
Lee, D., 7, *28*
Lee, G.S., 8, *28*, 93, 95, 101, 102, 108, *115*, 224, *250*
Lee, H.Y., 17, 18, 19, *31*, 61, *66*, 93, 94, 97, 98, 111, *115*, 224, *250*

Leenen, F.H., 142, *170*
Leff, J.A., 161, *181*
Lefkowitz, M.S., 149, *173*
Lefkowitz, R.J., 138, 139, *167, 168*
Le Gros, G., 42, *50*
Lehrer, P.M., 124, *132*, 214, *218*
Leiferman, K.M., 35, *48*
Leitner, J., 101, *117*, 123, *132*
Lejemtel, T., 104, *118*
Lemanske, R.F., 239, *255*
Leroux, M., 62, *67*
LeRoy, O., 225, *250*
Letts, L.G., 36, 43, *48, 50*
Levine, J.H., 146, *173*
Levine, M.A., 142, *170*
Levison, H., 56, 61, *65*
Liberman, U.A., 155, *176*
Lichtenstein, M.J., 205, *216*
Lieberman, P., 234, 241, *253*
Liippo, K., 160, *179*
Lilker, E.S., 105, *118*
Lim, K.H., 246, *258*
Limbird, L.E., 99, *116*, 137, *167*
Linden, A., 139, *167*
Lindgren, S., 146, 150, *173, 174*
Lipman, H.B., 240, *256*
Lipworth, B.J., 79, *91*, 139, 142,
    143, 157, *168, 170, 171, 178*,
    244, *257*
Littenberg, B., 150, *173*, 195, *201*
Liu, M.C., 36, *48*
Lockhart, A., 88, *92*
Lofdahl, C.G., 142, *170*
Logue, G., 153, *175*
Loh, R.K., 161, *180*
Lokshin, B., 146, *173*
Loudon, R.G., 105, *118*
Louis, R.E., 144, *172*
Love, L., 141, *170*, 212, *217*
Lovejoy, F.J., Jr., 146, 147, *173*
Lozewicz, S., 3, *26*
Lukert, B.P., 155, *176*

Lumsden, A., 57, *65*
Lyles, K.W., 154, *176*
Lyons, H.A., 190, 191, *201*

M

McCann, R.M., 238, 239, *255*
McCoy, R.A., 143, *171*
McDermott, M.F., 193, 196, *201*
McDevitt, D.G., 79, *91*, 139, 142,
    143, *168, 170, 171*
McDonald, A.F., 160, *179*
Macdonald, J.B., 113, 114, *120*
MacDonald, M.R., 16, *30*
McDowell, E.M., 56, *64*
McDuffie, H.H., 229, *252*
McFadden, E.R., Jr., 57, *65*, 113,
    120, 190, 194, *201*, 211, *217*,
    234, *253*
McGavin, D.D., 155, *177*
McGeady, S., 5, *27*
McGill, K., 161, *181*
McGregor, M., 142, *170*
Mackay, A., 146, *173*
MacKechnie, H.L.N., 244, *257*
McKenniff, M., 144, *172*
MacKenzie, E.J., 142, *171*
McKinney, B., 102, *117*
McKinney, W.P., 107, 111, *119*
Macklem, P.T., 3, *26*, 62, *67*
McLennan, L.A., 20, *31*
McManus, D.Q., 205, *216*
McNally, P., 159, *179*
McNicol, K., 5, 6, 20, *27*
McParland, C.P., 139, 161, *168, 180*
Mader, S.L., 137, 142, *166*
Maestrelli, P., 40, *50*
Mahesh, V.K., 151, *174*
Maikoe, T., 161, *180*
Majid, P.A., 142, *170*
Mak, J.C., 139, *168*
Mak, V.H., 160, *179*

Malik, S.K., 8, *28*, 93, 95, 101, 102,
  108, *115*, 224, *250*
Malo, J.L., 129, *133*, 210, *217*, 230, *252*
Manatunga, A.K., 158, *178*
Mandaleson, K., 93, *115*
Manfreda, J., 7, *28*
Manolio, T.A., *90*
Manton, K.G., 220, 223, *249*
Manzella, B.A., 125, *133*, 220, 224,
  225, 228, 229, 233, 239, 243, *249*
Marder, D., 98, *116*
Marin, J.M., 161, *180*
Marini, J.J., 197, *202*
Markov, A.E., 160, *179*
Markowe, H.L.J., 23, *31*
Marquette, C.H., 225, *250*
Marrie, T.J., 240, *256*
Marshall, D.H., 154, *176*
Marshall, N., 150, *174*
Marston, B.J., 240, *256*
Martelli, A.N., 113, *120*
Martin, A.J., 20, *31*
Martin, L.B., 35, *48*
Martin, R.J., 140, 151, *169*, *174*,
  237, *255*
Martineau, P., 233, *253*
Martinez, F., 5, *27*
Martinusen, S., 212, *217*
Mason, U.G., III, 108, *119*
Massarella, G.R., 56, 57, 61, *64*
Matera, M.G., 238, 240, *255*
Mathews, K.P., 8, *28*
Mathiseon, D.A., 107, *119*
Matran, R., 103, 104, *118*, 230,
  252
Matsuba, K., 60, *66*
Matsunga, S.K., 228, *251*
Matthay, R.A., 229, *252*
May, F.E., 223, *249*
Mayne, T., 214, *218*
Mayo, P.H., 114, *120*, 206, *216*
Mays, E.E., 241, *256*

Medici, T.C., 155, *176*
Meeker, D.P., 107, 111, *119*
Mekori, Y.A., 161, *180*
Melchor, R., 160, *179*
Meldrum, L.A., 137, *166*
Mellis, C.M., 8, *28*
Mellor, A.L., 36, *49*
Melmed, C.A., 237, *254*
Meltzer, E.O., 158, *178*
Meltzer, S.S., 162, *181*
Melzer, E., 242, *256*
Mengelers, H.J., 161, *180*
Mensinga, T.T., 80, *91*
Menter, R.R., 235, *254*
Mercer, G.D., 144, *172*
Mercik, S.A., 146, *172*
Mestecky, J., 36, *49*
Metcalfe, T., 236, *254*
Meuleman, J., 127, *133*
Meunier, P.J., 155, *176*
Meyer, J.W., 204, *215*
Meyer, S.M., 160, *179*
Michael, J.R., 146, *173*
Michaels, L., 55, *64*
Michel, F.B., 12, *29*, 239, 240,
  255
Mier, A., 245, *257*
Miesfeld, R.L., 152, *175*
Mikawa, K., 136, *166*
Miles, J.F., 106, 111, *118*
Miller, A., 79, *91*
Miller, T.D., 139, *168*
Minder, C.E., 156, *177*
Mitchell, D.M., *178*
Mitenko, P.A., 148, *173*
Miyajima, A., 37, *49*
Molema, J., 84, *92*
Molfino, N.A., 113, *120*
Montamat, S.C., 226, *250*
Montserrat, J.M., 156, *177*
Mootoosamy, I.M., 111, *119*
Moqbel, R., 36, *48*

Moran, M.B., 15, *30*, 94, *115*
Moreno, R.H., 58, 61, 62, *66*
Morice, R., 60, *66*
Morreale, A., 156, *178*
Morrell, R.W., 124, 127, *132*
Morris, A.H., 78, 79, *90*
Morris, H.G., 152, 153, *175*
Morris, J.C., 205, *216*
Morrison, N.J., 78, *90*
Mortensen, J., 137, *166*
Morton, A., 57, *65*
Moser, K.M., 108, *119*
Motta, J., 237, *255*
Moulton, S.B., 156, *177*
Mountina, R.D., 190, *201*
Muhlhauser, I., 206, *216*
Muiesan, G., 77, *90*
Mulder, M., 77, *90*
Mullally, D.I., 10, 11, 13, *29*
Mullarkey, M.F., 161, *181*
Mullee, M.A., 210, *217*
Muller-Lissner, S.A., *256*
Munoz, N.M., 43, *50*
Munroe, W.P., 162, *182*
Munt, P.W., 144, 148, *171*
Murdock, K.Y., 5, *27*, 161, *180*
Murphy, M.B., 142, *171*
Murphy, W.A., 155, *176*
Murray, A.M., 234, *253*
Murray, M.D., 158, *178*
Musher, D., 208, *216*
Myers, J.L., 107, 111, *119*

N

Nadeau, J., 99, *116*, 137, *167*
Nadel, J.A., 184, *199*
Nadel, J.M., 184, *200*
Nair, N.M., 99, *116*
Najjari, C., 224, *250*
Nakajima, H., 36, *49*
Nakatsu, K., 144, 148, *171*

Nannin, L.J., 113, *120*
Nassif, E.G., 150, *174*
Nathan, R.A., 140, *169*
Naylor, B., 56, *64*
Neas, L.M., 79, *91*
Neff, T.A., 146, *173*, 237, *254*
Neill, P., 161, *180*
Nejjari, C., 94, *115*, 123, *132*
Nelson, F.C., 3, *26*
Nelson, H.S., 136, 138, 139, 140,
    142, 143, *166*, *167*, *169*, 232,
    242, 244, *252*, *256*
Nelson, J., 13, *29*
Neugarten, B.L., 204, *215*
Neukirch, F., 16, 17, *30*, *31*
Newhouse, M.T., 140, 143, 157,
    169, *171*
Newman, G.B., 99, *116*, 138, 151,
    167, 185, *200*
Newman, K.B., 108, *119*
Newnham, D.M., 83, *91*, 139, *168*
Nickeson, D., 237, *255*
Nicklas, R.A., 219, 220, 225, 230,
    232, 237, 239, 240, 241, 242,
    243, 246, 247, *248*, 252
Nicodemus, C.F., 239, *256*
Niden, A.H., 14, *30*
Nielson, C.P., 99, *117*
Niewoehner, D.E., 60, 61, *66*, 74,
    90
Nijkamp, F.P., 41, *50*, 136, *166*
Nimmo, A.J., 136, *166*
Nimmo, C., 212, *217*
Nishikawa, M., 139, *168*
Nitta, Y., 46, *51*
Noble, W.H., 104, *118*
Nogradi, S., 84, *92*
Noonan, M., 157, *178*
Nordin, B.E., 154, *176*
Norman, A., 93, *115*
Northfield, M., 156, 160, 164,
    179

Noseda, A., 208, *217*
Nowak, D., 139, *167*
Nunan, L.M., 151, *174*
Nunn, A.J., 161, *181*

O

Obdrzalek, J., 104, *118*
O'Byrne, P.M., 161, *180*
Ocampo, E., 244, 245, *257*
O'Connell, E.J., 34, *47*, 227, 228, *251*
O'Connor, B.J., 139, *168*
O'Connor, G.T., 5, 16, *27*, *30*, 80, *91*, 99, *117*, 224, *249*
O'Connor, S.W., 137, *167*
Oehling, A., 36, *48*
Offord, K.P., 98, *116*
Ogilvie, R.I., 148, *173*
O'Hallaren, M.T., 98, *116*
Ohman, J.L., 16, *30*
Ohno, I., 46, *51*
Ohno, S., 43, *50*
Okabe, S., 101, *117*, 185, *200*, 225, *250*
Okayama, Y., 37, *49*
Okubo, M., 155, *176*
Oliver, J.S., 146, *173*
Ollerenshaw, S.L., 54, 55, 56, 57, *64*
Olson, D.E., 105, *118*
Onnelly-Fittingoff, M., 137, *167*
Onorato, D., 103, *118*
Opdycke, R.A., 127, 130, *133*
Orgel, H.A., 158, *178*
Orris, P., 98, *116*
Oryszezyn, M.P., 16, *30*
Osler, W., 11, *29*, 93, 103, *115*
Osman, J., 111, *119*
Osman, L.M., 210, *217*
Otten, M., 246, *258*
Ouslander, J.G., 219, 222, *248*, *249*
Overbeek, S.E., 84, *92*

Owens, G.R., 143, 148, 149, *171*

P

Pachana, N.A., 205, *215*
Packe, G.E., 160, *179*
Paganin, F., 45, *51*
Page, M.M., 243, *257*
Pain, M., 208, *217*
Pairolero, P.C., 108, *119*
Palmer, J.B., 150, *174*
Palmer, K.N.V., 191, *201*
Paoletti, P., 78, 80, *90*, *91*
Pare, P.D., 44, 45, *51*, 57, 58, 61, 62, *65*, *66*
Park, D.C., 124, 127, *132*
Parkin, D.H., 209, *217*
Paronetto, F., 57, *65*
Parson, G.H., 102, 104, 112, 113, *118*
Partridge, M.R., 62, *67*
Patel, A.K., 146, *173*
Paterson, R.W., 155, *177*
Patterson, D.R., 225, 228, 234, *250*
Patterson, R., 156, *177*, 225, 228, 234, 240, 241, *250*, *253*, *256*
Pearce, F.L., 161, *180*
Pearce, N., 140, *169*
Pearlman, D.S., 139, 140, *167*
Pearson, M.G., 163, *182*
Pearson, R.S.B., 53, 56, 57, 59, 60, 61, *64*
Peat, J.K., 5, 8, 22, 23, *27*, *28*, *31*, 80, 81, *91*, 96, *115*, 121, 123, *132*
Pedersen, B., 228, *251*
Pedersen, S., 152, 157, 158, 159, 160, *175*, 232, 234, 237, 241, *253*
Pelikan, Z., 160, *179*
Pennock, B.E., 143, 148, 149, *171*
Pepe, P.E., 197, *202*
Perret, C., 198, *202*
Perry, H.M., 154, *176*
Persson, C.G., 137, 144, 145, *166*, *172*

Pesci, A., 3, *26*
Peselow, E.D., 156, *178*
Peters, E.J., 60, *66*
Petheram, I.S., 100, 101, 113, *117*, 192, *201*
Petit-Frere, C., 37, *49*
Peto, R., 14, *30*
Petty, T.L., 105, *118*, 164, *182*, 189, *201*, 229, *251*
Pfeifer, M.A., 99, 101, *116*, 185, *200*
Phelan, P.D., 20, *31*
Phillips, J.H., 37, *49*
Phipps, B., 112, *119*
Picado, C., 156, *177*
Pierce, N., 235, *253*
Pierson, D.J., 102, *117*
Pieton, R., 243, *257*
Pingleton, S.K., 198, *202*, 237, 243, *254*
Pisani, R.J., 107, 111, *119*
Pison, C., 230, *252*
Pistelli, G., 78, *90*
Pitchenik, A., 190, *201*
Plezia, P.M., 228, *251*
Plikaytis, B.D., 240, *256*
Poe, R.H., 245, *257*
Poh, S.C., 245, 246, *258*
Pokrajac, M., 246, *258*
Polansky, M., 98, *116*
Pontoppidan, H., 106, *118*, 185, *200*
Popkin, M.K., *178*
Popplewell, P.Y., 222, *249*
Porter, J., 156, 164, *177*, 222, *249*
Posey, W.C., 139, *167*
Postma, D.S., 5, *27*, 80, 84, *91*, 140, *169*, 224, *250*
Potgieter, P.D., 196, *202*
Potter, J.F., 205, *216*
Powell, J.R., 146, *173*, 195, *201*
Powell, N., 238, *255*
Powell-Jackson, P.R., 241, *256*
Prakash, U.B.S., 236, *254*
Pratt, P.C., 58, *66*

Pratter, M.R., 5, *28*, 245, *257*
Pretolani, M., 36, *48*
Pride, N.B., 14, 16, *30*
Prideaux, D.J., 207, *216*
Prigogine, T., 208, *217*
Prince, D.S., 107, *119*
Print, C.G., 140, *169*
Prior, A., 141, *170*, 211, *217*, 234, *253*
Pulliam, C.C., 233, 234, *253*
Puolijoki, H., 160, *179*

Q

Quanjer, P.H., 70, 72, *89*, 139, 153, *168*
Quera-Salva, M.A., 238, *255*

R

Rabe, K.F., 139, 144, *167*, *172*
Rachelefsky, G.S., 146, *173*
Rackemann, F., 3, *26*
Radermecker, M.F., 144, *172*
Rado, V., 40, *50*
Rafferty, P., 239, 240, *255*
Raine, D., Jr., 139, *167*
Raisz, L.G., 155, *176*
Ramadan, F., 78, *90*
Ramage, L., 139, *168*
Ramsay, L.E., 146, *173*
Rand, C.S., 124, 130, *132*
Ranhosky, A., 232, *252*
Raps, E.C., 198, *202*
Raucci, J.C., 193, 196, *201*
Rea, H.H., 13, *29*, 225, 234, *250*
Rebuch, A.J., 195, *202*
Rebuck, A.S., 84, *92*, 151, *174*, 230, 231, 243, *252*
Rebuck, H.S., 194, *201*
Redpath, A.T., 78, 85, *90*
Reed, C.E., 5, 13, *27*, *29*, 34, *47*, 227, 228, 244, 245, 246, *251*, *257*
Reid, J.L., 142, *171*

Reid, L., 56, 59, 60, *64*, *66*
Reidy, M.A., 45, *51*
Reilly, P., 36, *48*
Rennard, S., 24, *31*
Renon, D., 157, *178*
Repsher, L.H., 139, *167*, *168*
Reynolds, C., 205, *216*
Reynolds, S., 160, *179*
Rezneck, R.H., 111, *119*
Rhoden, K.J., 137, *166*
Rich, L.F., 155, *177*
Richards, J.M., Jr., 101, *117*, 123, 124, 125, 126, *132*, *133*, 214, *218*, 220, 224, 225, 228, 229, 233, 239, 243, *249*
Richards, J.S., 235, *254*
Richman, J., 114, *120*, 206, *216*
Richmond, I., 60, *66*
Richter, B., 206, *216*
Richter, J.E., 112, *119*, 228, 242, *251*, *256*
Riekse, R., 211, *217*
Riendl, P., 107, 111, *119*
Riggs, B.L., 153, *175*
Rijcken, B., 80, *91*
Rindone, J.P., 162, *182*
Rivington, R.N., 150, *174*
Rizos, A.L., 156, *178*
Rizzon, P., 232, *252*
Roberts, J., 214, *218*
Roberts, J.A., 3, *26*, 184, *199*
Robertson, P.C., 71, *89*
Robin, E.D., 165, *182*
Robinson, D.R., 38, *50*
Robinson, D.S., 36, *48*, 159, *179*, 232, 234, 237, 241, 247, *253*
Roca, A., 237, *255*
Roche, W.R., 3, *26*, 55, 56, *64*, *65*, 184, *199*
Rodarte, J.R., 87, *92*
Roe, F.J.C., 60, *66*
Roehrs, T.A., 238, *255*

Rogers, D.F., 136, 153, *166*, *175*
Rogers, R.M., 143, 148, 149, *171*
Rogiers, P., 156, *177*
Rolla, G., 109, 110, *119*
Rollins, D.R., 164, *182*
Romagnoli, P., 62, *67*
Rona, R.J., 7, *28*
Roorda, R.J., 20, *31*
Rosen, R.I., 127, 130, *133*
Rosenberg, H.M., 227, *251*
Rosenberg, M., 162, *181*, 195, *202*
Rosenow, E.C., III, 107, 111, *119*, 236, *254*
Rosenstock, I.R., 122, 127, 130, *132*
Rosina, C., 57, *65*
Rosner, B., 99, *117*
Ross, I., 7, *28*
Rossi, A., 197, *202*
Rossi, F., 238, 240, *255*
Rossing, T.H., 190, 194, *201*
Roth, T.R., 238, *255*
Rothstein, M.S., 104, *118*
Rouby, J.J., 197, *202*
Rouleau, J., 230, *252*
Rowe, M.S., 244, *257*
Rowley, J.J., 101, 103, *117*, 137, *167*
Roy, K., 8, 17, 18, 19, *29*, 93, 97, 98, *115*
Rubaker, H., 141, *170*
Rubinfeld, A.R., 208, *217*
Ruegsegger, P., 155, *176*
Ruffie, C., 36, *48*
Russell, I.T., 210, *217*
Ryan, M., 78, 85, *90*
Ryder, K.W., 142, *171*
Rylander, R., 228, *251*
Ryo, U., 5, *27*
Ryssing, E., 20, *31*

S

Saag, K.G., 153, *175*

Saagles, M.T., 237, *255*
Sackner, M.A., 108, *119*
Saetta, M., 57, 58, *65, 66*
Sahn, S.A., 189, 190, 191, *201*
Sakula, A., 56, *64*
Salata, R.A., 156, *177*
Salome, C.M., 5, *27*, 80, 81, *91*
Salvato, G., 55, 57, *64*
Samanta, A., 159, *179*
Sambrook, P., 155, *176*
Sami, M.H., 142, *170*
Sampol, G., 237, *255*
Samuelson, G., 243, *257*
Sanders, G., 161, *181*
Sanderson, C.J., 36, *49*
Sargunaraj, D., 214, *218*
Sarkar, M.A., 145, *172*
Sarma, M., 207, *216*
Sasaki, H., 56, 61, *64*
Sato, A., 155, *176*
Saulnier, F., 225, *250*
Saunders, K.B., 62, *67*, 99, *116*, 138, 151, *167*, 185, *200*
Savelkoul, H.F., 36, *49*
Sbarbaro, J.A., 192, 193, *201*
Scali, M., 153, *175*
Scamagas, P., 206, *216*
Scarpace, P.J., 99, *116*, 137, 142, *166, 167*
Schachter, E.N., 22, 23, *31*
Schan, C.A., 106, 112, *118, 119*
Schatz, M., 156, *177*
Schein, J.R., 228, *251*
Scheitel, S.M., 235, 241, 244, 245, *254*
Schenker, M., 71, 76, 77, 85, *89*
Scher, D.L., 142, *171*
Scherr, P.A., 208, *216*
Schindlbeck, N.E., *256*
Schinnar, R., 11, *29*, 140, *168*
Schleimer, R.P., 36, *48*, 152, *175*
Schlichtig, R., 197, *202*

Schlueter, D.P., 107, 111, *119*
Schmaling, K.B., 108, *119*
Schmerber, J., 208, *217*
Schoenfeld, E., 244, 245, 246, *257*
Schouten, J.P., 80, 84, *91, 92*
Schrader, L., 36, *48*
Schrier, A.C., 208, *216*
Schulzer, M., 5, *28*
Schwartz, 79, *91*
Schwartz, J., 98, *116*
Schwartz, O., 237, 243, *254*
Scoggin, C.H., 189, *201*
Scragg, R., 225, 234, *250*
Sears, M.R., 5, 6, 13, *27, 29*, 140, *169*
Seaton, A., 93, 97, 98, 113, 114, *115, 120*, 195, *202*
Sebastian, J.L., 107, 111, *119*
Sedgwick, J.B., 36, *48*
Seeman, E., 153, *175*
Segal, M., 224, *249*
Segal, M.R., 80, *91*
Segel, D.P., 107, 111, *119*
Seidelman, M.J., 104, *118*
Seminario, M.C., 35, *48*
Semper, A., 37, *49*
Seneterre, E., 45, *51*
Serow, W.J., 204, *215*
Sessler, C.N., 146, 147, 148, *173*, 195, *202*
Settipane, G.A., 244, 245, 246, *257*
Shabb, J.B., 136, *166*
Shah, P., 236, *254*
Shannon, M., 146, 147, *173*
Shapiro, B.A., 77, *90*
Shapiro, G.G., 146, *173*
Shavit, G., 246, *258*
Shaw, G., 156, 160, 164, *179*
Sheldon, J.M., 57, *65*
Sheller, J.R., 184, *200*
Sheppard, D., 142, 149, *170*, 195, *201*

Sherry, M.K., 105, *118*
Shim, C., 140, *169*, 211, *217*
Shimp, L.A., 127, 130, *133*
Shimura, S., 56, 61, *64*
Shin, C.S., 190, *201*
Shiner, R.J., 161, *181*
Shipley, M.J., 23, *31*
Shirasaki, H., 139, *168*
Shulimzon, T., 161, *181*
Shuttleworth, D., 160, *179*
Siefkin, A.D., 232, *253*
Siegel, D., 142, 149, *170*, 195, *201*
Siegler, D., 191, 194, *201*
Sieradzski, J., 243, *257*
Siggard-Andersen, O., 77, *90*
Silverberg, J.D.H., 244, 245, 246, *257*
Silverstein, M.D., 13, *29*, 227, 228, *251*
Simic, D., 246, *258*
Simon, R.A., 107, *119*
Simons, F.E.R., 239, *255*
Simpson, W.G., 112, *119*, 242, *256*
Singh, A., 228, *251*
Skarpass, I., 7, *28*
Skatrud, J.B., 146, *173*
Skidmore, I.F., 137, *166*
Skorodin, M.S., 150, *174*
Slater, D., 98, *116*
Slavin, R.G., 239, *255*
Slutsky, A.S., 113, *120*
Sly, D.F., 204, *215*
Sly, R.M., 10, *29*, 165, *182*, 224, *250*
Smith, A.J., 7, *28*
Smith, D., 83, *92*
Smith, H.C., 229, *252*
Smith, J.A., 139, *167*
Smith, L., 161, *180*
Smith, L.J., 162, *181*
Smith, S., 139, *168*
Smith, T.C., 197, *202*
Smith, W.H., 151, *174*

Snadden, D., 126, *133*
Snashall, P.D., 103, *118*
Snider, G.L., 24, *31*
So, S.Y., 211, 212, *217*
Sobonya, R.E., 53, 54, 61, 63, *63*, *66*, 97, *116*, 185, *200*
Soler, N.G., 243, *257*
Solinas, E., 77, *90*
Soong, S., 124, *132*
Sorbini, C.A., 77, *90*
Sornet, C., 156, *177*
Souhrada, J.F., 242, *256*
Spagnolatti, L., 77, 78, *90*
Spain, D.M., 60, *66*
Sparrow, D., 5, 16, *27*, *30*, 80, *91*, 99, *117*, 224, *249*
Speare, A., 204, *215*
Spector, S.L., 149, 162, *173*, *181*, 219, 220, 225, 230, 232, 237, 239, 240, 241, 242, 243, 246, 247, *248*
Speight, A., 7, *28*
Speiser, B.L., 105, *118*
Speizer, F.E., 5, 11, 14, *27*, *29*, *30*, 93, *115*
Spiro, S.G., 160, *179*
Spitzer, W.O., 79, *91*, 140, 157, *169*, *178*
Spratling, L., 105, *118*
Springer, C., 7, *28*
Spungen, A.M., 235, 236, *254*
Stallard, E., 220, 223, *249*
Stammen, D., 155, *176*
Stanflin, N., 62, *67*
Starr-Schneidkraut, N.J., 122, *132*
Stas, K.J., 156, *177*
Staub, J.-J., 246, *258*
Stauffer, J.L., 105, *118*
Steele, D., 232, *253*
Steigman, D., 185, *200*
Stein, M., 243, 245, *257*
Stenger, R., 46, *51*

Sterk, P.J., 208, *216*
Stevenson, D.D., 107, *119*
Steward, R.B., 223, *249*
Stewart, A.G., 62, *67*
Stewart, G.A., 7, *28*
Stickney, S.K., *178*
Stierle, H., 44, *51*
Stivers, D.S.H., 245, *257*
Stogner, S., 211, 212, *217*
Stolley, P., 11, *29*
Stolley, P.D., 140, *168*
Stover, S.L., 235, *254*
Strachan, D.P., 10, *29*
Strath, M., 36, *49*
Streiner, D., 214, *218*
Stretton, T.B., 17, 18, 19, *31*, 61, *66*, 93, 94, 97, 98, 111, *115*, 224, *250*
Strickland, D., 142, *171*
Stromquist, A., 146, *173*
Strunk, R.C., 113, *120*, 150, *174*
Struthers, A.D., 142, 143, *171*
Stuck, A.E., 153, 156, *175*, *177*
Sue, M.A., 153, *175*, 234, 241, *253*
Suissa, S., 140, 157, *169*, *178*, 235, *253*
Sullivan, C.E., 237, 238, *255*
Sullivan, P., 144, *172*
Sur, S., 59, *66*
Surks, M.I., 244, 245, *257*
Sutherland, D., 11, 12, *29*
Sutton, F.D., Jr., 146, *173*, 237, *254*
Svedmyr, K., 142, *170*
Svedmyr, N., 139, 141, 142, *168*, *170*
Svensson, C., 137, *166*
Swanson, M.C., 36, *48*
Swenson, C.A., 239, *255*
Swenson, S.J., 107, 111, *119*
Synek, M., 57, *65*
Szalai, J.P., 140, *169*
Szczeklik, A., 243, *257*
Szefler, S.J., 140, 145, 157, *169*, *172*, *178*

Szymanski, D., 237, 243, *254*

T

Tack, C.M., 101, *117*
Taillandier, D., 156, *177*
Takagi, K., 136, *166*
Takizawa, T., 56, 60, 61, *64*, *66*
Talebi, Z., 229, *252*
Talseth, T., 146, *172*
Tammeling, G.J., 70, 72, *89*
Tamura, G., 101, *117*, 185, *200*, 225, *250*
Targonski, P., 98, *116*
Tashkin, D.P., 80, *91*, 139, *167-68*
Tattersfield, A.E., 161, *180*, 186, *200*
Taylor, D.R., 140, 142, *169*, *171*
Taylor, P.M., 144, 149, 150, *172*
Tazellar, H.D., 108, *119*
Teengs, J.P., 140, *169*
Teichman, S., 246, *258*
Temple, K., 5, *28*
Templin, R.K., 77, *90*
Teshima, T., 137, *166*
Tessier, J.F., 94, *115*, 123, *132*, 224, *250*
Teule, G.J., 142, *170*
Thakur, M.K., 153, *175*
Thieme, E.T., 57, *65*
Thiringer, G., 139, 141, *168*, *170*
Thom, T.G., 227, *251*
Thomas, A., 11, *29*
Thomas, C., 122, *132*
Thomas, T.P., *175*
Thompson, A., 141, *170*
Thompson, H., 2, 5, *26*
Thompson, H.C., 185, *200*
Thompson, L.W., 205, *215*
Thompson, R., 150, *174*
Thomsen, J.H., 146, *173*
Thomson, K., 56, 59, 61, *65*

Thornton, J.C., 79, *91*
Thurlbeck, W.M., 56, 60, 61, *64*, *66*
Tietze, K.J., 226, *250*
Timmers, M.C., 139, 161, *168*, *180*
Tinkelman, D., 244, *257*
Tinker, C., 14, *30*
Tockman, M.S., 229, *251*
Tolep, K., 77, *90*
Tollerud, D.J., 5, *27*
Tomita, D.K., 7, *28*
Tomlinson, P.R., 62, *67*
Tomoe, S., 36, *49*
Tonel, A.B., 161, *180*
Toogood, J.H., 154, 155, 157, 158,
    159, 160, *176*, *178*, *179*
Torcellini, C.A., 36, *48*
Toren, K., 4, *26*
Tornatore, K.M., 153, *175*
Torphy, T.J., 136, 137, *166*
Tousignant, P., 79, *91*
Tovey, E.R., 8, *28*
Townley, R., 5, *27*
Townley, R.G., 99, *116*
Townsend, M., 84, *92*
Tracey, M., 16, *31*
Tracy, R.P., 230, *249*
Trautlein, J.J., 142, *170*
Trautner, C., 206, *216*
Traver, G.A., 21, 22, *31*, 85, 86, *92*,
    97, *116*, 127, *133*, 141, *170*, 223,
    224, 227, *249*, *251*
Tregaskis, B.F., 142, *170*
Tremper-Mitchell, J., 141, *170*
Troyer, W.G., Jr., 146, *173*
Trudeau, C., 210, *217*
Tsicopoulos, A., 161, *180*
Tuck, M.L., 137, *167*
Tumer, N., 137, 142, *166*
Tun, C.G., 235, *254*
Turcotte, H., 113, *120*, 225, 234, *250*
Turner, K.J., 7, *28*
Tuuponen, T., 10, *29*

Twohig, K.J., 229, *252*

U

Ullah, M.I., 99, *116*, 138, 151, *167*,
    185, *200*
Ullman, A., 139, *168*
Ulrik, C.S., 22, 23, *31*, 44, *51*, 228,
    251
Ulstad, D.R., 197, *202*
Unger, L., 114, *120*
Urban, R.C., Jr., 155, *176*
Urley, F.J., 111, *119*

V

Vail, A., 162, *182*
Valenzuela, J.E., 187, *200*, 242,
    256
Vallon, A., 212, *217*, 234, *253*
Vamos, M., 214, *218*
Van Aalderen, W.M.C., 20, *31*
van Ark, I., 41, *50*
Vance, J.W., *172*
Van der Lende, R., 17, *31*
van der Schoot, T.A.W., 206, *216*
Vandewalker, M.L., 140, *169*
van Herwaarden, C.L., 44, *51*, 96,
    99, *116*, 140, *169*
Van Oosterhout, A.J., 36, 41, *49*, *50*,
    136, *166*
van Schayck, C.P., 44, *51*, 84, *92*,
    96, 99, *116*, 138, 140, 151, *167*,
    169, 185, 195, *200*
Varagic, V.M., 246, *258*
Vardey, C.J., 137, *166*
Vathenen, A.S., 161, *180*
Vaughan, L.M., 233, *253*
Vaughan, T.R., 161, *181*
Vaughn, J.H., 57, *65*
Vedal, S., 5, *28*
Vena, J.E., 229, *252*

Venuto, R.C., 153, *175*
Verbeek, P.R., 194, *201*
Vergnenegre, A., 5, *27*, 61, *66*
Verheyen, A., 41, *50*
Vermeire, P., 14, 16, *30*
Verweij, W., 77, *90*
Vestal, R.E., 144, *172*, 226, *250*
Vestbo, J., 228, *251*
Viegi, G., 78, 80, *90*, *91*
Vignola, M., 46, *51*
Villa, M.P., 243, *257*
Villar, A., 16, *31*
Violi, F., 232, *252*
Virchow, J.C., Jr., 36, *48*
Viskum, K., 22, 23, *31*
Vittadello, G., 153, *175*
Vittone, J., 229, *252*
Vollmer, W.M., 13, 16, *30*, 98, *116*
Vozeh, S., 146, *173*, 195, *201*, 246, *258*
Vuori, M.L., 162, *182*

W

Wagener, D.K., 12, *29*, 224, *250*
Wahner, H.W., 153, *175*
Wald, J.A., 242, *256*
Walker, C., 36, 40, *48-49*, *50*
Walsh, G.M., 36, *48*
Walters, E.H., 60, *66*, 101, 103, *117*
Wang, P.Z., 7, *28*
Wang, S.-P., 240, *256*
Wang, Y.T., 245, 246, *258*
Wanner, A., 99, 103, *117*, *118*, 140, *169*
Ward, A.J., 144, *172*
Ward, B.J., 230, *249*
Ward, C., 60, *66*
Ward, M.J., 151, 160, *174*, *179*
Wardlaw, A.J., 3, *26*, 36, 42, *48*
Warren, H.S., 37, *49*
Warringa, R.A., 161, *180*

Warshaw, R., 79, *91*
Washabau, R.J., 136, *166*
Wass, J.A.H., 245, *257*
Wasserman, S.I., 156, 160, 161, *179*, *180*
Wasterman, D.E., 196, *202*
Watkins, P.J., 243, *257*
Watson, W.T.A., 239, *255*
Watters, J.M., 156, *177*
Weber, A.L., 105, 112, *118*
Weber, R.W., 139, 140, 161, *167*, *169*, *181*
Weber, S.N., 103, 104, *118*, 230, *252*
Webster, J.R., 15, *30*, 94, *115*
Wegner, C.D., 36, 43, *48*, *50*
Weiler, D.A., 36, *48*
Weinberg, C.R., 99, 101, *116*, 185, *200*
Weinberg, P.F., 142, 149, *170*
Weinberger, M., 143, 144, 145, 150, *171*, *172*, *174*, 226, 228, 231, 236, 241, *251*
Weiss, K.B., 10, 11, 12, *29*, 98, 114, *116*, *120*, 123, *132*, 224, *250*
Weiss, S.R., 155, *176*
Weiss, S.T., 5, *27*, 80, *91*, 99, *117*, 224, *249*
Welch, M.J., 158, *178*
Weller, P.F., 56, 61, *64*
West, J.B., 74, *90*
West, R., 143, *171*
West, R.L., 205, *216*
Whang, R., 142, *171*
Wheeldon, A., 137, *166*
White, D.P., 237, *254*
White, J.G., 194, *201*
White, S.R., 43, *50*
Whitelaw, W.A., 12, *29*
Whitfield, M., 208, *217*
Wible, D.A., 246, *258*
Wick, K.A., 211, 212, *217*

Wiedemann, H.P., 107, 111, *119*
Wiest, P.M., 156, *177*
Wiggs, B.R., 58, *66*
Wilkins, G.T., 142, *171*
Williams, D.A., 11, *29*, 113, 114, *120*
Williams, D.M., 233, 234, *253*
Williams, H., 5, 6, 20, *27*
Williams, J.H., 56, *65*
Williams, M.H., Jr., 140, *169*, 211, *217*
Williams, S., 211, 212, *217*
Williams, S.J., 141, *170*, 233, *253*
Williamson, J., 155, *177*, 222, *249*
Willians, H.M., 190, *201*
Wilson, J., 3, 11, *26*, *29*, 55, 62, *64*, *67*
Wilson, R.W., 10, 11, 13, *29*
Wilson, S.R., 206, *216*
Wimberley, P.D., 77, *90*
Windsor, R.A., 214, *218*
Winner, S.J., 141, *170*
Winter, J.H., 83, *91*
Wise, R.A., 124, 130, *132*
Wo, J., 146, *173*
Wolf, K.M., 99, *116*, 138, *167*
Wolff, M., 105, *118*
Wong, B., 112, *119*
Wong, C.S., 161, *180*
Wood, K.A., 156, *178*
Wood, P.J., 143, *171*
Wood, R.P., II, 108, *119*
Wood-Baker, R., 239, *256*
Woodcock, A.J., 96, *115*
Woodhouse, A., 194, *201*
Woods, K.L., 99, *116*

Woolcock, A.J., 5, 22, 23, *27*, *28*, *31*, 54, 55, 56, 57, *64*, 80, 81, 88, *91*, *92*, 123, *132*, 157, *178*, 237, 238, *255*
Worth, H., 155, *176*, 206, *216*
Wright, E.C., 15, *30*, 84, *92*, 229, *251*
Wright, J.L., 58, *66*
Wrigley, J.M., 204, *215*
Wu, W.C., 242, 243, *256*
Wyatt, R.A., 228, 230, *251*

Y

Yamauchi, K., 46, *51*
Yarnell, P.R., 237, *254*
Yarnold, P.R., 247, *258*
Yernault, J., 208, *217*
Ying, S., 37, 38, *49*, *50*
Young, M.J., 107, 111, *119*
Yukawa, T., 144, *172*
Yunginger, J.W., 34, *47*, 98, *116*

Z

Zagelbaum, G., 190, 193, *201*
Zawacki, J.K., 111, *119*, 241, 242, *256*
Zeitz, H.J., 232, 233, *252*
Zell, M., 146, *173*
Ziment, I., 230, *252*
Zitnik, R.J., 230, 231, 232, *252*
Zocchi, L., 197, *202*
Zoia, M.C., 77, 78, *90*
Zwillich, C.W., 146, *173*, 237, *254*
Zwinderman, A.H., 139, *168*

SUBJECT INDEX

A

Acute respiratory failure (*see also* Mechanical ventilation)
    ICU management, 196–199
    pharmacologic management, 193–196
Adhesion molecules
    intercellular adhesion molecule-1, 36
    vascular cell adhesion molecule-1, 36
Adrenocortical insufficiency, 246–247
Airways
    effects of aging, 60–61
    irreversible obstruction, 44, 96–97
    nonspecific reactivity, 80
    remodeling, 44, 61–62
Airways hyperresponsiveness, 42
Allergens, environmental, 33, 46
Allergic bronchopulmonary aspergillosis, 240–241
Allergy, 46, 98
    occupational, 34
    skin testing, 34
Ambulatory monitoring, 87

Anticholinergics, 150–152 (*see also* Bronchodilators)
Anti-inflammatory agents, 152–161
    cromolyn sodium, 160–161
    glucocorticoids, 152–160
    inhaled, 157–160
    nedocromil sodium, 160–161
Arterial blood gases, 76–77
Arthritis, 233–234
Asthma (*see also* Coexisting conditions)
    acute exacerbations
        assessment of, 188–191
        differential diagnosis, 187–188
        hospital care, 194–196
        physiologic measurements, 190
    course and prognosis of, 21–23
    definition of, 2–3, 54, 95–96
    disease prevalence in elderly, 223–224
    elderly, clinical features of, 16–19
    fatal, 113–114
    inflammation in, 57
    natural history, 19–23

[Asthma]
  pathology of epithelial sloughing, 56
  pathology of mucus plugging in, 56
  pathology of small airways in, 57
  pathology of subepithelial fibrosis,
    56–57
  pathophysiology, 184–186
  relapses of, 21
  remission of, 20–21
Asthmatic bronchitis, 23–24, 55 (*see
  also* Bronchitis)

B

Beta-adrenergic agonists (*see also*
  Bronchodilators)
  adverse effects, 142–143
  clinical problems, 140
  mechanisms of action, 136–137
  route of administration, 140–141
  tolerance, 139
Beta-adrenergic receptors, 136–138
  function, 99, 137–138
  localization, 137
Bronchial hyperreactivity, 80–82
Bronchitis
  asthmatic, 23–24, 55
  chronic, 11
  simple, 54–55
  obstructive, 57–58 (*see also* Small
    airways disease)
Bronchodilator response, 79, 83–84
Bronchodilators, 136–152
  anticholinergic, 150–152
  beta-adrenergic agonists, 136–143
  theophylline, 143–150

C

Cancer, bronchogenic, 228–229
Cardiovascular disease, 229–233
Chronic obstructive pulmonary disease
    (COPD), 226–227
  definition of, 54
  relationship to asthma, 25
  small airways disease in, 58

Coexisting conditions
  adrenocortical insufficiency, 246–247
  arthritis, 233–234
  bronchogenic cancer, 228–229
  cardiovascular disease, 229–231
  COPD, 226–227
  diabetes mellitus, 243–244
  neurologic and psychiatric conditions,
    234–237
  pulmonary embolism, 232–233
  sleep apnea, 237–238
  thyroid disease, 244–246
Cough
  in COPD, 111 (*see also* Asthmatic
    bronchitis)
  drug induced, 111
  in gastroesophageal reflux disease
    (GERD), 111
  as symptom of asthma, 108–111
Cytokines, 35–36
  granulocyte-macrophage colony-
    stimulating factor, 36–38
  interferon-gamma, 36, 40–41
  interleukin-3, 36–38
  interleukin-4, 38, 40, 46
  interleukin-5, 36–38, 40–41, 46
  tumor necrosis factor-alpha, 36

D

Depression, 205
Diabetes mellitus, 243–244
Diaphragm, 75 (*see also* Muscles)
Diffusing capacity, 77–79, 84 (*see also*
    Pulmonary function tests)
Drug interactions, 236–237
Dyspnea, 112
  impaired perception of, 101

E

Environmental control, 128
Eosinophils, 35–36, 46
  major basic protein in, 42–44
  peroxidase, 43–44
Epidemiology questionnaires, 4–5
  reliability, 4–5

[Epidemiology questionnaires]
sensitivity, 4
specificity, 4
validity, 4

F

Forced expiratory volume in 1 second
(FEV$_1$), 73–75, 82–83, 85–88,
96 (*see also* Pulmonary function
tests)
Forced vital capacity, 73–75, 82, 87–88
(*see also* Pulmonary function
tests)
Functional residual capacity, 72, 74 (*see
also* Pulmonary function tests)

G

Gastroesophageal reflux disease
(GERD), 241–243
Glucocorticoids (*see also* Anti-
inflammatory agents)
adverse effects of systemic therapy,
153–156
inhaled, 157–160
adverse effects, 158–160
pharmacokinetics, 157–158
mechanism of action, 152
pharmacokinetics, 153, 157–158

I

ICD-9
definition of, 10
effects on morbidity, 10
effects on mortality, 10
Immunoglubulin E, 34, 46
Incidence, 8
Inflammation, 44
allergic, 35, 46
Inhaled medication, patient education in
use of, 211–213

L

Lower respiratory infections, 240–241
Lung Health Study, 86

M

Management care plan, 214–215
Management, nonpharmacological
effects of
economic factors, 122–123
environmental factors, 123
factors related to adherence, 126–128
physical factors, 123
psychological factors, 124
social factors, 122
Maximal expiratory flow, 72 (*see also*
Pulmonary function tests)
Maximal inspiratory pressure, 76 (*see
also* Pulmonary function tests)
Mechanical ventilation, 197–199
Medication, patient education, 210–213
Metered dose inhalers, 141
physical problems with, 127
Morbidity, 9–11
Mortality, 9–13, 224
death certificate diagnosis of, 12–13
Mucociliary function, 99
Muscarinic receptors, 43, 150–151
Muscles
diaphragm, 75
respiratory, 75, 88

N

Neurological and psychiatric conditions, 234

P

Patient education (*see* Management,
nonpharmacological effects of)
Peak expiratory flow, 72, 85, 88, 190
(*see also* Pulmonary function
tests)
meters, 87
monitoring, 208–210
Peak flow monitoring, 129
Pharmacological therapy, 135–182
approach to, 162–165
Psychosocial factors, 204–205
Pulmonary embolism, 233
Pulmonary function tests, 70–79, 82–88

R

Receptors
  beta-adrenergic, 99, 136–138
  muscarinic, 43, 150–151
Residual volume, 71, 74 (*see also*
    Pulmonary function tests)

S

Sinusitis, 238–240
Sleep apnea, 237–238
Small airways disease, 55
Smoking, 227–228
Socioeconomic factors, 98
Spirometry, 85
Status asthmaticus, pathology of, 53–
    54

T

Theophylline (*see also* Bronchodilators)
  indications, 149, 150
  mechanism of action, 144
  pharmacokinetics of, 144–146
  toxicity, 146–149
Thyroid disease, 244–246

Tidal volume, 72 (*see also* Pulmonary
    function tests)
T lymphocytes
  CD4+, 37, 40, 42, 46
  CD8+, 37–38, 40–42, 46
  TH2-like, 38
Total lung capacity, 70, 71, 73 (*see also*
    Pulmonary function tests)

U

Upper respiratory infections, 238–240

V

Vital capacity, 72

W

Wheeze
  airway obstruction, 105–106
  differential diagnosis of, 102–108
  drug induced, 107
  in congestive heart failure, 103–105
  secondary aspiration, 106–107 (*see
    also* Gastroesophageal reflux
    disease)